Sports Cardiology Essentials

Christine E. Lawless, MD, MBA
Editor

Sports Cardiology Essentials

Evaluation, Management and Case Studies

Springer

Editor
Christine E. Lawless, MD, MBA
President, Sports Cardiology Consultants, LLC
Clinical Associate Faculty
University of Chicago
Consulting Cardiologist, Major League Soccer
Team Physician, US Figure Skating
Chicago, IL, USA
christine.lawless@yahoo.com

ISBN 978-0-387-92774-9 e-ISBN 978-0-387-92775-6
DOI 10.1007/978-0-387-92775-6
Springer New York Dordrecht Heidelberg London

Library of Congress Control Number: 2010937776

Printed on acid-free paper

Springer is part of Springer Science+Business Media (www.springer.com)

Contents

Contributors

Michael J. Ackerman, MD/PhD
Division of Pediatric Cardiology, Department of Pediatrics and Adolescent Medicine, Mayo Clinic, Rochester, MN, USA

Shafeeq Ahmed, MD
Cardiovascular Services Hospitalist, Hartford Hospital, Hartford, CT, USA

Paolo Angelini, MD
Staff Cardiologist, Texas Heart Institute at St. Luke's Episcopal Hospital, Houston, TX, USA

Chad A. Asplund, MD, FACSM
Primary Care Sports Medicine, Department of Family Medicine, Eisenhower Army Medical Center, Fort Gordon, GA 30905

Aaron L. Baggish, MD
Division of Cardiology, Harvard University, Boston, MA, USA

Holly J. Benjamin, MD, FAAP, FACSM
Associate Professor of Pediatrics and Surgery, Section of Academic Pediatrics, Section of Orthopedic Surgery and Rehabilitation Medicine, Director of Primary Care Sports Medicine, The University of Chicago, 5841 S. Maryland Ave. Chicago, IL 60637

George Chiampas, DO
Clinical Instructor, Department of Emergency Medicine, Feinberg School of Medicine, Northwestern University: Medical Director, Bank of America Chicago Marathon; Team Physician, Northwestern University, Chicago, IL, USA

Joseph A. Congeni, MD
Akron Children's Hospital, Akron, OH, USA

Eric E. Coris, MD
Associate Professor, Departments of Family Medicine and Orthopaedics and Sports Medicine, University of South Florida College of Medicine, Tampa, FL, USA

Anne B. Curtis, MD
Chair, Department of Cardiology, University of South Florida
College of Medicine, Tampa, FL, USA

Iwona Cygankiewicz, MD/PhD
Visiting Assistant Professor of Cardiology, University of Rochester Medical Center; Heart Research Follow-up Program, Rochester, NY, USA

Rakesh Gopinathannair, M.D., M.A.
Assistant Professor of Medicine, Division of Cardiology,
Section of Electrophysiology, University of Louisville Hospitals, Louisville, KY 40202

Adolph M. Hutter, MD
Division of Cardiology, Harvard University, Boston, MA, USA

Steven J. Keteyian, PhD
Division of Cardiovascular Medicine, Department of Internal Medicine, Henry Ford Hospital, Detroit, MI, USA

Rachel Lampert, MD
Section of Cardiology, Yale University School of Medicine, New Haven, CT, USA

Andrew P. Landstrom, BS
Department of Molecular Pharmacology and Experimental Therapeutics, Mayo Clinic, Rochester, MN, USA

Christine E. Lawless, MD, MBA
President, Sports Cardiology Consultants, LLC, Clinical Associate Faculty, University of Chicago Consulting Cardiologist, Major League Soccer Team Physician, US Figure Skating World Teams, 360 West Illinois Street #7D, Chicago, IL 60654, USA

Benjamin D. Levine, MD
Director, Institute for Exercise and Environmental Medicine; S. Finley Ewing Jr. Chair for Wellness, Presbyterian Hospital of Dallas; Harry S. Moss Heart Chair for Cardiovascular Research and Professor of Medicine, University of Texas Southwestern Medical Center at Dallas, Dallas, TX, USA

Mark S. Link, MD
Professor of Medicine, Tufts University School of Medicine, Boston, MA, USA

John M. MacKnight, MD
Associate Professor, Clinical Internal Medicine and Orthopaedic Surgery; Team Physician and Co-Medical Director, University of Virginia Sports Medicine, University of Virginia Health System, Charlottesville, VA, USA

Sanjeev Malik, MD
Assistant Medical Director, Department of Emergency Medicine, Feinberg School of Medicine, Northwestern University, Chicago, IL, USA

Marla A. Mendelson, MD/FACC
Director, Northwestern Adult Congenital Heart Center and Marfan Syndrome Program, Department of Cardiology, Chicago, IL, USA

Dilaawar J. Mistry, MD
Co-Medical Director and Primary Care Team Physician, University of Virginia Sports Medicine, Charlottesville, VA, USA

Francis G. O'Connor, MD/MPH/COL/MC/USA
Associate Professor of Military and Emergency Medicine; Medical Director, USUHS Consortium for Health and Military Performance, Uniformed Services University of Health Sciences, Bethesda, MD, USA

Brian Olshansky, MD
Professor of Medicine, Department of Internal Medicine – Cardiology, University of Iowa Hospitals and Clinics, Iowa City, IA, USA

Steve R. Ommen, MD
Division of Cardiovascular Diseases and Internal Medicine, Mayo Clinic, Rochester, MN, USA

Jonathan P. Parsons, MD/MSc
Assistant Professor of Internal Medicine; Associate Director, OSU Asthma Center, The Ohio State University Medical Center, Columbus, OH, USA

Robert E. Poley, MD/MS/BS
Staff Physician, Private Practice; Division of Sports Medicine, William Beaumont Hospital, Macomb, MI, USA

William O. Roberts, MD/MS
Professor, Department of Family Medicine, University of Minnesota Medical School; Medical Director, Twin Cities Marathon Inc., Minneapolis-St. Paul, MN, USA

Frances Sahebzamani, ARNP/PhD
Director, Nursing Residency Program, College of Nursing, The University of South Florida, Tampa, FL, USA

J. Philip Saul, MD
Department of Pediatrics, Medical University of South Carolina, Charleston, SC, USA

John R. Schairer, DO
Division of Cardiovascular Medicine, Department of Internal Medicine, Henry Ford Hospital, Detroit, MI, USA

Paul Sorajja, MD
Assistant Professor of Medicine, Consultant, Cardiovascular Diseases and Internal Medicine, Mayo Clinic, Rochester, MN, USA

David J. Tester, BS
Division of Cardiovascular Diseases, Department of Medicine, Mayo Clinic, Rochester, MN, USA

Paul D. Thompson, MD
Director, Cardiology; Director, Athlete's Heart Program, Hartford Hospital, Hartford, CT, USA

Steve Walz, MS/ATC
Head Athletic Trainer, Director of Sports Medicine and Assistant Athletic Director, USF Department of Athletics, The University of South Florida, Tampa, FL, USA

Bryan M. White, MD
Medical Corps, USAF, Wright Paterson Cardiology, Wright Patterson Air Force Base, Dayton, OH, USA

Malissa J. Wood, MD
Division of Cardiology, Harvard University, Boston, MA, USA

Kibar Yared, MD/FRCPC
Division of Cardiology, Harvard University, Boston, MA, USA

Wojciech Zareba, MD/PhD
Heart Research Follow-up Program, University of Rochester Medical Center, Rochester, NY, USA

Kira Zwygart, MD
Assistant Professor, Department of Family Medicine; Director, Ambulatory Care Clerkship, The University of South Florida College of Medicine, Tampa, FL, USA

Part I
Prevention of Sudden Cardiac Arrest in Athletes: Application of appropriate cardiac evaluation and treatments

Chapter 1
Sudden Cardiac Death in Athletes: Scope of the Problem and Emergency Response

Eric E. Coris, Steve Walz, Anne B. Curtis, Frances Sahebzamani, and Kira Zwygart

Incidence

Introduction

Exceeding 300,000 cases annually, sudden cardiac death (SCD) is the leading cause of death in the USA [1, 2]. SCD is also the leading cause of death in athletes [3]. Defined as occurring within 1 h of participation in sports [4], exercise-related SCD occurs in one to five cases per one million athletes per year. Of the approximately 25 million competitive athletes in the USA, there are 25–125 documented cases of SCD per year, likely a significant underestimation [5]. The National Federation of High School Coaches estimates 10–25 cases of SCD per year in individuals younger than 30 years [6]. A study of Minnesota high schools revealed three deaths due to SCD in a period of 12 years, translating to a risk of one death per 200,000 athletes/year [6]. The overall occurrence rate of SCD in high school athletes is estimated to be 1:100,000–1:300,000 athletes/year [7]. Despite significant efforts nationally to identify the ideal mechanism for detecting and preventing these events, cardiovascular collapse as the cause of athletic fatalities in high school and collegiate athletes outnumbers death by trauma by 2:1 [8].

SCD in older athletes (>35 years of age) is most often related to atherosclerotic coronary arterial disease with myocardial infarction. However, in young athletes (<35 years of age), the majority of these cases are caused by defined and hereditary cardiovascular disorders. Cardiac electrical instability, due to these underlying pathologies, deteriorating into fatal ventricular tachycardia or ventricular fibrillation, appears to be the most common immediate cause of death [1, 5, 9, 10].

E.E. Coris (✉)
Department of Family Medicine, University of South Florida College of Medicine, Tampa, FL, USA
and
Department of Orthopaedics and Sports Medicine, University of South Florida College of Medicine, Tampa, FL, USA
e-mail: ecoris@health.usf.edu

C.E. Lawless (ed.), *Sports Cardiology Essentials: Evaluation, Management and Case Studies*, DOI 10.1007/978-0-387-92775-6_1,

A retrospective review, by Maron, of sudden deaths of competitive athletes from 1985 to 1995 found that 134 deaths (85%) were due to cardiovascular disorders [11]. The majority of these athletes were involved in high school sports (62%), with collegiate athletes a distant second (22%), and professional athletes ranking third (7%). Of the athletes who experienced sudden death, 90% were male. From a sport-specific standpoint, 68% of these deaths occurred during football and basketball participation, likely a population-participation-based statistic, but also potentially an intensity-related phenomenon. Ninety percent of these athletes collapsed during or immediately after a training session or competition.

Unfortunately, although symptoms or family history of SCD may precede the event, most episodes of arrest are the first manifestation of disease in an "apparently healthy" individual. Many athletes are capable of exceptionally high levels of performance for long periods of time, even while harboring occult and potentially lethal cardiovascular malformations [11]. Traumatic to the family and the surrounding community, such events are typically excruciating, prompting public outcry and ever-increasing efforts by sports medicine professionals to detect, prevent, and respond aggressively to these rare but catastrophic events.

To further complicate the issue, one response to this difficult problem has been to focus significant energy and resources on the preparticipation examination. This, however, has yielded modest benefits at best [12]. The ability of the preparticipation examination alone to optimally identify all athletes with these underlying cardiovascular predispositions to sudden cardiac arrest has been limited, and noninvasive cardiovascular screening techniques have not yet been adopted on a broad scale in the US [7, 13–16]. Particularly, the relative rarity of actual events, approximately 1:200,000 US athletes/year, demands an extremely sensitive and specific screening test, and clear indications for definitive action, to be deemed a "cost-effective" intervention [17].

Another approach has been to aggressively implement emergency response protocols to optimally respond to a sudden cardiac arrest event [18]. While there has been significant success in the development of nationally standardized recommendations in emergency action planning [19], particularly from the National Athletic Trainer's Association [20], the success of defibrillation in the young athlete may be lower than that of defibrillation in the general population [21]. We discuss these studies later in the chapter.

Ultimately, successful efforts to save every young athlete will require further understanding of the optimal preparticipation evaluation, considerable expanded research in the detection and management of the various underlying cardiac pathologies commonly associated with arrest in active youth, and continued pursuit of optimal response to arrest episodes.

Causes

Greater than 20 cardiac pathologies have been identified as causes of SCD in athletes. In a retrospective review from 1985 to 1995 of SCD in US athletes [11], Maron

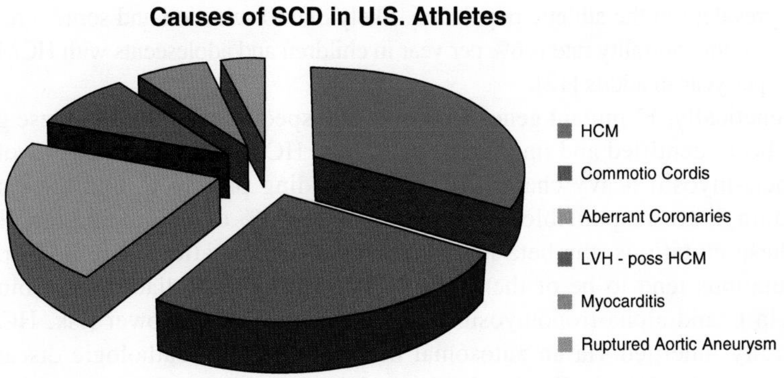

Fig. 1.1 Causes of SCD in U.S. Athletes (data from Maron, JACC, 2005 [46])

reported pathological findings at autopsy revealing a predominance of hypertrophic cardiomyopathy (HCM) (26%) and aberrant coronary arteries (13%) as the underlying cause of death. Only 18% of these patients had symptoms attributed to the cardiovascular system in the preceding 36 months prior to death (i.e., chest pain, exertional dyspnea, syncope, or dizziness). Further, 115 of these athletes had standard preparticipation examinations performed. Of these, only 3% were suspected of having cardiovascular disease and only one athlete (0.9%) had the correct cardiovascular abnormality identified (see Fig. 1.1) [11].

The lack of standardization in the quality and type of preparticipation physical examination performed on these athletes as well as the high rate of unrecognized cardiovascular disease illustrates the need for health care professionals, particularly in the sports medicine community, to explore adjunctive means for preventing and/or treating SCD [23].

SCD in older athletes (>35 years old) is most often related to coronary artery disease [4], with the incidence of SCD increasing with age [24]. Including this older population of vigorous exercisers, estimates of SCD incidence approach 1:15,000–1:18,000 [25]. Most of these deaths, of young and old athletes, are thought to be related to electrical instability leading to ventricular tachycardia and, eventually, ventricular fibrillation [4, 26].

Specific Causes

Hypertrophic Cardiomyopathy

The single most common cardiac abnormality leading to SCD in the USA in athletes is hypertrophic cardiomyopathy or HCM [11]. Responsible for approximately 26% of all SCD events in US athletes, it is the most significant cardiac pathology with which we as a sports medicine community struggle. Affecting approximately one in every 500 adults in the US, it seems to have a fairly equal male:female genetic distribution ratio.

Less prevalent in the athletic population, likely due to selection and some screening practices, the mortality rate is 6% per year in children and adolescents with HCM, and 1–3% per year in adults [12].

Genetically, 11 mutant genes with over 200 specific mutations in these genes have been identified and implicated in clinical HCM [27]. Mutations involving the beta-myosin heavy chain, the myosin-binding protein C, and the cardiac troponin T are responsible for approximately 50% of the population HCM. Of these mutations, the beta-myosin heavy chain mutations and the troponin T mutations tend to be of the highest risk, while the cardiac myosin-binding protein C and alpha-tropomyosin mutations tend to be of lower risk. HCM is generally inherited via an autosomal dominant pattern. Pathologic disease of the myocardium typically develops in adolescence in conjunction with rapid growth of the body [27]. Only 60% of all individuals with HCM have an affected first degree relative, due in large part to the occurrence of spontaneous mutations [28].

Pathologic evaluation of the heart with HCM reveals a larger than normal heart with a particularly enlarged left ventricle [27]. Total left ventricular mass is increased without compensatory dilation of the chamber; thus, ventricular filling is decreased in diastole. Thickness of the ventricular septum is typically markedly increased from 15 to 50 mm, with less than 13 mm considered normal [5, 27]. The marked septal hypertrophy is particularly asymmetric when compared to the left ventricular free wall, causing the characteristic left ventricular outflow tract obstruction [22]. Also commonly seen in the setting of HCM is significant anterior motion of the mitral valve during systole [29]. Microscopic pathology reveals abnormal small arteries, with "myocardial disarray" and a complex, disorganized arrangement of the myocytes with interstitial fibrosis [30].

On clinical evaluation, HCM can be asymptomatic [31], or patients may present, with exertional chest pain, shortness of breath, dizziness, or syncope with exertion. On examination, one may find a laterally displaced, enlarged point of maximal impulse. A systolic murmur may be heard, typically at the left lateral sternal border, and is characteristically increased by maneuvers that decrease preload. The Valsalva maneuver or a squatting-to-standing position change should make the murmur audibly louder. This is in contrast to more flow-dependent benign murmurs, which will often become quiet or disappear with these maneuvers.

ECG testing is fairly sensitive for HCM, likely greater than 90% [31, 32]. Characteristic findings include left ventricular hypertrophy, abnormal axis, q waves, and ST-T wave changes [22, 31, 32]. The ECG, however, can be normal, particularly in cases of nonobstructive or less obstructive disease. In cases of nonobstructive HCM, the sensitivity of ECG drops to approximately 75%. Asymmetric septal hypertrophy, systolic anterior motion of the mitral valve, abnormal diastolic filling, and often, diminished left ventricular cavity size can all be seen on echocardiogram [16, 33, 34]. Cardiac MRI, particularly with contrast, can often identify the abnormal myocardium if the diagnosis is in doubt. Genetic testing is available but can cost up to $4,500 [31, 35]. (See Chapter 5 for further information on role of genetic testing.)

Commotio Cordis

Responsible for 20% of all SCD in US athletes, commotio cordis is particularly concerning in high-velocity ball sports [36, 37]. A sudden forceful impact to the chest wall during ventricular repolarization can elicit electrical instability leading to asystole or ventricular fibrillation [37]. The mean age of victims is 13 years of age. No symptoms are present prior to the event [37]. No underlying cardiac abnormalities are found at autopsy. Unfortunately, although rapid defibrillation is the treatment of choice, defibrillation attempts are often unsuccessful, due to the fact that some athletes deteriorate immediately into asystole [21, 22]. The resuscitation rate is 15%, even with rapid response. A commotio cordis registry is tracking injuries and response, and hopefully it will provide important information in furthering our understanding of this deadly condition (see Chapter 14).

Coronary Arterial Abnormalities

The second leading cause of nontraumatic SCD is actually a group of disorders of the coronary arteries [1, 4, 18, 22, 34, 38, 39]. Anomalous origin of the left anterior descending from the right sinus of Valsalva is considered the most lethal of a variety of congenital anomalies of the coronary vessels [11]. Tunneled coronaries, myocardial bridging, single coronary arteries, and others have been found to contribute to transient myocardial ischemia during intense activity, that then induces malignant arrhythmia, often ventricular tachycardia/ventricular fibrillation [10, 40].

Most often asymptomatic, some one-third of athletes will experience angina, syncope, or exertional dyspnea prior to an SCD event [41]. In one study in the USA and Italy, 10 of 12 athletes with underlying coronary abnormalities had symptoms prior to death [42]. Physical examination is typically unremarkable [26].

The ECG is typically normal [7, 12, 31, 40], the resting echocardiogram is typically normal [23, 42], and even exercise treadmill stress testing is often normal [4, 42]. All nine of the athletes in the above study who had ECGs had normal findings, including six individuals who had completed exercise stress testing in addition to routine ECG [42]. One may see segmental wall motion abnormalities on stress echocardiography, but definitive diagnosis is often made by coronary angiography, computed tomography of the coronary arteries, or magnetic resonance imaging [31, 34, 42] (see Chapter 3 and 15).

Myocarditis

Inflammation or infection in the myocardial tissue can lead to electrical instability and SCD in athletes. Involvement of the conduction system can also lead to fatal complete heart block [10, 26, 34]. Typically related to Coxsackie B virus infection (approximately 50%), cardiac inflammation can be due to a great number of organisms [45, 46]. Affected individuals may present with chest pain, dyspnea, syncope, and/or dizziness, but they may also present with more systemic symptoms related to the infectious process [45]. Fever, chills, nausea, vomiting, upper respiratory symptoms, diarrhea, and/or sore throat may be present. Often, however, an athlete's presenting symptom is the SCD event [5, 18, 21, 46].

Clinically, athletes at risk may be identified by symptoms of infection as mentioned above or of cardiac involvement with chest pain, dyspnea, syncope, or dizziness [46]. On exam, they may have evidence of congestive heart failure such as distended neck veins, a laterally displaced enlarged PMI, audible S3 gallop, rales, peripheral edema, and/or hepatojugular reflux [34, 45, 46].

Chest X-ray is typically normal, but it could reveal cardiomegaly or pulmonary edema [45]. ECG may indicate myocarditis with ST segment elevation, but sensitivity is relatively low and variable (10–50%) [34, 45, 46]. Echocardiogram may reveal hypokinesis, depressed ejection fraction, or may be normal. Cardiac MRI with contrast may be helpful in demonstrating myocardial inflammation [46].

Definitive diagnosis depends on myocardial biopsy [46]. Pathologic analysis typically demonstrates myocardial inflammation but may reveal only idiopathic myocardial scarring [46, 47]. It may be this scarring that generates the arrhythmogenic focus in some asymptomatic athletes with SCD events [5, 10, 45]. Treatment for myocarditis is geared toward the clinical cardiac disease, treating any underlying heart failure, and protecting from excessive stress during the active phase of the disease. Echocardiography, electrophysiology, and stress testing may be utilized to document resolution of the condition and lack of arrhythmogenic potential [1, 5, 26, 45].

Marfan's Syndrome

Accounting for only 2% of SCD in US athletes, Marfan's syndrome is an important underlying problem for the sports physician and cardiologist to be familiar with, as it is one of the more recognizable pathologies with a largely clinical diagnosis. It is an autosomal dominant inherited connective tissue disorder occurring in approximately one in 10,000 individuals [46]. An athlete with this condition will often have a family history significant for Marfan's syndrome. The physician's ability to diagnose and subsequently monitor Marfanoid athletes to reduce their risk of SCD is unique among the pathologies here and warrants some attention. Marfan's is one of the family of connective tissue disorders that leads to increased risk of progressive dilatation of the aortic root, potentially leading to dissection and/or rupture of the aorta with massive hemorrhage, pericardial tamponade, coronary artery dissection, acute aortic valve insufficiency, and congestive heart failure [46, 48].

Marfan's syndrome is typically asymptomatic but does have characteristic morphologic/clinical findings related to the connective tissue pathology [48]. Athletes are characteristically very tall and thin. They often have disproportionately long limbs, with an arm span greater than their height and an upper body to lower body ratio more than one standard deviation below the mean, as well as long thin facies [46]. They often have an arm span greater than their height.

Hyperextension and significant overlap of the thumb and fifth digit when circumferentially wrapped around the thin wrist is also common [46, 48, 49]. Kyphoscoliosis and anterior thoracic deformities such as pectus excavatum and carinatum are often present [49].

Once identified clinically, the typical athlete with Marfan's syndrome is evaluated via echocardiogram for dilation of the aortic root, evaluated by ophthalmology for ectopia lentis, and limited appropriately from activity, depending on the sport [49]. Athletes are then typically studied via echocardiogram every 6 months to 1 year for aortic dilatation [46, 48]. See Chapter 16 for a complete discussion of this important syndrome.

Long QT Syndrome and Wolff–Parkinson–White Syndrome

Long QT Syndrome

A reported rare (1% of all SCD episodes in US) but dramatic group of congenital ion channel defects may lead to SCD in an athlete [3]. Approximately one in 10,000 Americans have prolonged QT syndrome by current estimations [3, 50]. In this syndrome, the period of the cardiac cycle between ventricular firing and repolarization known as the QT interval is longer than normal. In men, this period is considered prolonged if the interval, after correction for rate, is greater than or equal to 440 ms. In women, the corrected QT interval is considered prolonged if it is greater than or equal to 460 ms.

Of those individuals with long QT syndrome, 60% have a positive family history of long QT or SCD [3, 50]. One-third of all patients present with symptoms referable to the disorder, with palpitations, seizures, and syncope being most common [23, 51]. Statistically, these syndromes are likely very underreported due to the inconclusive autopsy findings that are common in these disorders [50]. Because the heart is structurally normal in most patients, with the primary abnormality being a tendency toward life-threatening ventricular arrhythmias as a result of an ion channel defect, these syndromes are often asymptomatic leading up to a catecholamine surge and SCD under extreme stress [3, 9, 48].

If long QT syndrome is suspected, the ECG is almost always abnormal, displaying the prolonged QT interval [1, 3, 31, 32]. Occasionally, only an atypical U wave is seen. In the related Brugada syndrome, ECG shows incomplete right bundle branch block and ST segment elevations in the right precordial leads, with a structurally normal heart. Genetic testing may allow identification of the disease and the underlying subtype. The testing typically will detect up to 75% of the most common genetic mutations leading to prolonged QT syndrome (QT1, QT2, QT3, QT5, QT6). The three major types of testing for this condition are focused on slightly different genetic tendencies. The Comprehensive Cardiac Ion Channel Analysis provides analysis for variants in all five genes and is the most comprehensive test. Sodium Channel Analysis tests only for the SCN5A gene and is appropriate in cases of suspected Brugada syndrome. There is also a family-specific analysis looking to the specific subtype of prolonged QT syndrome that is carried in the family genome [3, 31, 48].

This testing, however, can be very expensive and often requires repeated negotiation with the patient's insurance company to get the test reimbursed by their insurance. Testing can be further investigated through http://www.familion.com.

Interestingly, of the four major subtypes of long QT syndrome that account for the majority of mutations, each has a different predictable trigger that precedes a SCD episode [3, 27, 31, 50]. In QT1, the common trigger is swimming. Although these athletes may tolerate an extreme level of exertion of most types, the unique cardiovascular demands of swimming typically produce a sudden death event due to malignant tachyarrhythmia, often ventricular tachycardia decompensating into ventricular fibrillation. In QT2, the most common trigger is extreme emotion. Often a frightening surprise sends those athletes with prolonged QT2 into the aberrant tachyarrhythmia and SCD. Interestingly, in QT3 the most common trigger is not activity at all, but inactivity. The malignant tachyarrhythmia seems to erupt almost spontaneously during low levels of activity. In QT4, the most common trigger of a SCD episode is a sudden malignant tachyarrhythmia precipitated by a loud noise, such as an alarm clock.

Treatment often involves therapy with B-blockers, a pacemaker, and/or implantable cardiac defibrillator, typically then refraining from activity. There are, however, a growing number of athletes, after extensive consultation and assessment, who are returning to competitive sport even with an ICD in place [31, 52]. Please see Chapter 18 and 19.

Unlike the channelopathies, Wolff–Parkinson–White Syndrome (WPW) is a result of an accessory pathway connecting the atrium to the ventricule that can promote the development of "reentrant tachycardias." Typically manifesting as a relatively benign intermittent supraventricular tachycardia, or SVT, patients will often present with symptoms of palpitations, dizziness, or lightheadedness [26, 34, 53]. The ECG during an episode may reveal a narrow complex tachycardia. Once the rhythm is back to normal sinus rhythm, a characteristic "delta wave," a slurred, early upstroke in the QRS complex, can typically be seen [26, 31] (see Fig. 1.2). The acute episode of SVT can often be terminated with stimulation of the vagal system. Maneuvers such as unilateral carotid sinus massage, the Valsalva maneuver,

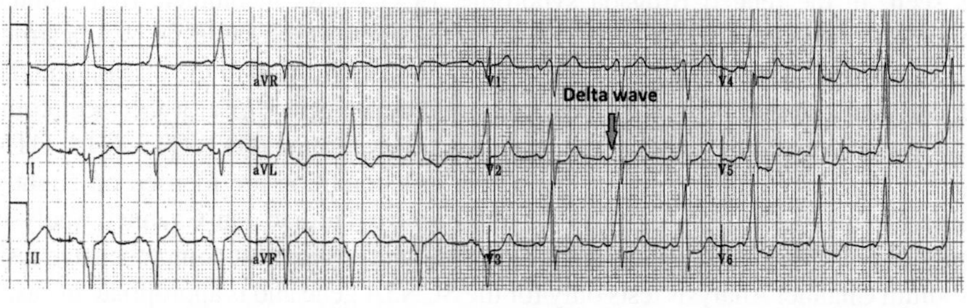

Fig. 1.2 Classic WPW ECG with deltawave (arrow)

or even facial immersion in ice water will often break the tachycardia and return the patient to normal sinus rhythm [53]. If not, often a calcium channel blocker or even adenosine can break the abnormal rhythm medically.

SCD is rare in WPW syndrome, but it can occur, particularly with rapid ventricular rates during atrial fibrillation that may degenerate into ventricular fibrillation. In cases of aborted SCD in WPW, or for patients with recurrent or severe symptoms, an electrophysiology study with radiofrequency catheter ablation of the abnormal accessory pathway will be performed [53].

Arrhythmogenic Right Ventricular Dysplasia

Arrhythmogenic right ventricular dysplasia (ARVD), also known as arrhythmogenic right ventricular cardiomyopathy, is a genetic disorder characterized by right ventricular enlargement and dysfunction as well as potentially life-threatening ventricular arrhythmias. The incidence of SCD in athletes with ARVD is estimated to be 0.5/100,000 persons/year [54]. Typically, the disease becomes manifest during adolescence and early adulthood, with a male predominance. ARVD is the most common pathological finding in athletes who have died suddenly in the Veneto region of Italy, accounting for approximately one-fourth of fatal events. The identification of ARVD as the cause of SCD in the USA is much less frequent, with an estimated incidence of 3% [46].

ARVD is a genetic disorder with autosomal dominant transmission in about one-third of cases. In many cases it is recognized to be a desmosomal disease caused by defective cell adhesion proteins such as desmoplakin, plakoglobin, and others [55]. There is also a mutation in the cardiac ryanodine receptor that has been identified as the cause of ARVD in other patients. Progressive myocyte death occurs with fibro-fatty infiltration. Thinning of the right ensues occurs along with localized aneurysmal dilatation. The disease affects the right ventricle primarily, with a much lower incidence of left ventricular dysfunction.

Athletes with ARVD have a 5.4-fold higher risk of dying during competitive sports than when they are sedentary [54]. The reasons for this observation are not known but may relate to increases in right ventricular afterload during exertion along with denervation hypersensitivity to catecholamines that may lead to an increase in ventricular arrhythmias during exercise.

Athletes with ARVD may present with palpitations or syncope, but others may be asymptomatic when first evaluated. Physical examination is usually normal unless extensive disease and right ventricular failure is present. The typical ECG abnormality in an individual with ARVD is T-wave inversions in the right precordial leads beyond V1. Ventricular arrhythmias, including premature ventricular beats and ventricular tachycardia, are frequent and usually have a left bundle branch block morphology. Signal-averaged electrocardiography is typically abnormal as well. The diagnosis may be confirmed by noninvasive imaging studies such as echocardiography, angiography, or magnetic resonance imaging. In some cases, endomyocardial biopsy is used to demonstrate fibro-fatty infiltration of the right ventricle. The diagnosis of ARVD in an athlete would lead to disqualification from sports participation, given the high risk of SCD during competition. ICDs are often implanted in symptomatic individuals.

Immediate Treatment

Following a thorough preparticipation exam, the next step in prevention of SCD is the implementation of a well thought out emergency action plan (EAP). Careful planning and consideration must be taken into account when developing the EAP. Several factors must be considered including, but not limited to, the physical facilities, emergency equipment requirements, designated personnel, communication strategies, and the local hospital settings. Because of its high participation levels and variety of venues, athletics has become a key EAP target, not only for athletes, but for coaches, staff, and spectators as well [21, 56]. The National Athletic Trainers' Association (NATA) and the National Collegiate Athletic Association (NCAA) have developed statements and positions regarding the EAP and its utilization for sporting events [20, 56].

The following components have been identified as fundamental to the organization and development of a comprehensive EAP [20]:

(a) Personnel – mandating personnel trained in cardiopulmonary resuscitation (CPR), AED, and first aid. It is imperative to have all key personnel who are directly involved with the athletes trained in emergency care. Key personnel may include coaches, athletes, administrators, equipment managers, and officials. The implementation of the EAP is not limited to only those who are certified in emergency care. Personnel not trained in emergency care can be instrumental in coordinating communication, directing emergency medical response teams to the correct location, and in helping to maintain the area around the emergency situation. These individuals need to be accounted for in your EAP.
(b) Equipment – Having the appropriate equipment on-site, or nearby, assists in the smooth implementation of the EAP [18]. One of the most essential pieces of emergency equipment is the Automated External Defibrillator (AED) [57]. Access to an AED is critical in many SCD cases and can make the difference between saving or losing a life [18, 20, 21]. Other equipment needed for CPR would include masks and oxygen supplies. Personnel participating in the EAP must be familiar with and trained to use the necessary equipment [18].
(c) Communication – A communication device could easily be listed in the equipment section as the most essential piece of emergency rescue equipment. Access to communications in the event of an emergency including SCDs should be the first step in initiating your EAP. The EAP should clearly identify where the closest land line is located, who should have cell phones on site, and/or who is in charge of radio communication. In the event of utilizing radio communication,

the plan must be clear on the duties of the person receiving the emergency message and how they should proceed as well. It is important that the person being identified to make the emergency call know the correct information to give on a 911 call and to make sure they are calm and listening to the dispatcher so that the information is clear and action can be taken quickly. Key elements of a 911 call include the nature of emergency, the patient's symptoms, care being given currently, approximate age of patient, and any medical history you can ascertain from the patient, or those involved in his/her care. Specifically, concern regarding a cardiac event must be relayed to the dispatcher as, often, it is possible to expedite AED arrival to the scene, even prior to full EMS response.

(d) Venue – The EAP should be specific for each venue in which sporting activities take place. For example, in an intercollegiate athletics program, you will need to have an EAP for each sport and for each site in which athletes may compete or practice. Even when practicing at a site for a short period of time, it is imperative to have a plan in place for an emergency. Items that should be considered for each venue include communication (are there any land lines for telephone), access to the field/court, the location and number of gates around the venue that may require keys in order to unlock them to allow emergency access, and the location of the nearest AED. Hospital access from the site is another consideration and should be included in the plan.

(e) Emergency Care Facilities – Access to the emergency room facilities and personnel are additional key components to a comprehensive EAP. It is important to communicate beforehand with the emergency facility closest to your venue and to establish how information can best be relayed to these emergency providers during an emergency event. Making contact with the hospital and local EMTs/paramedics can help establish improved implementation of the EAP and its efficacy when applied in an emotionally charged setting.

(f) Practice and Review – The EAP should not only be reviewed but should also be practiced at each site. The importance of practicing the EAP prior to an event cannot be overstated. A verbal review of the EAP procedures with personnel involved in the emergency plan is important, but implementing a practice run with selected scenarios for the EAP at specific venues will enhance the ultimate performance and plan. The results of these reviews should be well documented and indicate any changes in the plan.

The NATA consensus statement on Emergency Planning in Athletics is a thorough, detailed document that forms a comprehensive blueprint on customizing an EAP for any venue for athletics. The NCAA guidelines for Emergency Care and Coverage (*NCAA Sports Medicine Handbook*) is another source for universities and colleges to help design, construct, and implement an EAP. While the statistics show that the survival rate of a SCD is low, especially in cases of young, otherwise healthy athletes, the numbers also show that there have been successful outcomes with revival attempts. Well-planned EAP procedures play an integral part in those successful cases of survival.

AED Utilization: NCAA Collegiate Experience

In 2002, Coris et al. examined current AED access, ownership, and utilization among NCAA Division 1 athletic departments [18]. Of the 186 (61%) of 303 institutions responding to the survey, 72% (133) reported having access to AED units for their athletic programs, either through departmental ownership of the units or through the university system or local emergency medical services, while slightly more than half, 54% (101), reported departmental ownership of AED units for their programs. The mean number of total students attending the responding departments' institutions was 16,360 (SD = 11,026.00) with a reported 498 (SD = 222) mean number of varsity athletes per institution [18].

At the time of the survey, 8.6% (16) of the 133 programs with either access to, or ownership, of AED units reported having had to use the AED in an SCD event since purchase (see Fig. 1.3).

Reported recipients of the AED interventions included 62.5% (ten) officials, fans, and athletic department staff; 18.7% (three) athletes; and 6.25% (one) events involving a department's coach. Twelve and one-half percent (two) reported having had to use their AED units multiple times since purchase [21] (see Fig. 1.4).

Cases of AED utilization reported by athletic departments are outlined in the table above. Twenty percent of AED uses were attributed to student athletes, with 33% of utilizations for athletic department staff, and 47% for fans. Defibrillation was actually administered in 53% of AED unit applications. Time to shock was an average of 3.4 min, with average EMS response time of 8.2 min for those events without EMS on site (see Fig. 1.5).

Reported survival in this university athletic department setting for SCD was 0% for students, 75% for staff, 57% for fans, and 61% overall [21]. Eighty-eight percent of the reported AED interventions occurred during athletic events or training venues, with the exception of two events which occurred on campus locations unrelated to the athletic department. Of departments directly involved with the AED unit intervention (67%), 56% reported the AED units as easy to use, with all 16 respondents denying problems specifically with the units during the SCD event (see Fig. 1.6).

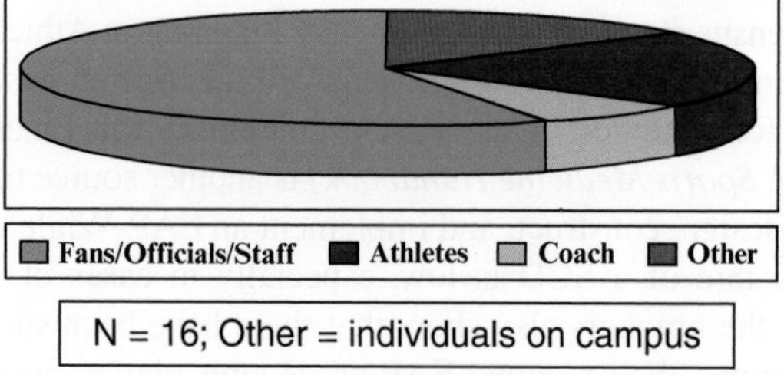

Fig. 1.3 Sudden cardiac death in collegiate sports medicine programs – victims

Case #	Patient	Outcome	Time to Shock	Location	EMS response time
1	Student-athlete	Head athletic trainer notified 5-10 minutes after event, defibrillator applied within 9 minutes, non-shockable, deceased	No shock	Student weight room	11 min
2	Student-athlete	Pt with cardiac history, reported chest pain, monitored within 30 seconds, survived, diagnosis: non-cardiac chest pain	No shock	Practice field	8-10 min
3	Student-athlete	Defibrillator applied within 90 seconds, non-shockable rhythm (PEA), deceased, diagnosis: hypertrophic cardiomyopathy	No shock	Campus recctr	8 min
4	Coach	Defibrillator applied within 2 minutes, non-shockable rhythm, deceased, diagnosis: myocardial infarction	No shock	Bleachers	Unknown
5	Graduation attendee	Suspected MI, Defibrillator applied in 5-7 min, no shock advised, survived to hospital discharge	No shock	Gymnasium	10 minutes
6	Lecture attendee	Defibrillator x 3, once more by EMS, survived to discharge, diagnosis: MI	2 min	Lecture hall	5-10 min
7	Staff	Monitored, survived to discharge	No shock	Training room	7 min
8	Football official	Defibrillator applied within one minute, ventricular fibrillation noted, defibrillated x1, survived to hospital discharge, diagnosis: myocardial infarction	55 sec	Football stadium	Immediate, on site
9	Fan	Defibrillated x1, survived to discharge	≤ 5 min	Arena	Immediate, on site
10	Fan	Defibrillated x2, resumed normal sinus rhythm, survived to hospital discharge	≤ 2.5 min	Basketball arena	Within 5 min
11	Fan	CPR provided until EMS arrival, no defibrillation prior, patient did not survive, diagnosis: MI	5-10 min	Basketball arena	5-10 min
12	Fan	VF/VT, Defibrillated x3, resumed normal sinus rhythm, survived to hospital discharge	4 min	Parking area	Within 5 min
13	Fan	VF/VT, Defibrillated x1, resumed normal sinus rhythm, survived to hospital discharge	2 min	Unknown	15 min
14	Fan	Notified within minutes, Defibrillated x1, presumed VF/VT, precipitated non-shockable rhythm, did not survive	3 min	Stadium	5 min
15	Fan	Hockey trainer notified, EMS on site, CPR immediately, Defibrillator applied in 7-8 min due to crowd related delay, non shockable rhythm, did not survive, diagnosis: massive MI	No shock	Hockey arena	On site

Fig. 1.4 Sudden cardiac death experience in NCAA Division I Sports Medicine Programs

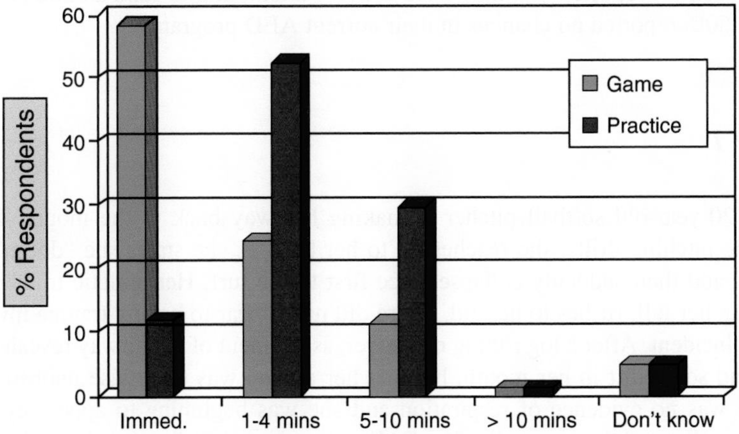

Fig. 1.5 NCAA Division I – EMS response time to collegiate SCD episode

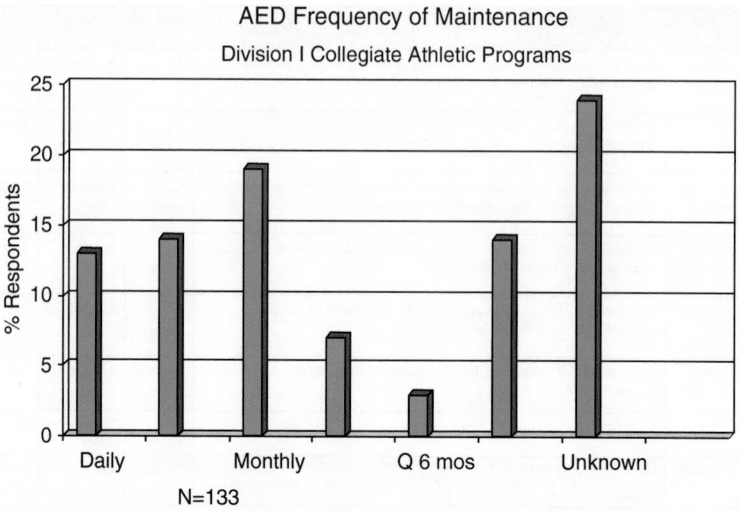

Fig. 1.6 AED frequency of maintenance Division I Collegiate Athletic Programs

Figures 1.6 and 1.7 illustrate the AED unit program utilization and maintenance policies for the subsample, which were not significantly different from the total sample of NCAA respondents. When compared with the total sample of Division I Athletic departments reporting access to or ownership of AED units (n = 133), departments reporting having experienced an SCD event were significantly more likely to report a greater number of units per department (4.5 SD = 2.7 vs. 2.84 SD = 2.4; $t = -2.32$, $p = 0.03$) at a greater per unit cost ($2,568.00 SD = $1,115.00 vs. $1,872.00 SD = $1,597.00, $t = -2.21$, $p < 0.03$) than departments without an SCD event. Five (31%) of departments reported purchasing additional AED units to expand their program since their initial implementation of their AED programs, three (18.5%) reported that they were actively attempting to fund additional units, while 50% reported no changes in their current AED programs.

Case 1

As a 20-year-old softball pitcher is making her way back to the mound during routine pitching drills, she reaches up to her head as she states she "doesn't feel good" and then suddenly collapses face first to the turf. Her athletic trainer, witnessing her fall, rushes to her aid. There did not appear to be any trauma involved in the incident. After a log rolling maneuver, assessment of her airway revealed that she had some dirt in her mouth, but that her airway was otherwise unobstructed. There was no evidence of respiration and she was beginning to appear cyanotic peripherally, and then centrally. The EAP was activated. Following the look, listen, and feel protocol, no respiration or pulse could be found and CPR was immediately initiated. The AED was called for and chest compressions and rescue breaths were begun by one person CPR while awaiting the AED. Upon arrival of the AED, approximately 1½ min later, chest pads were applied and a shock was advised. All were cleared and one shock was delivered. Return of color was witnessed in the athlete and gasping respirations were observed. A pulse was palpated and the patient was placed on her side in the recovery position. Two minutes later, the AED advised another shock, but the patient was alert and responsive at the time, and the AED pads were removed. After the initial shock event, she converted to a sinus tachycardia with a right bundle branch block.

EMS arrived approximately 5 min after the initial shock event. At this time, she was still responsive and found to be in a normal sinus tachycardia rhythm with a right bundle branch block. The patient was placed on oxygen, an IV was started, and she was placed on a transport gurney and subsequently taken to the nearest ER. In the emergency room, her ECG showed a mild U wave and a right bundle branch block, but it was otherwise normal. The chest X-ray was normal and her lab reports revealed mild hypokalemia. The rest of her lab reports was normal, and the patient was admitted to a cardiac care unit for observation.

No further ectopy or ventricular arrhythmia was noted. Echocardiogram was normal, cardiac MRI was normal, with normal muscle signal and normal takeoff of the coronary arteries. Given the patient's SCD event, extensive discussion with the patient and her parents was completed, and an implantable cardiac defibrillator was placed. The patient tolerated the procedure well and was discharged to home after hospital day 3 (see Fig. 1.7).

Summary

There are significant concerns with the rare, but catastrophic case of SCD in athletes. There are a variety of conditions, many asymptomatic, which can lead to sudden death. Preparticipation examinations can identify some athletes at risk and should be done in accordance with the AHA guidelines [7] for preparticipation examination and by the recommendations for the Preparticipation Physical Evaluation endorsed by the American Academy of Family Physicians, the American Academy of Pediatrics, The American College of Sports Medicine, the American Medical Society for Sports Medicine, the American Orthopaedic Society for Sports Medicine, and the American Osteopathic Academy of Sports Medicine [17].

Many cardiovascular abnormalities will not be identified by even the most thorough preparticipation evaluation. As more data becomes available in the US population, the role of noninvasive cardiovascular screening in the large scale preparticipation examination, particularly the screening ECG, may become more clear. Further research into the underlying causes of SCD in athletes is also ongoing and should provide invaluable insights into the detection and treatment of underlying cardiac disease in athletes.

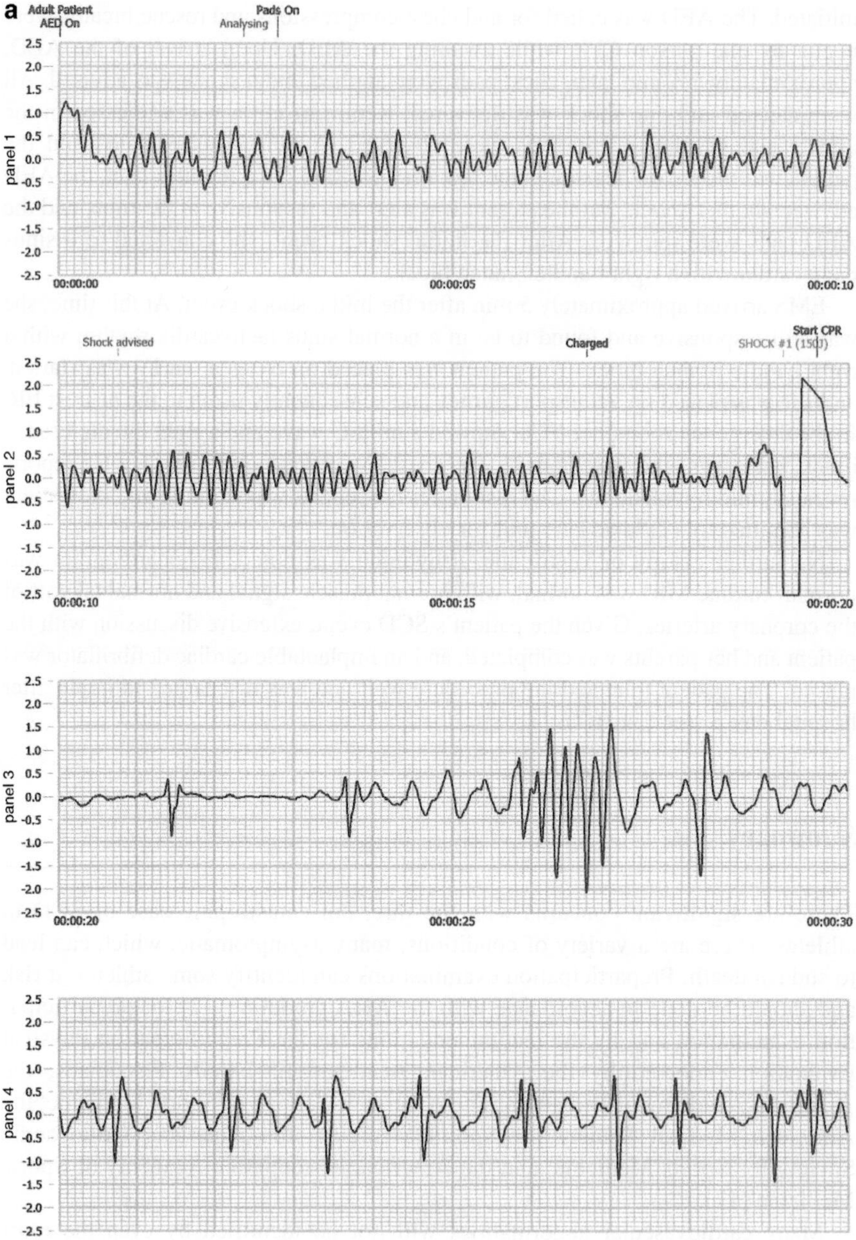

Fig. 1.7 (**a**) AED tracing of case 1: Ventricular fibrillation resulting in SCD. (**b**) Post defibrillation tracing

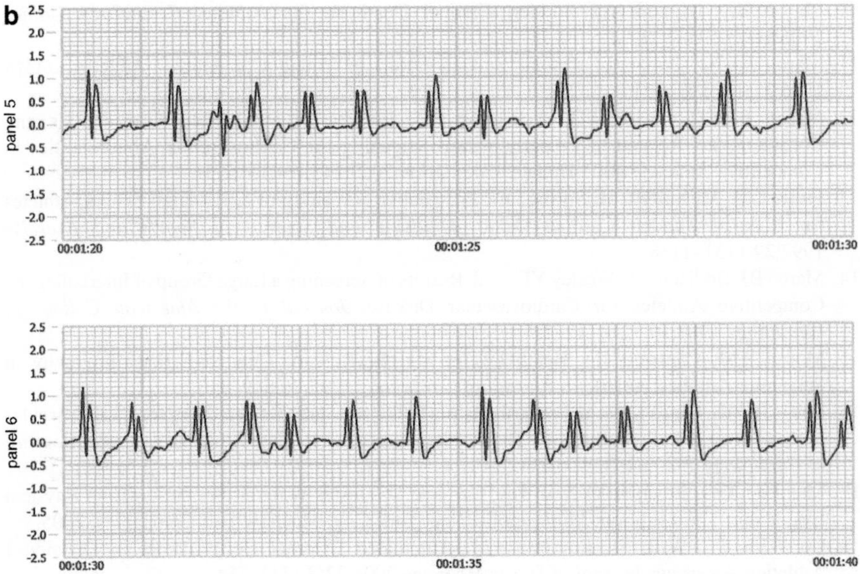

Fig. 1.7 (continued)

Finally, a robust EAP is imperative to optimally respond to the inevitable emergencies that will infrequently, but emergently, present themselves to the sports medicine team. Establishing, teaching, and practicing this plan may save lives that otherwise would be lost to this difficult collection of hidden disorders.

References

1. Huikuri HV, Agustin C, Myerburg RJ. Sudden Death Due to Cardiac Arrhythmias. *New England Journal of Medicine* 2001;**345**(20):1473–1482.
2. Gillum RF. Sudden Coronary Death in the United States. *Circulation* 1989;**79**:756–765.
3. Ackerman MJ. The Long QT Syndrome: Ion Channel Diseases of the Heart. *Mayo Clinic Proceedings* 1998;**73**:250–269.
4. Basilico F. Current Concepts: Cardiovascular Disease in Athletes. *American Journal of Sports Medicine* 1999;**27**(1):108–121.
5. Futterman LG MR. Sudden Death in Athletes: An Update. *Sports Medicine* 1998;**26**(5):335–350.
6. Van Camp SP. Sudden Death. *Clinics in Sports Medicine* 1992;**11**(4):273–289.
7. Maron BJ, Thompson PD, Puffer JC, et al. Cardiovascular Pre-Participation Screening of Competitive Athletes. *Circulation* 1996;**94**(4):850–856.
8. Cantu RC. Congenital Cardiovascular Disease: The Major Cause of Athletic Death in High School and College. *Medicine and Science in Sports and Exercise* 1992;**24**:279–280.
9. Myerburg RJ, Kessler KM, Castellanos A. Sudden Cardiac Death: Structure, Function, and Time-Dependence of Risk. *Circulation* 1992;**85**(Suppl I):I2–I10.

10. Maron BJ. Triggers for Sudden Cardiac Death in the Athlete. *Cardiology Clinics* 1996;**14**(2):195–210.
11. Maron BJ SJ, Poliac LC, et al. Sudden Death in Young Competitive Athletes. *JAMA* 1996;**276**(3):199–204.
12. Maron BJ, Thompson PD, Ackerman MJ, Balady G, et al. Recommendations and Considerations Related to Preparticipation Screening for Cardiovascular Abnormalities in Competitive Athletes: 2007 Update. *Circulation* 2007;**115**:1643–1655.
13. Fuller CM, McNulty CM, Spring DA. Prospective Screening of 5,615 High School Athletes for Risk of Sudden Cardiac Death. *Medicine and Science in Sports and Exercise* 1997;**29**:1131–1138.
14. Maron BJ, Bodison SA, Wesley YE, et al. Results of Screening a Large Group of Intercollegiate Competitive Athletes for Cardiovascular Disease. *Journal of the American College of Cardiology* 1987;**10**:1214–1221.
15. Murray PM, Cantwell JD, Heath DL, et al. The Role of Limited Echocardiography in Screening Athletes. *American Journal of Cardiology* 1995;**76**:849–850.
16. Lewis JF MB, Diggs JA, et al. Preparticipation Echocardiographic Screening for Cardiovascular Disease in a Large Predominantly Black Population of Collegiate Athletes. *American Journal of Cardiology* 1989;**64**:1029–1033.
17. Matheson GO, Boyajian-O'Neill LA, Cardone D, Dexter W, et al. Preparticipation Physical Evaluation: Third Edition. Minneapolis, New York City: McGraw-Hill Companies, 2005.
18. Coris EE SF, Walz SJ, Ramirez AM. Automated External Defibrillators in Division I Athletics. *American Journal of Sports Medicine* 2004;**32**(3):744–754.
19. White RD, Hankins DG, Bugliosi TF. Seven Years' Experience with Early Defibrillation by Police and paramedics in an Emergency Medical Services System. *Resuscitation* 1998;**39**:145–151.
20. Drezner JA, Courson RW, Roberts WO, Mosesso VN, et al. Interassociation Task Force Recommendations on Emergency Preparedness and Management of Sudden Cardiac Arrest in High School and College Athletic Programs: A Consensus Statement. *Journal of Athletic Training* 2007;**41**(1):143–158.
21. Coris EE, Miller E, Sahebzamani F. Sudden Cardiac Death in Division I Collegiate Athletics. *Clinical Journal of Sports Medicine* 2005;**15**(2):89–91.
22. Bille K, Figueiras D, Schamasch P, Kappenberger L, et al. Sudden Cardiac Death in Athletes: the Lausanne Recommendations. *European Journal of Cardiovascular Prevention and Rehabilitation* 2006;**13**:859–875.
23. Wingfield K, Matheson GO, Meeuwisse WH. Preparticipation Evaluation: An Evidence-Based Review. *Clinical Journal of Sports Medicine* 2004;**14**(3):109–122.
24. Maron BJ, Poliac LC, Roberts WO. Risk of Sudden Cardiac Death Associated with Marathon Running. *Journal of the American College of Cardiology* 1996;**28**:428–431.
25. Siscovick DS, Weiss NS, Fletcher RH, et al. The Incidence of Primary Cardiac Arrest During Vigorous Exercise. *New England Journal of Medicine* 1984;**311**:874–877.
26. Link MS, Homoud MK, Wang PJ, Estes NAM. Cardiac Arrhythmias in the Athlete. *Cardiology in Review* 2001;**9**(1):21–30.
27. Maron BJ, Towbin JA, Thiene G, Antzelevitch G, et al.. Contemporary definitions and classification of the cardiomyopathies: an American Heart Association Scientific Statement from the Council on Clinical Cardiology, Heart Failure and Transplantation Committee; Quality of Care and Outcomes Research and Functional Genomics and Translational Biology Interdisciplinary Working Groups; and Council on Epidemiology and Prevention. *Circulation* 2006;**113**(14):1807–1816.
28. Maron BJ, Roberts WC, Epstein SE. Sudden Death in Hypertrophic Cardiomyopathy: a Profile of 78 Patients. *Circulation* 1982;**65**:1388–1394.
29. Shah JS, Tome Esteban MT, Thaman R, Sharma R, et al. Prevalence of Exercise Induced Left Ventricular Outflow Tract Obstruction in Symptomatic Patients with Non-obstructive Hypertrophic Cardiomyopathy. *Heart* 2008;**94**:1288–1294.

30. Maron BJ, Gohman TE, Aeppli D. Prevalence of Sudden Cardiac Death During Competitive Sports Activities in Minnesota High School Athletes. *Journal of the American College of Cardiology* 1998;**32**:1881–1884.
31. Lawless CE, Best TM. Electrocardiograms in Athletes: Interpretation and Diagnostic Accuracy. *Medicine and Science in Sports and Exercise* 2008;**40**(5):787–798.
32. Corrado D, Basso C, Pavei A, Michieli P, Schiavon M, Gaetano T. Trends in Sudden Cardiovascular Death in Young Competitive Athletes After Implementation of a Preparticipation Screening Program. *JAMA* 2006;**296**(13):1593–1601.
33. Feinstein RA, Colvin E, Oh MK. Echocardiographic Screening as Part of a Preparticipation Examination. *Clinical Journal of Sports Medicine* 1993;**3**:149–152.
34. Koester MC. A Review of Sudden Cardiac Death in Young Athletes and Strategies for Preparticipation Cardiovascular Screening. *Journal of Athletic Training* 2001;**36**(2):197–204.
35. Cardiology ACo. ACC/ESC Clinical Expert Consensus Document on HCM. *Journal of the American College of Cardiology* 2003;**42**(9):1687–1713.
36. Orliaguet G, Ferjani M, Riou B. The Heart in Blunt Trauma. *Anesthesiology* 2001;**95**(2).
37. Perron AD, Brady WJ, Erling BF. Commotio Cordis: An Underappreciated Cause of Sudden Cardiac Death in Young Patients: Assessment and Management in the ED. *American Journal of Emergency Medicine* 2001;**19**(5):406–409.
38. Kyle JM, Leaman J, Elkins G. Planning for Scholastic Cardiac Emergencies: The Ripley Project. *The West Virginia Medical Journal* 1999;**95**(September/October):258–260.
39. Berger, S Dhala A, Friedberg DZ. Sudden Cardiac Death in Infants, Children, and Adolescents. *Pediatric Clinics of North America* 1999;**46**(2):221–227.
40. Thiene G, Basso C, Corrado D. Is Prevention of Sudden Death in Young Athletes Feasible. *Cardiologia* 1999;**44**:497–505.
41. Liberthson RR, Dinsmore RE, Fallon JT. Aberrant Coronary Artery Origin from the Aorta: Report of 18 Patients, Review of the Literature and Delineation of Natural History and Management. *Circulation* 1979;**59**:748–754.
42. Basso C, Maron BJ, Corrado D, Thiene G. Clinical Profile of Congenital Coronary Artery Anomalies with Origin from the Wrong Aortic Sinus Leading to Sudden Death in Young Competitive Athletes. *Journal of the American College of Cardiology* 2000;**35**:1493–1501.
43. Moss AJ. Sudden Cardiac Death and National Health. *Pacing and Clinical Electrophysiology* 1993;**16**:2190–2191.
44. Weidenbener EJ, Krauss MD, Waller BF, et al. Incorporation of Screening Echocardiography in the Preparticipation Examination. *Clinical Journal of Sports Medicine* 1995;**5**:86–89.
45. Bresler MJ. Acute Pericarditis and Myocarditis. *Emergency Medicine* 1992;**24**:35–51.
46. Maron BJ, Ackerman MJ, Nishimura RA, Pyeritz RE, Towbin JA, Udelson JE. Task Force 4: HCM and Other Cardiomyopathies, Mitral Valve Prolapse, Myocarditis, and Marfan Syndrome. *Journal of the American College of Cardiology* 2005;**45**(8):1340–1345.
47. Lecomte D, Fornes P, Fouret P, Nicholas G. Isolated Myocardial Fibrosis as a Cause of Sudden Cardiac Death and Its Possible Relation to Myocarditis. *Journal of Forensic Science* 1993;**38**:617–621.
48. Maron BJ, Chaitman BR, Ackerman MJ, Bayés de Luna A, et al., Working Groups of the American Heart Association Committee on Exercise, Cardiac Rehabilitation, and Prevention; Councils on Clinical Cardiology and Cardiovascular Disease in the Young. Recommendations for Physical Activity and Recreational Sports Participation for Young Patients with Genetic Cardiovascular Diseases. *Circulation* 2004;**109**(22):2807–2816.
49. McKeag DB. Preparticipation Screening of the Potential Athlete. *Clinics in Sports Medicine* 1989;**8**:373–397.
50. Kapetanopoulos A, Kluger J, Maron BJ, Thompson PD. The Congenital Long QT Syndrome and Implications for Young Athletes. *Medicine and Science in Sports Exercise* 2006;**35**(5):816–825.
51. Reiserdorff EJ, Prodinger RJ. Sudden Cardiac Death in the Athlete. *Emergency Medical Clinics of North America* 1998;**16**:281–294.

52. Lawless CE. Implantable Cardiac Defibrillators in Athletes. *Current Sports Medicine Reports* 2008;**7**(2):79–85.
53. Sarubbi B. The Wolff–Parkinson–White Electrocardiogram Pattern in Athletes: How and When to Evaluate the Risk for Dangerous Arrhythmias. The Opinion of the Paediatric Cardiologist. *The Journal of Cardiovascular Medicine* 2006;**7**(4):271–278.
54. Basso C, Corrado D, Thiene G. Arrhythmogenic Right Ventricular Cardiomyopathy in Athletes: Diagnosis, Management, and Recommendations for Sport Activity. *Cardiology Clinics* 2007;**25**:415–422.
55. Rampazzo A, Nava A, Malacrida S, et al. Mutation in Human Desmoplakin Domain Binding to Plakoglobin Causes a Dominant Form of Arrhythmogenic Right Ventricular Cardiomyopathy. *American Journal of Human Genetics* 2002;**71**:1200–6.
56. Anderson JC, Courson RW, Kleiner DM, McLoda TA. National Athletic Trainers' Association Position Statement: Emergency Planning in Athletics. *Journal of Athletic Training* 2002;**37**(1):99–104.
57. Cummins RO, Ornato JP, Thies WH, et al. Improving Survival From Sudden Cardiac Arrest: The Chain of Survival Concept. *Circulation* 1991;**83**:1832–1847.

Chapter 2
Cardiovascular Screening of Athletes: Focused Exam, Electrocardiograms, and Limited Echocardiograms

Christine E. Lawless

Introduction

The incidence of sudden cardiac death (SCD) in athletes is estimated to occur at a frequency of 1/200,000 athletes per year [1]. It is postulated that intense exercise predisposes the competitive athlete with previously undetected cardiac disease to lethal rhythm disturbances, and that the risk can be diminished if the athlete is withheld from sports participation.

This chapter explores the rationale for preparticipation cardiovascular screening with and without cardiovascular testing such as electrocardiograms (ECGs) and echocardiograms (echoes); workup of athletes with past history of heart disease, symptoms, abnormal findings or family history; barriers to routine ECG-based screening in the USA; how to implement ECG-based screening programs; how to interpret ECGs in athletes; the role of echo in screening of athletes; and what questions need to be addressed before widespread screening can be implemented in the USA.

Rationale for Pre-participation Cardiovascular Screening with and Without ECG

Attempts to reduce or eliminate the risk of SCD have led to intense screening efforts to detect the underlying potentially lethal cardiac conditions, with the primary screening tool being the preparticipation history and physical examination (PPE). The true sensitivity and specificity of the PPE is not known, but early retrospective studies suggest that the sensitivity of the PPE to detect underlying cardiac disease appears to be quite low, in the range of 2.5–6% [2]. In a registry study published in

---

C.E. Lawless (✉)
Sports Cardiology Consultants, LLC, Clinical Associate Faculty, University of Chicago Consulting Cardiologist, Major League Soccer Team Physician, US Figure Skating World Teams, 360 West Illinois Street #7D, Chicago, IL 60654, USA
e-mail: christine.lawless@yahoo.com

C.E. Lawless (ed.), *Sports Cardiology Essentials: Evaluation, Management and Case Studies*, DOI 10.1007/978-0-387-92775-6_2,

1996, 4 of 115 athletes who had undergone PPE were successfully diagnosed with underlying cardiovascular disease, suggesting a sensitivity of 2.5% for PPE alone in detecting previously unsuspected heart disease. However, in another 15 athletes who underwent PPE plus cardiac testing (ECG, echo, stress testing), the correct underlying diagnosis was made in 7 of 15 athletes, thus increasing the sensitivity of the PPE to correctly identify heart disease to about 50% [2]. Two recent studies of PPE in collegiate athletes suggest that careful history and physical examination contribute to a PPE sensitivity of approximately 40–50% [3, 4]. Reasons for increased sensitivity of PPE in recent years may include increased awareness of SCD in athletes, increasing requirements for and standardization of PPE forms at the state level, growing experience and skill of the US physician workforce in administration of the PPE, and increased use of the 2007 AHA guidelines describing a focused cardiovascular PPE [5]. However, despite improvements in the PPE over the last 15 years, the incidence and epidemiology of SCD in athletes, based on the latest report from the SCD registry, appears unchanged in the last decade [6].

Assuming that the PPE alone has a sensitivity between 2.5 and 40% in the athletic population, it has been suggested that routine cardiac testing such as ECG or echo be added to the standard PPE [7–9]. This approach appears to be effective, based on retrospective epidemiologic data obtained from Italy, where ECG-based screening has been in place long enough to determine long-term effects on mortality. The incidence of SCD in athletes appears to have decreased by 89% over the past 25 years. Italian researchers are convinced that this has been primarily due to ECG-based screening rather than administration of the PPE alone [10]. American critics of the Italian data have suggested that as multiple interventions were introduced in Italy over the past 25 years, and this is not randomized prospective data one cannot be certain that the reduction in SCD was solely due to the addition of ECG to the PPE.

The American Heart Association (AHA) consensus document on preparticipation screening of athletes published in March 2007 states that ECG-based screening protocols are not encouraged in the USA for several important reasons: (1) There is a lack of specialized practitioners carefully trained in screening and interpretation of ECGs in the athletic population; (2) The cost of conducting such screening in such a large number of eligible athletes may be prohibitive; (3) The mortality rate from SCD in athletes in the USA is already quite low, in fact, at the level achieved by the Italians after over 20 years of performing ECG-based screening; (4) Randomized trials with outcomes demonstrating clear superiority of the ECG-based screening over a standardized PPE without ECG are lacking; (5) There is a lack of standardization for interpretation of ECGs in athletes; and (6) There is a lack of normative data in certain demographic and ethnic groups [5]. At present, US athletic governing bodies such as the NCAA have not endorsed use of the ECG for routine screening of athletes. However, organized professional sports such as the NBA, NFL, and MLS have embraced the practice, with some including echocardiography and stress testing as well the ECG [11].

In lieu of widespread ECG-based screening for athletes, AHA consensus writers have recommended that the AHA 12 points or elements ought to be included in the focused cardiac portion of the PPE [5] (Table 2.1), and that cardiac signs and symptoms, and significant family history be promptly and thoroughly evaluated.

Table 2.1 The 12-element AHA recommendations for preparticipation cardiovascular screening of competitive athletes (reprinted with permission)

Medical history[a]
Personal history
1. Exertional chest pain/discomfort
2. Unexplained syncope/near-syncope[b]
3. Excessive exertional and unexplained dyspnea/fatigue, associated with exercise
4. Prior recognition of a heart murmur
5. Elevated systemic blood pressure
Family history
6. Premature death (sudden and unexpected, or otherwise) before age 50 years due to heart disease, in ≥1 relative
7. Disability from heart disease in a close relative <50 years of age
8. Specific knowledge of certain cardiac conditions in family members: hypertrophic or dilated cardiomyopathy, long-QT syndrome or other ion channelopathies, Marfan's syndrome, or clinically important arrhythmias
Physical examination
9. Heart murmur[c]
10. Femoral pulses to exclude aortic coarctation
11. Physical stigmata of Marfan's syndrome
12. Brachial artery blood pressure (sitting position)[d]

Reprinted with permission
[a]Parental verification is recommended for high school and middle school athletes
[b]Judged not to be neurocardiogenic (vasovagal); of particular concern when related to exertion
[c]Auscultation should be performed in both supine and standing positions (or with Valsalva maneuver), specifically to identify murmurs of dynamic left ventricular outflow tract obstruction
[d]Preferably taken in both arms

Appropriate Workup of Athletes with Past History of Heart Disease, Symptoms, Positive Family History, or Abnormal Physical Examination

The main point of the cardiac portion of the PPE is to establish the risk of participation in those with prior history of heart disease, and to detect previously undetected lethal cardiac conditions. On occasion, the athlete may present with a prior history of heart disease or a prior workup for heart disease. The clinician is obliged to confirm the diagnosis and determine the risk of participation. Multiple sets of published guidelines, especially the 36th Bethesda Guidelines, provide a framework as to whether to allow such an athlete to participate [12]. Clinicians need to be aware that not all healthcare practitioners adhere to published guidelines, and that there may be differences of opinion as to whether play should be allowed [13, 14].

It is absolutely crucial that clinicians understand the common causes of SCD in athletes and know how to identify these conditions. For example, as hypertrophic cardiomyopathy (HCM) is the most common cause of SCD in athletes, the clinician must be aware that the cardinal features of HCM are syncope, chest pain, shortness of breath, palpitations, fatigue, family history, and presence of a cardiac murmur. Anomalous coronary artery, the second most common underlying cardiac cause of SCD in athletes, may or may not be symptomatic. If symptoms are present, they will most likely consist of syncope, shortness of breath, chest pain with exertion, and palpitations.

Chest Pain

The differential diagnosis of chest pain is lengthy; cardiac causes probably account for less than 5%, with the majority of chest pain in athletes being caused by musculoskeletal conditions, gastrointestinal reflux, or pulmonary causes [15]. It is crucial that the clinician think of a cardiac cause before all others; once a significant cardiac condition is ruled out or deemed unlikely, other causes should be entertained.

Dyspnea

Shortness of breath is more likely to be pulmonary, but clinicians must carefully consider cardiac causes before assuming a pulmonary cause. Although not all physicians might agree with the practice, it is common for the physician to try empiric inhalers in a dyspneic athlete. However, if the athlete fails to improve, cardiac investigation is warranted.

Syncope, Near-Syncope, and Dizziness

Syncope *during exercise* necessitates a cardiac workup, while syncope occurring *at rest* may be of a benign nature [16]. Keep in mind that not all patient-athletes follow these widely held perceptions. Similarly, palpitations occurring with exercise are likely to be rhythm disturbances exacerbated or unmasked by catecholamines or enhanced adrenergic tone, while those occurring at rest are more likely to be of a benign nature. However, as with syncope, not all patient-athletes follow these common beliefs, and numerous examples to the contrary have been reported at sports medicine meetings and in small case studies [17]. This author strongly recommends that a recording of the underlying ECG rhythm *during the symptoms* be obtained in all athletes presenting with symptoms of palpitations, regardless of the symptoms occur at rest or with exercise [18]. If the rhythm is indeed benign, such as premature atrial beats, then no further workup is indicated. Some athletes present with either symptomatic or asymptomatic premature ventricular beats or contractions (PVCs). Biffi and colleagues have shown that the PVC burden correlates with the likelihood of underlying heart disease; the greater the PVC burden, the more likely the athlete is to have underlying disease [19]. Specifically, more than 2,000 PVCs/24 h indicates a 30% risk of underlying heart disease, but less than

2,000 PVCs/24 h correlates with a risk of less than 5%. More serious rhythms such as ventricular tachycardias or short runs require appropriate investigation [20].

Family History

Athletes with a family history of SCD prior to the age of 50 must be evaluated for inheritable forms of heart disease such as cardiomyopathy or channelopathy. It is more likely that athletes with a positive family history will have a relative who succumbed to coronary artery disease (CAD) rather than cardiomyopathy, as CAD is far more common in the general population. However, the PPE represents an opportunity to identify young people who are either carriers of cardiomyopathy genes or genes known to be associated with the development of premature CAD. Since there is an exhausting differential diagnosis for premature CAD, readers are referred to an excellent review of this subject from the AHA [21]. To illustrate that the concern for premature CAD is real among athletes, recall the case of Olympic figure skater Sergei Grinkov. He suffered fatal acute thrombosis of the left anterior descending artery during a practice session when he was 28 years old; postmortem analysis of his blood revealed a defect in a platelet proteoglycan, which is known to lead to premature coronary events [22].

Aside from history, physical examination may reveal clues to the presence of underlying heart disease. Blood pressure measurement, any delay in femoral pulses (indicative of coarctation of the aorta), presence of a cardiac murmur (consider HCM or valvular disease), or features of Marfan's syndrome may lead one to suspect an underlying cardiac condition (see chapters on murmurs 11, HCM 13, and Marfan's syndrome 16).

Once the PPE has been completed, any prior history of cardiac disease has been addressed, and any signs or symptoms have been satisfactorily explained, there are multiple sets of useful guidelines that suggest proper levels of participation and activity for the athlete. The most commonly used guideline is the 36th Bethesda Guidelines, updated in 2005 and summarized in Table 2.2 [12]. See chapter 21 for a comprehensive list and discussion of all existing guidelines.

Case Study of Positive Family History

On PPE, a 16–year-old high school basketball player had a significant family cardiac history. His father had a diagnosis of HCM since age 36 and suffered a cardiac arrest at the age of 42. After this happened, family members were evaluated for phenotypic and genotypic evidence of HCM. The player had no symptoms and no cardiac murmur. ECG, echo, and cardiac MRI were all normal, showing no hypertrophy or scar. Genetic blood testing revealed that the player carried the same HCM gene that his father carried. The player was allowed to participate in basketball, according to the recommendation of the 36th Bethesda Guidelines (genotype positive, phenotype negative HCM) [12]. However, the European guidelines would

Table 2.2 Summary of 36th Bethesda guidelines (adapted and reprinted with permission form reference [2])

	HCM	Anomalous coronary	ARVC	DCM	Long QT syndrome	Marfan's syndrome
Participation in all sports allowed	No	No	No	No	No	IA–IIA sports, with certain restrictions, depending on size of aorta (≤40 mm), absence of family history of dissection, and absence of significant valve disease)
Participation allowed if genotype +, phenotype –	Yes	N/A	Not specified in Bethesda guidelines	Not addressed	Yes, but no swimming allowed for Long QT1	Not specified
Participation allowed after corrective surgery	No	Yes	N/A	Yes, post heart transplant, provided no coronary luminal narrowing or ischemia	N/A	Low intensity (IA) sports only
Participation allowed with ICD	No	No	No	No	No	N/A
Participation allowed with beta blockers	No	Not specifically addressed	Not specifically addressed	Not addressed. If ejection fraction has normalized, no specific comment made	Not specifically addressed	Not specifically addressed

HCM = hypertrophic cardiomyopathy; ARVC = arrhythmogenic right ventricular cardiomyopathy; DCM = dilated cardiomyopathy not allow play in this instance [23]. Follow-up: The athlete has been playing without incidence for 4 years; annual ECG, echo, and MRI show no evidence of phenotypic expression of the disease.

ECG-Based Screening

Despite the limitations of the PPE alone, and the limitations of the ECG as a screening tool, some authors and professional organizations have recommended that ECG be added to routine PPE to enhance its ability to detect disease [8, 24]. In 2004, the International Olympic Committee recommended that an ECG be performed on all elite athletes prior to Olympic sports participation [23] and in 2005, the European Society of Cardiology recommended implementation of a common European ECG-based screening protocol [8]. Concurrently, the authors of the AHA/American College of Cardiology 36th Bethesda Guidelines for Sports Participation concluded that "ECG's are a practical and a cost effective strategic alternate to routine echocardiography for population based pre-participation screening," assuming that the ECG would be 75–95% sensitive in detecting HCM [12].

The true sensitivity and true specificity of the ECG in the athletic population is not known. However, Pelliccia has attempted to estimate such statistics by correlating surface ECG with underlying echocardiography in 1,005 consecutive elite athletes and categorizing the ECGs into three categories: normal, mildly abnormal, and distinctly abnormal, with the distinctly abnormal pattern being associated with a greater chance of underlying heart disease [24]. The combination of mildly abnormal and distinctly abnormal ECGs demonstrates a sensitivity of 51%, a specificity of 61%, a positive predictive accuracy of 7%, and a very high negative predictive accuracy of 96%. In the last decade, a number of investigators have evaluated the utility of ECG for screening of athletes, with varying results (Table 2.3).

Surface ECG patterns vary according to gender and sport, with distinctly abnormal patterns more likely to occur in males than in females and more likely to occur in endurance sports [24]. This may become clinically relevant when interpreting ECGs in specific athlete groups. For instance, if a distinctly abnormal pattern is seen in a female equestrian athlete, pathology is more likely than athletic adaptation.

In a study of 32,652 athletes, distinct ECG abnormalities included deeply inverted T waves (2.3%), significant LV hypertrophy (0.8%), right bundle branch block (1.0%), left anterior fascicular block (0.5%), left bundle branch block (0.1%), cardiac preexcitation pattern (WPW; 0.1%), and prolonged QTc interval (0.03%) [25]. Deeply inverted T waves may be particularly ominous, perhaps a precursor of cardiomyopathy, and may represent the earliest form of phenotypic expression [26]. The Italian authors note that the prevalence of markedly abnormal ECG patterns suggestive for structural cardiac disease is actually quite low (<5% in the general population) and should not represent an obstacle for implementation of 12-lead ECG-based screening program [25].

In 1999, Sharma and colleagues compared the ECGs of 1,000 junior elite British athletes (mean age 15 years) with the ECGs of 300 control, nonathletic,

Table 2.3 Studies of ECG as part of preparticipation examination for sports participation

Authors	Population	N	Incidence ECG abnormalities
Baggish et al. 2010	Collegiate athletes	510	2.2% had relevant cardiac abnormalities; ECG doubled sensitivity of screening over exam and history alone (45.5–90.9%)
Le et al. 2010	Collegiate athletes	658	10% distinctly abnormal ECG
Thunenkotter et al. 2010	Professional soccer players	605	4.8% pathological ECG
Crouse et al. 2009	NCAA football players	77	79% had ≥1 abnormal ECG finding
Sofi et al. 2008	General population seeking eligibility for sports participation	30,065	4.9% abnormal pattern on exercise ECG; 0.6% considered ineligible for sports
Basavarajaiah et al. 2008	Asymptomatic elite athletes in UK	3,500	0.08% LV hypertrophy consistent with HCM
Pelliccia et al. 2008	Trained athletes seeking eligibility for sports participation	From 12,550 tracings: $n = 81$ with ECG abnormalities; $n = 229$ matched controls	6% of athletes with abnormal ECG had cardiomyopathies
Wilson et al. 2008	National and international junior athletes	1,074 junior athletes; 1,646 active schoolchildren	0.3% had positive diagnosis of disease associated with SCD
Magalski et al. 2008	Elite American football players	1,959	25% had abnormal ECG; 30% among black players vs. 13% among white players; ECG abnormalities suggestive of cardiac disease: 6% vs. 2% in black and white athletes, respectively
Pelliccia et al. 2007	General population seeking eligibility for sports participation	32,652	11.8% had abnormal ECG; <5% had marked changes suggestive of cardiac disease
Pelliccia et al. 2006	Professional athletes	4,450	0.3% had cardiac abnormalities
Pelliccia et al. 2000	Competitive athletes	1,005	14% had distinctly abnormal ECG; 5% had structural cardiac deficits

See text for abbreviations cardiomyopathy

age-matched individuals [27]. Junior athletes were more likely to demonstrate sinus bradycardia (80%), sinus arrhythmia (52%), first degree A–V block (5%), incomplete right bundle branch blocks (29%), left atrial enlargement (14%), right atrial enlargement (16%), S–T segment elevation (45%), tall-peaked T waves (22%), and isolated Sokolow voltage criteria for LVH (45%). Corrected Q–T interval and the QRS duration were longer in the athletes than in the non-athletes. The authors concluded that the following might be indicative of underlying pathology in a highly trained junior athlete: ST depression or deep T inversion, minor T-wave inversions in any lead except V2–V3 when the athlete is less than 16 years old, Romhilt–Estes voltage criteria for LVH in female athletes, pathological Q wave, left axis deviation, and complete left bundle branch block.

American athletes have not been studied to the same degree as European athletes have been. However, isolated studies performed over the past 10 years illustrate the challenges faced in the USA. In 1997, Fuller et al. prospectively screened 5,615 high school athletes in northern Nevada with a PPE and ECG [7]. Five percent of subjects were found to have R or S waves greater than 30 mm; 6% had T-wave flattening or inversion in two or more leads; 2% had abnormal Q waves; and the axis was deviated greater than –30 or 120° in 1%. ECG abnormalities were present in 15.7% of the entire cohort. Fuller correlated findings on PPE and ECG with outcomes, defined as detection of any cardiovascular disease during the screening process that would preclude sports participation according to the 16th Bethesda guidelines. The sensitivity of the PPE to detect the abnormality was only 6%, whereas, ECG significantly increased the sensitivity to 70%.

Fuller's study was conducted primarily in Caucasian high school athletes in Reno, Nevada. However, based on early studies conducted in nonathletic African American subjects, there is reason to suspect that there are substantial ethnic differences in the appearance of the ECG in athletes [28, 29]. Two studies reported in 2008 shed light on this issue [30, 31]. Magalski et al. reported that the most abnormal ECG patterns (increased voltage, diffuse T inversion, deep Q waves) were found in 5.8% of blacks compared to only 1.8% of whites [30]. Concurrently, Basavarajaiah et al. showed that Sokolow–Lyon voltage criteria for LVH were more common in blacks than in whites with echocardiographic features of LVH, 68 vs. 40% [31]. Deep T-wave inversions in the precordial leads were also more prevalent (12 vs. 0%). Two recent studies of collegiate athletes suggest that ECG interpretation may lead to false-positive identification of athlete's cardiovascular risk [3, 4]. Baggish et al. screened 510 athletes at Harvard University [3]. The addition of ECG to physical examination and history improved the sensitivity of PPE to approximately 90%; however, inclusion of ECG reduced specificity and was associated with a false-positive rate of 16.9%. Le et al. evaluated the use of ECG in 658 athletes presenting for PPE at Stanford University [4]. Although 68% of female athletes had normal ECGs, only 38% of men had normal tracings. In all, 10% of athletes were considered to have distinctly abnormal ECG and were subjected to further testing. These studies are highly illustrative of the pitfalls of ECG interpretation in athletes in the USA; false positives are common, especially in the black population.

None of the above studies reflect the true impact of the PPE alone vs. the value added by the ECG in the prevention of SCD in athletes. Such an analysis would require a prospective randomized study, comparing standardized PPE with the 12 AHA questions to the standardized PPE with AHA questions plus the 12-lead ECG. Such a study would also require a "gold standard" such as echocardiography, advanced cardiac imaging, or genetic testing on all athletes to determine whether or not underlying heart disease was present and would include a certain percentage of known abnormals such that sensitivity and specificity could be determined. Such a study would also demand that endpoints include the impact of diagnosing and treating possible underlying disease such that the true effect on overall mortality and SCD could be determined. Given the low incidence of SCD in athletes in the USA, and the potential morbidity of cardiac procedures it is entirely possible that cardiac screening and further testing might actually result in worse outcomes [32].

Barriers to Routine ECG-Based Screening in the USA

Large Numbers of Athletes and Size of Appropriate Physician Workforce to Conduct the Screenings

The population of Italy is about one-fifth that of the USA, and Italian athletes are seen in one of several screening clinics by a highly trained Italian screening physician. The training program for screening physicians consists of 4 years of specialized sports medicine training, including rotations like sports traumatology, sports dermatology, and sports cardiology. During the sports cardiology rotation, trainees spend a significant amount of time performing ECGs and echoes, evaluating symptomatic athletes, and making participation decisions for all athletes. Thus, upon completion of their 4-year training, Italian sports medicine physicians are very familiar with the discipline of sports cardiology. The Italian approach to screening athletes is illustrated in Fig. 2.1. It should be noted that in Europe there has been a shift from the three-category Pelliccia criteria to the two-category Corrado criteria, with or without a recommended cutoff for degree of LVH voltage [8, 33].

In contrast, in the USA, the number of athletes, the training programs for sports medicine physicians, and the types of clinicians clearing athletes are vastly different from the Italian model. An estimated 40 million athletes participate at the professional, collegiate, high school, middle school, club, and recreational levels in some type of organized sport. At the professional level, athletes typically undergo PPE by contracted team physicians who are granted the authority to make participation determinations. A recent survey indicated that 92% of professional athletes underwent ECG screening, with a smaller percentage undergoing additional cardiac testing such as echocardiography and stress testing [11]. This approach is possible because of the small numbers of athletes, the ability of the sports organization to pay for such testing, and the training of the specialized team physicians caring for these athletes. The current US approach to PPE for athletes is illustrated in Fig. 2.2.

According to the NCAA, 300,000 athletes participate at the collegiate level. The PPE is required and generally conducted by team physicians contracted by

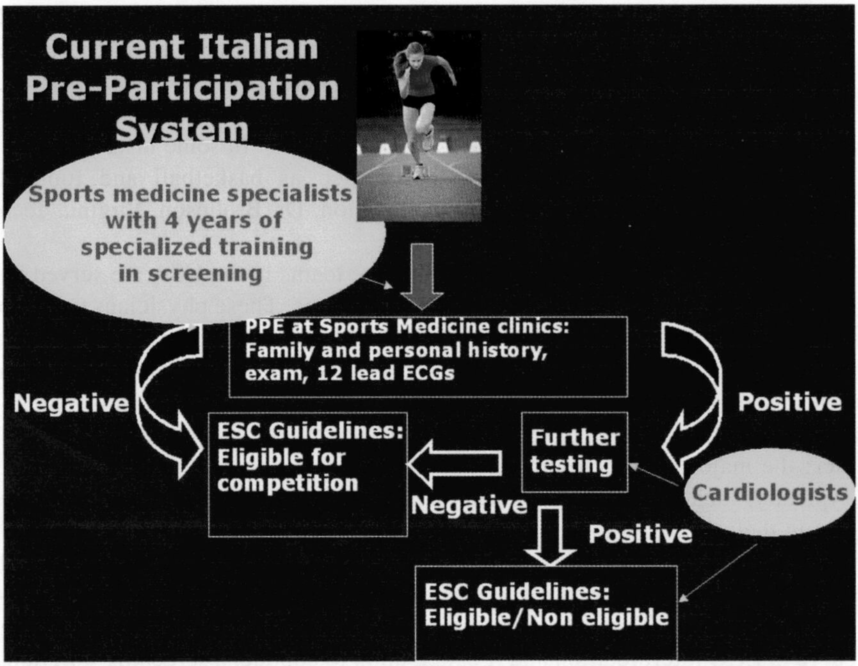

Fig. 2.1 The Italian approach to PPE screening for athletes, including the use of ECG

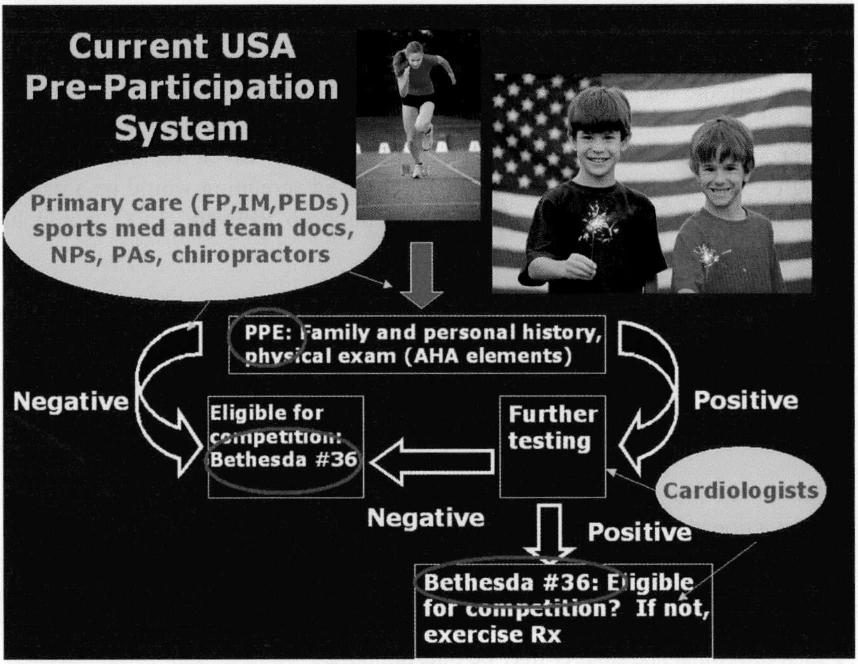

Fig. 2.2 The current US approach to PPE screening for athletes

the athletic departments. However, ECG in addition to the PPE is not mandated by the NCAA. Nonetheless, individual collegiate programs have chosen to include ECG based on the strength of the Italian data (personal communication, team physicians at University of South Florida, University of Georgia, University of Nevada, University of Florida, St. Louis University). In some instances, only athletes participating in high-risk sports such as basketball and football undergo cardiac testing (personal communication, Dr. Brolinson, Virginia Tech University).

The majority of professional and collegiate teams in the USA are served by sports medicine fellowship-trained team physicians. These physicians undergo a training program that is vastly different from that undergone by their European counterparts. In the USA, sports medicine physicians complete a 1-year sports medicine fellowship after 3 years of generalized family medicine, internal medicine, physiatry, pediatrics, emergency medicine, or orthopedics; the majority completing the fellowship are family medicine physicians. Typically, such physicians have had just 1 or 2 months of cardiology exposure during their family practice training and may have limited experience in ECG interpretation. During the sports medicine fellowship, trainees are not exposed to sports cardiology to any significant degree, as this does not exist as a specialty in the USA. Thus, sports medicine physicians have a substantial learning curve in ECG interpretation and if called upon to conduct a screening program, they often partner with the local cardiology consultant. Thus, it is crucial that the partnering cardiologist has a working knowledge of ECG interpretation in athletes.

At the high school level, the PPE may be conducted by a variety of clinicians, including sports medicine physicians, primary care physicians with no sports medicine background, nurse practitioners, and chiropractors. The quality of the PPE may be variable, exposure to cardiology may be extremely limited, and the ability to read an ECG may be highly variable. Given the large numbers of high school athletes, application of ECG-based screening would be a daunting task. Requiring club sport athletes to undergo PPE and ECG would be equally challenging.

Cost of Conducting Such Screening in Such a Large Number of Eligible Athletes

Although not the primary issue, the cost for conducting ECG-based screening is often mentioned in debates regarding such screening. For example, in a high school with 500 athletes and at a cost of $20 per ECG, theoretically it may cost up to $10,000 to conduct such a program. Despite the costs, some high schools have adopted ECG-based screening due to the efforts of volunteers, but the sustainability of such programs and quality may be questionable.

Mortality Rate from SCD in Athletes is Already Quite Low

One of the more compelling arguments against ECG-based screening in the USA is the unlikely possibility of improving upon the already low rates of SCD in US athletes. When the Italians embarked on their program in the early 1980s, the SCD rate in athletes was 3.5/100,000, but this declined to 1/200,000 approximately 25 years after ECG-based screening was initiated [10]. This figure is remarkably similar to what the USA already has achieved [6], opening to question whether ECG-based screening ought to be considered at all [32].

Lack of a Randomized Trial Demonstrating Clear Superiority of the ECG-Based Screening over a Standardized PPE Without ECG

Although the Italian data are compelling, the report published in 2007 was a retrospective analysis, and one cannot conclude with certainty that the results observed were due to the ECG alone. The program was implemented in 1981, but several interventions were implemented at once: enhanced history and physical by specially trained clinicians, ECG, and algorithms for work up and return to play. Over the years, protocols underwent gradual refinement. Thus, it cannot be concluded that the decline in SCD rate in athletes was due to the ECG alone; rather, one would have to conclude that the combination of practices allowed for the improvement.

Lack of Standardization for Interpretation of ECGs in Athletes

Computerized ECG interpretation algorithms have been derived from studies conducted in the general population many years ago. It has been well documented that athletes demonstrate distinctive 12-lead surface ECG patterns, which are more prevalent among endurance athletes and in male gender [24]. Interpretation criteria have been published by the Europeans, but these criteria have not yet been shown to have the ability to reliably identify underlying heart disease in a prospective, controlled trial. There are also the issues of false positives and overreading. As there is more hypertrophy, bradycardia, early repolarization, and ST–T alterations in athlete ECGs, there exists a false-positive rate of up to 40% among inexperienced readers [13, 30] to 1–2% among experienced readers [33]. This degree of variance would certainly justify aids such as algorithms or benchmarks for voltage or T waves that would trigger workups. At the moment, there are no such aids.

Lack of Normative Data in Certain Demographic and Ethnic Groups

It is important to note that the Italian ECG patterns are based on results obtained in elite Caucasian European athletes with a mean age of 23 years, and that rules of ECG interpretation derived from the Italian data may not necessarily be applied to younger athletes, to the recreational athlete, or to athletes of other ethnic groups. One such group is the African American athlete.

An early study in nonathletes of age 11–17 years indicated that black males ($n = 27$) demonstrated statistically higher voltage measurements in lead 1 (15 vs. 10 mm), V4 (50 vs. 36 mm), V5 (44 vs. 39 mm) and V6 (30 vs. 24 mm) than their white counterparts of the same gender ($n = 27$) [34]. Black males also had higher voltage than black females ($n = 34$) in lead V4 (50 vs. 47 mm), V5 (44 vs. 25 mm), and V6 (30 vs. 22 mm). In contrast, black females did not demonstrate significant differences from white females with the exception of the S wave in V1 (26 vs. 16 mm).

Recently, Magalski reported ECG findings of 1959 collegiate football players (67% black) [30]. The most abnormal patterns (distinctly abnormal, high voltage, diffuse deep T waves or Q waves) were found in 5.8% of blacks compared with 1.8% of whites. After adjustment for all other variables, black race was the only independent predictor of a distinctly abnormal ECG. Basavarajaiah reported in a group of British athletes that Sokolow–Lyon voltage criteria were more common in black athletes with echo evidence of LV hypertrophy than in white athletes (68 vs. 40%) [31]. Deep T-wave inversions in the precordial leads were seen in 12% of black athletes compared with none of the white athletes. These data suggest that screening large numbers of American athletes, especially if they are black, may not be practical due to the inability to distinguish normal athletic adaptation or normal ethnic variants from true pathology.

As there is currently no standard for ECG interpretation in the athlete, the ECG is subject to marked variation in interpretation by cardiologists and others involved in athlete care. As ECG is not 100% sensitive for the detection of underlying heart disease, the possibility of false negatives exists. Table 2.4 summarizes the sensitivity and specificity of the ECG for conditions known to predispose to SCD in athletes [35]. For some diagnoses, such as anomalous coronary artery, the sensitivity of the ECG will be extremely low, whereas for others, such as HCM, the ECG ought to be an excellent screening tool. False positives exist as well, as normal athletic adaptation to exercise can result in marked alterations of the surface ECG, resulting in delays due to the time it takes to follow-up and perform further cardiac evaluation.

How to Implement ECG-Based Screening Programs

Despite the critiques and limitations of the ECG, for those clinicians who choose to use an ECG-based approach in their preparticipation screening of athletes, the decision tree shown in Fig. 2.3 may be a useful guide [35]. This proposed approach

Table 2.4 Sensitivity and specificity of ECG for specific cardiovascular diagnoses (reproduced with permission)from reference #35

CV disease	Likelihood of being detected with ECG	ECG findings	Sensitivity	Specificity
Hypertrophic CM	High	LVH, abnormal axis, Q waves, ST-T changes	73–98%	Low
ARVD	Low to intermediate	T-wave inversions V leads	25–94%	Low, with exception of the epsilon wave
Dilated CM	High	May have infarct pattern, left anterior hemiblock, RBBB or LBBB, or LBBB, LVH, or ST-T abnormalities, LAE, or atrial fibrillation	Probably high ≤1% are normal	Low
Myocarditis	Low to intermediate	ST elevation	10–54%	Low
Long QT syndrome	High	Q–T c >440 ms males Q–T c >460 in females	83–100%	Intermediate
Brugada syndrome	Low	RBBB, and "coved" ST elevation in V1 and V2	At least 20%	High
Coronary anomalies	Low	None characteristic	Low	Low
Myocardial bridging	Low	None characteristic	Low	Low
Aortic stenosis	High	LVH, ST-T abnormalities	80%	Low
Mitral valve prolapse	Low	ST-T changes, PVCs	66%	Low
Marfan's syndrome	Low	None characteristic	Unknown	Unknown

CM cardiomyopathy, *LVH* left ventricular hypertrophy, *LBBB* left bundle branch block, *PVCs* premature ventricular contractions, *RBBB* right bundle branch block, *ARVD* arrhythmogenic right ventricular dysplasia/cardiomyopathy

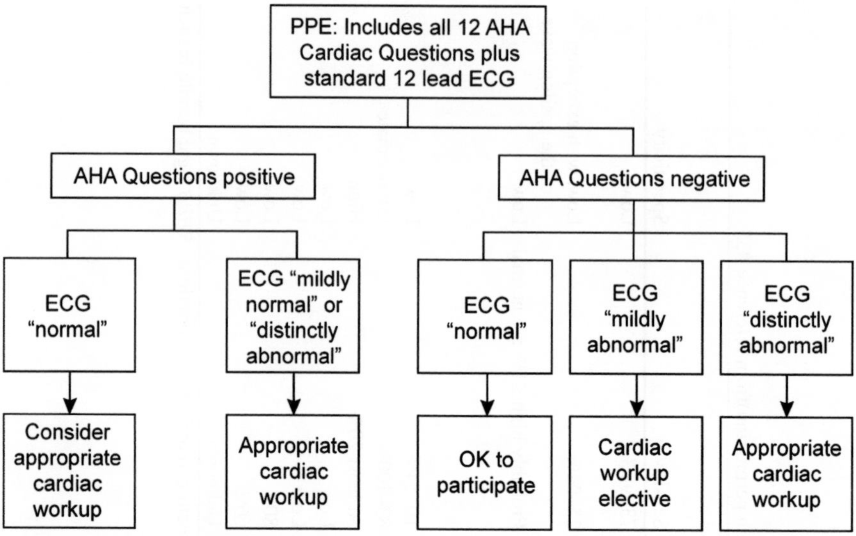

Fig. 2.3 Decision tree for ECG-based screening program (reproduced with permission from reference [35])

is consistent with what the Europeans have recommended [10]. The athlete with the distinctly abnormal ECG requires further investigation, regardless of symptoms. Cardiac workup is considered optional for the athlete without symptoms and mildly abnormal ECG or athletes with positive answers to the AHA questions but normal ECG. An alternative approach is to determine normative ECG data for the population one is screening and work up significant deviations from normal. This approach has been used by the NFL for years and has recently been adopted by MLS (personal communication, Dr. Christine Lawless, consulting cardiologist to MLS).

How to Interpret ECGs in Athletes

Although there is no uniform algorithm for interpretation of the ECG in asymptomatic athletes, the Europeans have proposed some simple rules that appear to reliably detect the majority of heart disease in young athletic populations (Table 2.5) [10, 30, 35]. It is important to note that the Italian ECG patterns are based on results obtained in elite, Caucasian, European athletes with a mean age of 24 years and that rules of ECG interpretation derived from the Italian data may not necessarily be applied to younger athletes, to the recreational athlete, or to athletes of other ethnic groups. One such group is likely the African American athlete. Based on published data in nonathletic African American populations, there is reason to suspect that ECGs in athletic African Americans may be markedly different from that in their white European counterparts [30, 31, 34]. Further study is necessary to determine normative data in this group of athletes. As there is currently no standard for ECG interpretation in the American

Table 2.5 Classification of abnormalities of the athlete's ECG (reproduced with permission from the European Society of Cardiology) [33]

Group 1: common and training-related ECG changes	Group 2: uncommon and training-unrelated ECG changes
Sinus bradycardia	T-wave inversion
First-degree AV block	ST-segment depression
Incomplete RBBB	Pathological Q waves
Early repolarization	Left atrial enlargement
Isolated QRS voltage criteria for left ventricular hypertrophy	Left-axis deviation/left posterior hemiblock
	Right ventricular hypertrophy
	Ventricular preexcitation
	Complete LBBB or RBBB
	Long- or short-QT interval
	Brugada-like early repolarization

RBBB right bundle branch block, *LBBB* left bundle branch block
Adapted from [33]

athlete, the ECG is subject to marked variation in interpretation by cardiologists and others involved in athlete care. It is not 100% sensitive for the detection of underlying heart disease; therefore, the possibility of false negatives exists. For some diagnoses, such as anomalous coronary artery, the sensitivity of the ECG will be extremely low, whereas for others, the ECG ought to be an excellent screening tool.

The Role of Echocardiography in Screening of Athletes

Because ECGs are not 100% sensitive, some authors advocate the addition of echo to the screening. However, there are many problematic issues inherent in this approach. Echo requires special equipment and training, is less portable, and more costly than ECG. Some would argue that there are quality concerns, since it is not likely that accredited echocardiographers would either perform and/or interpret all the screening tests. Given the number of athletes in the USA, widespread use of this technique does not seem practical. Nonetheless there are some who advocate this approach. Some collegiate programs have adopted an abbreviated echo for incoming athletes the first year they join their respective programs. Such abbreviated echoes tend not to be complete studies but are performed and interpreted by accredited laboratories and physicians and screen for the major causes of SCD in athletes. Wyman et al. reported results of a 5-min screening echo for collegiate athletes [9]. In 395 athletes studied, no athlete was found to have evidence of HCM. However, 19.5% were found to have trivial or mild mitral regurgitation, 13.4% trivial or mild tricuspid regurgitation, 3.9% trivial, mild, or moderate aortic insufficiency, 0.5% bicuspid aortic valve prolapse, and 1.3% mitral valve prolapse. Origin of the left coronary artery was identified in 99%, and origin of the right in 96%. This implies that anomalous coronary artery can be detected in the majority of cases, but not all authorities agree that the echocardiogram is this sensitive for detecting this anomaly. Further study is warranted.

In a survey conducted in 2005 among 122 North American professional sports teams from the MLB, NHL, and NFL, 13% performed preparticipation echo [11]. There are a number of charitable organizations whose members are parents who have lost their teen-age athletes from sudden death during athletics. These groups promote echo screening of high school athletes and go as far as to advocate training of nonprofessionals in performance of inexpensive "screening" echo [36]. The quality of such screening programs, and the sensitivity and specificity of the echo in this model has not yet been validated. Momentum appears to have shifted in favor of the ECG because of ease of administration, cost, relatively low cost, and its ability to detect both HCM and long QT.

What Issues Still Need to be Addressed Before Wide-Spread Screening Can be Implemented in the USA

Efficacy of ECG Screening

Efficacy, cost, ability of the physician workforce to interpret the ECGs, and health-care disparities are cited as the main reasons that ECGs are not indicated in the USA [37]. In the USA, SCD rates in athletes may be as low as what Italy achieved after several decades of screening. At a rate of 1/200,000, the SCD rate amounts to 150–200 athletes per year. However, these figures are based on data gleaned from years of combing newspaper reports and internet reports of SCD in young athletes. Such data may be subject to selection bias. A well-designed epidemiologic study in Minnesota, which collected details of all deaths over time, showed that the rate of SCD was comparable to that in Padua Italy [38]. Thus, one is hard pressed to conclude that ECG screening would improve upon these rates. Some argue that the additional cardiac testing and use of cardiac procedures would actually add to the morbidity and mortality, resulting in higher rates of death [32]. Given the incidence of HCM in the general population of 1/500, of long QT 1/3,000, and of anomalous coronary 1/1,000, screening is unlikely to have impact.

If the question of efficacy were to be resolved by a large multicenter trial, huge numbers of participants would be necessary to power the study to detect differences. Supposing such a trial could be conducted, the next step is to determine who would pay for the cost of ECGs. If left to the individual, even a $20 ECG may prove cost prohibitive for certain demographics.

Lastly, the Italian program has been conducted by specially trained sports medicine physicians. These clinicians have learnt how to perform ECGs and echoes in athletes and are skilled in their interpretation. In contrast, the sports medicine physician workforce in the USA is small in number; the majority is trained for 3 years in general family practice, receiving only 1–2 months of cardiology training in the hospital setting. Thus, the physicians trained to perform PPEs with ECGs are very small in number and inadequately trained in cardiology. As there are more than 40 million athletes in the USA, many athletes remain in the care of their primary doctor, who is unlikely to have significant experience in interpreting ECGs. Some authorities feel that the physician workforce is the greatest barrier to implementation of ECG-based screening in the USA. A recent abstract presented at the AHA meeting in November 2009 illustrates the challenge [13]. Surveys conducted in five physician specialties that screen athletes showed that up to 60% of physicians would overread the ECG (false positive) and up to 20–30% may miss pathology. Large-scale physician education would be required. Given these numbers and the low incidence of SCD in athletes in the USA, it is doubtful that a well-designed outcomes study would demonstrate the superiority of ECG-based screening over PPE alone.

Summary

In summary, the goal of PPE cardiovascular screening in athletes is to detect underlying, potentially lethal heart disease. With focused examination and increased awareness of the cardiovascular needs of the athlete, the sensitivity of the PPE alone appears to be increasing. The role of ECG is evolving as an adjunct to the standard PPE, and although well-controlled prospective trials are lacking, the ECG does appear to increase the sensitivity of the PPE alone to detect underlying cardiac disease. Because many of the conditions that cause SCD in athletes demonstrate ECG findings similar to what is seen in normal athletic adaptation, clinicians should follow some simple rules for ECG interpretation in athletes, and need to be prepared for the consequences of both over- and underinterpretation of the ECG in athletes. Although ECG-based screening has gained wide acceptance in Europe, ECG-based cardiovascular screening of young athletes is currently not recommended in the USA. However, future studies designed specifically for the American athlete at all levels may assist in evolving this field in the USA.

References

1. Maron BJ, Pelliccia A. The heart of trained athletes: cardiac remodeling and the risks of sports, including sudden death. *Circulation*. 2006;114:1633–44.
2. Maron BJ, Shirani J, Poliac LC, Mathenge R, Roberts WC, Mueller FO. Sudden death in young competitive athletes. Clinical, demographic, and pathological profiles. *JAMA*. 1996;276:199–204.
3. Baggish AL, Hutter AM Jr, Wang F, et al. Cardiovascular screening in college athletes with and without electrocardiography: a cross-sectional study. *Ann Intern Med*. 2010;152:269–75.
4. Le VV, Wheeler MT, Mandic S, et al. Addition of the electrocardiogram to the preparticipation examination of college athletes. *Clin J Sport Med*. 2010;20:98–105.

5. Maron BJ, Thompson PD, Ackerman MJ, et al. Recommendations and considerations related to preparticipation screening for cardiovascular abnormalities in competitive athletes: 2007 update: a scientific statement from the American Heart Association Council on Nutrition, Physical Activity, and Metabolism: endorsed by the American College of Cardiology Foundation. *Circulation*. 2007;115:1643–455.
6. Maron BJ, Doerer JJ, Haas TS, Tierney DM, Mueller FO. Sudden deaths in young competitive athletes: analysis of 1866 deaths in the United States, 1980–2006. *Circulation*. 2009;119: 1085–92.
7. Fuller CM, McNulty CM, Spring DA, et al. Prospective screening of 5,615 high school athletes for risk of sudden cardiac death. *Med Sci Sports Exerc*. 1997;29:1131–8.
8. Corrado D, Pelliccia A, Bjornstad HH, et al. Cardiovascular pre-participation screening of young competitive athletes for prevention of sudden death: proposal for a common European protocol. Consensus Statement of the Study Group of Sport Cardiology of the Working Group of Cardiac Rehabilitation and Exercise Physiology and the Working Group of Myocardial and Pericardial Diseases of the European Society of Cardiology. *Eur Heart J*. 2005;26:516–24.
9. Wyman RA, Chiu RY, Rahko PS. The 5-minute screening echocardiogram for athletes. *J Am Soc Echocardiogr*. 2008;21:786–8.
10. Corrado D, Basso C, Pavei A, Michieli P, Schiavon M, Thiene G. Trends in sudden cardiovascular death in young competitive athletes after implementation of a preparticipation screening program. *JAMA*. 2006;296:1593–601.
11. Harris KM, Sponsel A, Hutter AM Jr, Maron BJ. Brief communication: cardiovascular screening practices of major North American professional sports teams. *Ann Intern Med*. 2006; 145:507–11.
12. Maron BJ, Zipes DP. Introduction: eligibility recommendations for competitive athletes with cardiovascular abnormalities-general considerations. *J Am Coll Cardiol*. 2005;45:1318–21.
13. Lawless CE, Winicur ZM, Bellande BJ. Preparedness of US physician workforce to screen competitive athletes for sports participation. American Heart Association, 2009 Annual Meeting: Orlando, Florida, 2009.
14. Pelliccia A, Zipes DP, Maron BJ. Bethesda Conference #36 and the European Society of Cardiology Consensus Recommendations revisited a comparison of U.S. and European criteria for eligibility and disqualification of competitive athletes with cardiovascular abnormalities. *J Am Coll Cardiol*. 2008;52:1990–6.
15. Singh AM, McGregor RS. Differential diagnosis of chest symptoms in the athlete. *Clin Rev Allergy Immunol*. 2005;29:87–96.
16. Link MS, Estes NA 3rd. How to manage athletes with syncope. *Cardiol Clin*. 2007;25:457–66, vii.
17. Lawless CE, Lampert R, Olshansky B, Cannom D. Safety and efficacy of implantable defibrillators and automatic external defibrillators in athletes: results of a nationwide survey among AMSSM members. *Clin J Sports Med*. 2005;15:386–91.
18. Lawless CE, Briner W. Palpitations in athletes. *Sports Med*. 2008;38:687–702.
19. Biffi A, Pelliccia A, Verdile L, et al. Long-term clinical significance of frequent and complex ventricular tachyarrhythmias in trained athletes. *J Am Coll Cardiol*. 2002;40:446–52.
20. Estes NA 3rd, Link MS, Cannom D, et al. Report of the NASPE policy conference on arrhythmias and the athlete. *J Cardiovasc Electrophysiol*. 2001;12:1208–19.
21. Morey SS. AHA assesses the impact of genotyping on diagnosis of genetic cardiac disease. American Heart Association. *Am Fam Physician*. 1999;59:2915–6, 2918.
22. Goldschmidt-Clermont PJ, Shear WS, Schwartzberg J, Varga CF, Bray PF. Clues to the death of an Olympic champion. *Lancet*. 1996;347:1833.
23. Bille K, Figueiras D, Schamasch P, et al. Sudden cardiac death in athletes: the Lausanne recommendations. *Eur J Cardiovasc Prev Rehabil*. 2006;13:859–75.
24. Pelliccia A, Maron BJ, Culasso F, et al. Clinical significance of abnormal electrocardiographic patterns in trained athletes. *Circulation*. 2000;102:278–84.
25. Pelliccia A, Culasso F, Di Paolo FM, et al. Prevalence of abnormal electrocardiograms in a large, unselected population undergoing pre-participation cardiovascular screening. *Eur Heart J*. 2007;28:2006–10.

26. Pelliccia A, Di Paolo FM, Quattrini FM, et al. Outcomes in athletes with marked ECG repolarization abnormalities. *N Engl J Med*. 2008;358:152–61.
27. Sharma S, Whyte G, Elliott P, et al. Electrocardiographic changes in 1000 highly trained junior elite athletes. *Br J Sports Med*. 1999;33:319–24.
28. Rao PS, Thapar MK, Harp RJ. Racial variations in electrocardiograms and vectorcardiograms between black and white children and their genesis. *J Electrocardiol*. 1984;17:239–52.
29. Rao PS. Racial differences in electrocardiograms and vectorcardiograms between black and white adolescents. *J Electrocardiol*. 1985;18:309–13.
30. Magalski A, Maron BJ, Main ML, et al. Relation of race to electrocardiographic patterns in elite American football players. *J Am Coll Cardiol*. 2008;51:2250–5.
31. Basavarajaiah S, Wilson M, Whyte G, Shah A, McKenna W, Sharma S. Prevalence of hypertrophic cardiomyopathy in highly trained athletes: relevance to pre-participation screening. *J Am Coll Cardiol*. 2008;51:1033–9.
32. Thompson PD, Levine BD. Protecting athletes from sudden cardiac death. *JAMA*. 2006;296:1648–50.
33. Corrado D, Pelliccia A, Heidbuchel H, et al. Recommendations for interpretation of 12-lead electrocardiogram in the athlete. *Eur Heart J*. 2010;31:243–59.
34. Reiley MA, Su JJ, Guller B. Racial and sexual differences in the standard electrocardiogram of black vs white adolescents. *Chest*. 1979;75:474–80.
35. Lawless CE, Best TM. Electrocardiograms in athletes: interpretation and diagnostic accuracy. *Med Sci Sports Exerc*. 2008;40:787–98.
36. A Heart for Sports. 2207; Accessed May 7, 2010. Web Page. Available at: http://www.aheartforsports.org/.
37. Maron BJ. National electrocardiography screening for competitive athletes: feasible in the United States? *Ann Intern Med*. 2010;152:324–6.
38. Maron BJ, Haas TS, Doerer JJ, Thompson PD, Hodges JS. Comparison of U.S. and Italian experiences with sudden cardiac deaths in young competitive athletes and implications for preparticipation screening strategies. *Am J Cardiol*. 2009;104:276–80.
39. Thunenkotter T, Schmied C, Dvorak J, Kindermann W. Benefits and limitations of cardiovascular pre-competition screening in international football. *Clin Res Cardiol*. 2010;99:29–35.
40. Crouse SF, Meade T, Hansen BE, Green JS, Martin SE. Electrocardiograms of collegiate football athletes. *Clin Cardiol*. 2009;32:37–42.
41. Sofi F, Capalbo A, Pucci N, et al. Cardiovascular evaluation, including resting and exercise electrocardiography, before participation in competitive sports: cross sectional study. *BMJ*. 2008;337:a346.
42. Wilson MG, Basavarajaiah S, Whyte GP, Cox S, Loosemore M, Sharma S. Efficacy of personal symptom and family history questionnaires when screening for inherited cardiac pathologies: the role of electrocardiography. *Br J Sports Med*. 2008;42:207–11.
43. Pelliccia A, Di Paolo FM, Corrado D, et al. Evidence for efficacy of the Italian national pre-participation screening programme for identification of hypertrophic cardiomyopathy in competitive athletes. *Eur Heart J*. 2006;27:2196–200.

Chapter 3
Echocardiography and Advanced Cardiac Imaging in Athletes

Aaron L. Baggish, Kibar Yared, Malissa J. Wood, and Adolph M. Hutter

The association between abnormalities of cardiac morphology and participation in athletic activity is well established. Initial reports of cardiac silhouette enlargement date back to the late 1890s when Eugene Darling at Harvard used the rudimentary yet elegant physical examination skills of auscultation and percussion to demonstrate increased cardiac dimensions in Harvard rowers. Similar observations were made by the Swedish clinician Henschen in elite Nordic skiers. Over the last century, advances in our understanding of the relationship between athletic activity and cardiac structure and function have paralleled developments in cardiovascular diagnostic technology. Noninvasive cardiac imaging is an important component of the comprehensive approach to the athlete with suspected cardiovascular pathology. This chapter focuses on the use of available imaging modalities including transthoracic echocardiography (TTE), computed tomography (CT), and magnetic resonance imaging (MRI) for the cardiac evaluation of athletic individuals.

Case 1: Electrocardiographic Evidence of Left Ventricular Hypertrophy

A 21-year-old male is seen for preparticipation clearance prior to the start of a university football season. His past medical history is unremarkable while his family history is notable for paternal hypertension but no unexplained sudden death, cardiomyopathy, or premature atherosclerotic disease. His physical examination reveals normal vital signs without orthostatic changes, a prominent and sustained point of maximal impulse, and a 2/6 early systolic murmur audible only at the left upper sternal border that was unchanged during the Valsalva maneuver. A 12-lead ECG is performed. The tracing demonstrates sinus bradycardia, increased QRS voltage meeting criteria for left ventricular hypertrophy, and diffuse precordial T-wave inversions. What is the next step in the evaluation of this athlete?

A.L. Baggish (✉)
Division of Cardiology, Harvard University, Boston, MA, USA
e-mail: abaggish@partners.org

C.E. Lawless (ed.), *Sports Cardiology Essentials: Evaluation, Management and Case Studies*, DOI 10.1007/978-0-387-92775-6_3,

Twelve-lead electrocardiography (ECG) has been in widespread use in the evaluation of athletes for several decades, and common abnormalities including early repolarization patterns, increased QRS voltage, bradyarrhythmia, ST-segment deviation, T-wave abnormalities, and QRS complex widening have been documented repeatedly. The vast majority of athletes have no underlying cardiovascular disease, and thus the presence of such ECG findings is commonly attributed to the adaptive or physiologic cardiac remodeling that can occur in response to exercise training. However, ECG patterns common among athletes are also encountered in individuals with true underlying cardiovascular disease, and this overlap between the ECG findings of adaptive remodeling and those of true cardiac pathology is the source of considerable diagnostic uncertainty [1].

Perhaps the most commonly encountered ECG-based diagnostic dilemma is that of increased QRS voltage which occurs both in healthy athletes and in those with pathologic cardiac hypertrophy. A number of echocardiographic studies have documented increases in left ventricular (LV) chamber dimensions, wall thickness, and mass among healthy, highly trained individuals [2–5]. The increase in LV wall thickness that can result from exercise training has received particular attention because it can share similarities with that caused by hypertrophic cardiomyopathy (HCM).

HCM is a well-recognized cause of exercise-related sudden cardiac death among athletes. This condition is the most common cardiovascular cause of sudden death among athletes in the USA and has the propensity to affect individuals at all levels of competition [6, 7]. Histologic inspection of myocardium from afflicted individuals reveals characteristic myofibrillar disarray, while gross analysis demonstrates left ventricular hypertrophy with increased wall thickness of either symmetric or asymmetric distribution. Roughly 80% of individuals with HCM have ECG abnormalities including interventricular conduction delay, voltage criteria for left ventricular hypertrophy, ST-segment depression, T-wave inversion, and anterior/inferior Q-waves producing a "pseudo-infarct" pattern [8, 9]. While such findings are typical of HCM, they are encountered commonly among trained athletes with no underlying structural heart disease [10].

TTE is the preferred test for confirming or excluding the diagnosis of HCM. Echocardiographic findings in HCM include increased wall thickness, normal or reduced LV cavity dimensions, altered indices of diastolic filling, and mitral valve abnormalities including systolic anterior motion and regurgitation [11]. The magnitude of wall thickness increase varies considerably among individuals with HCM [12, 13]. Severity classification schemes based on wall thickness have been proposed, and this metric has been shown to provide important prognostic information [14, 15]. Mild phenotypic expression of HCM can lead to wall thickness that exceeds sedentary population-based limits of normal (<12 mm) by only several millimeters. Similarly appearing hypertrophy can also be a component of adaptive remodeling in athletes without HCM.

Several studies provide important data defining the magnitude of LV wall thickness increase that typically occurs in athletes without HCM. Pelliccia et al. performed echocardiographic assessment of LV wall thicknesses among 947 elite athletes. Within this cohort, a small but significant percentage of athletes (1.7%) had LV wall thicknesses greater than or equal to 13 mm, and all of these individuals had concomitant LV cavity dilation, a combination not typically found among individuals with HCM [16]. A similar study by Sharma et al. also reported relatively low incidence of LV wall thickness increase among elite junior athletes and again confirmed the pairing of increased LV chamber size and wall thickness increase among those with adaptive remodeling [17].

Although studies such as these demonstrate a relatively low incidence of increased wall thickness measurements among athletes, a small but significant number of individuals do have wall thickness values in the 13–15 mm range. This finding may be particularly common among elite athletes such as American National Football League players [4]. Such athletes are often termed "gray zone" individuals, a term used to reflect the uncertainty of the cause of their LV hypertrophy. Evaluation of the gray zone athlete can present a clinical challenge. The first step in the workup of an athletic individual with LV enlargement is to define the magnitude of abnormality and to consider it in the context of other cardiac structural and functional imaging data. LV wall thickness greater or equal to 16 mm is very rare among healthy athletes, and this finding must be considered as highly suggestive of HCM. For individuals with mild LV wall thickness increase, the work by Pelliccia and Sharma suggests that adaptive remodeling can be differentiated from structural heart disease by concomitant consideration of LV cavity dimensions [16, 17]. The finding of either isolated LV wall thickness increase or LV dilation should prompt further assessment for potential pathology.

Further steps in the assessment of the gray zone athlete have traditionally included exercise stress testing, Holter-monitoring, and prescribed deconditioning. While these complementary approaches retain their diagnostic value, several recently developed echocardiographic imaging techniques provide additive information. One such technique is tissue Doppler which provides a direct measure of tissue velocities, and thus tissue function, during the systolic and diastolic phases of the cardiac cycle. Several studies have shown that diastolic tissue velocities are reduced among individuals with HCM [18–20]. In contrast, a number of authors have independently shown that diastolic tissue velocities are normal or elevated among athletic individuals even in the context of LV enlargement and low–normal LV ejection fraction [21, 22]. The use of tissue Doppler imaging for the evaluation of indeterminate left ventricular hypertrophy is shown in Fig. 3.1. Echocardiographic strain and strain rate imaging also provide valuable information about tissue function. Strain measurements define changes in muscle fiber length as they contract and relax during the cardiac cycle, while strain rate measures these length changes as a function of time. A recent study by Serri et al. demonstrated that individuals with HCM have lower LV systolic strain values than normal controls [23]. In contrast, individuals with adaptive remodeling have strain values that are normal or higher than those found in sedentary healthy controls [24, 25]. Both tissue Doppler and strain imaging can be performed during routine echocardiographic examination and should be performed in all athletes with LV hypertrophy of indeterminate cause.

Occasionally, TTE does not provide sufficient information for a definitive determination of LV hypertrophy etiology. MRI has emerged as a valuable option in such cases [26]. Although the cost and time commitment of MRI do not compare

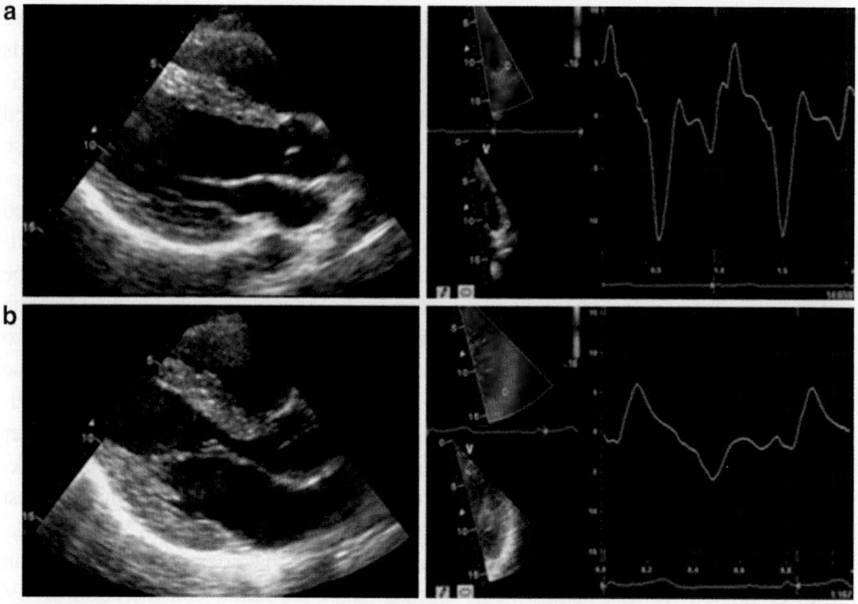

Fig. 3.1 Standard two-dimensional echocardiography and tissue Doppler imaging of a 26-year-old elite level male rower with physiologic hypertrophy (**a**) and a 32-year-old recreational runner with hypertrophic cardiomyopathy (**b**). Parasternal long-axis 2-dimensional images reveal similar left ventricular wall thickness increases and normal left ventricular cavity dimensions, while tissue Doppler images reveal the markedly different functional characteristics of physiologic remodeling (**a**) and hypertrophic cardiomyopathy (**b**)

favorably with TTE, it may serve as a valuable step in the assessment of athletes with suboptimal echocardiographic acoustic windows or in those with concerning ECGs and indeterminate echocardiograms. Further work is needed to define the optimal role of MRI in this context.

Summary

In the preceding case presentation, a young athlete demonstrates ECG findings suggestive of LV hypertrophy. A transthoracic echocardiogram confirmed mild concentric LV hypertrophy, mild LV dilation, and slightly elevated diastolic tissue Doppler velocities all consistent with adaptive remodeling. A 1-year follow-up echocardiogram was recommended and the athlete was cleared for sports participation. Signs of left ventricular hypertrophy on ECG are extremely common in high-level athletes. With an increasing number of ECGs being performed in athletes this promises to be an increasingly common diagnostic dilemma. Newer echocardiographic techniques have shown promise for assisting in the differentiation between physiological and pathological remodeling.

Case 2: Exertional Myocardial Ischemia in the Young Athlete

A 16 year-old female presents following several episodes of chest fullness which occurred during recent running workouts. She is participating in her first season of varsity track and field. There is no history of prior syncope, palpitations, or previous exertional chest discomfort. Her family history is unremarkable and there are no abnormalities on physical examination. A resting 12-lead ECG is notable only for sinus bradycardia and ST-segment elevation consistent with benign early repolarization in leads V2–4. She is referred for an exercise treadmill test during which she experiences her presenting symptoms and has ischemic ECG changes during stage 8 of standard Bruce protocol. What is the next step in her management?

The most common cause of exertional myocardial ischemia in young athletes (<35 years of age) is congenital anomalies of the coronary artery circulation. This condition accounts for approximately 15–20% of sudden death among athletes [7, 27, 28]. Sudden death attributed to a coronary artery anomaly is caused by transient myocardial ischemia occurring during vigorous physical exertion. An origin of either the left or right coronary artery from the contralateral sinus of Valsalva has been associated with sudden death in athletes [29, 30]. A left coronary artery originating from the right sinus of Valsalva or the proximal right coronary artery is the most common anomaly found in athletes. In this setting, the left main coronary artery has several possible routes to the left heart: (1) Anterior to the pulmonary artery; (2) Posterior to the aorta; (3) Within the intraventricular septum beneath the right ventricular infundibulum; (4) Between the great vessels. The first three are generally benign and have not been associated with exercise-related death, whereas passage of the left main coronary artery between the great vessels is a well-established cause of exercise-related death [31–34].

The diagnosis of anomalous coronary circulation in athletes is challenging and requires a high index of suspicion. This condition should be considered in young athletes presenting with symptoms of possible exercise-induced myocardial ischemia including exertional chest discomfort, exercise intolerance, palpitations, and exercise-induced syncope. Preparticipation screening with resting ECG cannot accurately detect this condition [30]. Conventional coronary artery angiography and aortography has long been the gold standard for the diagnosis of coronary anomalies and remains a useful diagnostic option when this condition is suspected. However, newer noninvasive imaging techniques including TTE, coronary artery CT, and MRI have gained recent popularity.

The widespread availability and relatively low cost of TTE make it an attractive option for the detection of coronary anomalies, and this modality has been examined in two large population screening studies. Pelliccia et al. performed two-dimensional TTE in 1,360 national caliber Italian athletes to screen for anomalies of coronary artery origin [35]. These authors reported a 6% subject exclusion rate due to technically unsatisfactory echocardiograms. Among the 1,273 individuals with adequate ultrasound images, 6/1,273 (0.5%) were found to have anomalous coronary origin. In a considerably larger study, Zeppilli and colleagues screened 3,150 athletes. They obtained technically usable images in 96% of subjects and found that three (0.09%) had a coronary artery which originated from the incorrect aortic sinus [36]. In aggregate, these two studies suggest that proximal coronary artery anatomy is determinable in roughly 95% of individuals using TTE.

Occasional inability to obtain definitive imaging and the limited capacity to visualize either coronary artery course or relationship to adjacent structures have led to interest in alternatives to TTE. Transesophageal echocardiography (TEE) is a reasonable option for confirming the diagnosis of coronary anomaly [37, 38]. TEE is an alternative form of ultrasound imaging during which the camera is placed in the esophagus. This procedure requires conscious sedation but has the advantage of providing superior images to those obtained by TTE. TEE provides the added benefits of direct visualization of blood flow direction, blood velocity, and characterization of coronary artery relationship to adjacent structures.

CT of the coronary circulation has emerged as a robust method of defining coronary artery origin and course (Fig. 3.2a, b). A number of small studies demonstrate comparable diagnostic accuracy between conventional angiography and CT angiography [39–43]. MRI has also been shown to be a viable modality for the detection of coronary anomalies [44–46]. At the present time, no imaging modality has emerged as the single best option for the evaluation of coronary anatomy. A comparative summary of available techniques is provided to assist with decision making on an individual patient basis (Table 3.1).

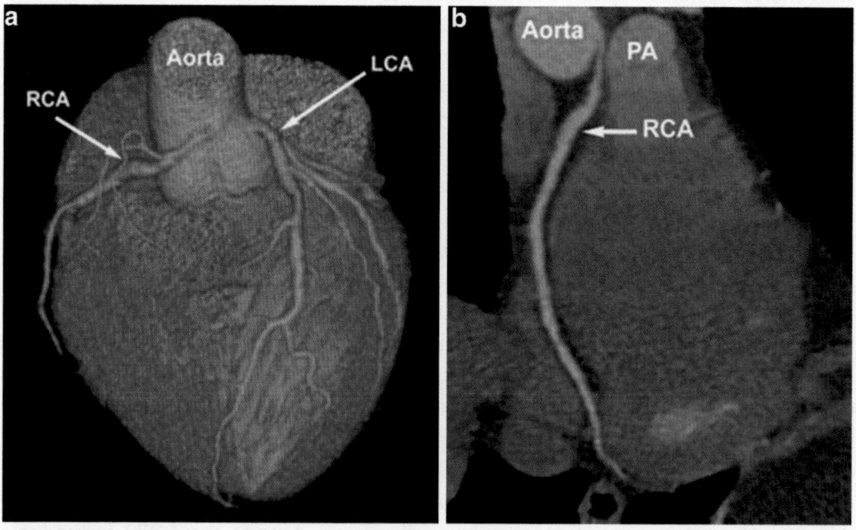

Fig. 3.2 Computed tomography (CT) three-dimensional reconstruction demonstrating an anomalous right coronary artery (RCA) arising from the left sinus of Valsalva (Panel (**a**)) and coursing between the aorta and pulmonary artery (PA) (Panel (**b**)). *LCA* left coronary artery

Table 3.1 Comparison of noninvasive imaging modalities for the evaluation of suspected coronary arterial anomalies

Modality	Cost	Contrast	Radiation	Diagnostic accuracy	Time of procedure	Time of recovery	Other
CA	++	I+	+	++	<1–2	2–4 days	Historical gold standard, significant radiation
TTE	+	None	None	+	<1 h	Minimal	Widely available, ~5% of studies indeterminate due to technical limitations
TEE	++	None	None	++	<1–2 h	6–8 h	Requires conscious sedation
CT	++	I+	+	+++	<1	Minimal	Rapid, significant radiation
MRI	+++	I–	None	+++	1–2 h	Minimal	Limited availability, numerous contraindications

CA conventional angiography, *TTE* transthoracic echocardiography, *TEE* transesophageal echocardiography, *CT* computed tomography, *MRI* magnetic resonance imaging, + least favorable, ++ intermediate favorability, +++ most favorable, I+ iodinated contrast, I– noniodinated contrast

Summary

In the preceding case presentation, the young athlete underwent CT coronary angiography and was found to have a right coronary artery originating from the left sinus of Valsalva and coursing between the aorta and the pulmonary artery. Further athletic participation was prohibited and surgical consultation for expectant reimplantation of the right coronary artery was recommended. Although rare, anomalies of the coronary circulation remain in the differential diagnosis in an athlete presenting with ischemic chest pain or exercise-induced syncope. TTE and TEE provide adequate means of screening for coronary artery anomalies. However, CT angiography and MRI provide superior imaging of both the origin and the course of the coronary arterial tree.

Case 3: Arrhythmia and Right Ventricular Dilation

A 23-year-old male cross-country skier presents with palpitations. He has been skiing competitively for 4 years and has no past medical or relevant family history. He recounts both exertional and rest palpitations lasting approximately 15–30s in duration occurring two to three times per week. Episodes are accompanied by occasional feelings of dizziness and presyncope. Physical exam is normal but a resting ECG demonstrates normal sinus rhythm, an incomplete right bundle branch block, and left ventricular hypertrophy by voltage criteria. An echocardiogram reveals normal LV size, function, and moderate right ventricular (RV) dilation with preserved systolic function. A 48-h Holter monitor reveals several runs of wide complex tachycardia of left bundle branch morphology. What is the next step in the assessment of this athlete?

The most common and potentially serious cause of paroxysmal ventricular tachycardia originating from the right heart in otherwise healthy athletes is arrhythmogenic right ventricular dysplasia/cardiomyopathy (ARVD/C). ARVD/C is a form of cardiomyopathy that can present with left bundle branch block (LBBB) morphology ventricular arrhythmia leading to cardiac arrest and sudden cardiac death [47, 48]. Morphologically, this disease entity is characterized by a combination of fatty or fibrofatty infiltration of the RV myocardium and RV dilation with or without the presence of sacculations or aneurysms (Fig. 3.3) [49–52]. According to the 1994 Task Force Report on ARVD/C, the diagnosis of ARVD/C is based on the presence of structural, histological, electrocardiographic, arrhythmic, and genetic factors, and specific criteria for diagnosis have been proposed [53]. Characterization of RV structure and function is of paramount importance when a diagnosis of ARVD/C is considered.

TTE, by virtue of its widespread availability, low cost, and ease of performance and interpretation, is a useful tool for establishing the diagnosis of ARVD. In 2005, Yoerger et al. quantified echocardiographic abnormalities in 29 probands newly

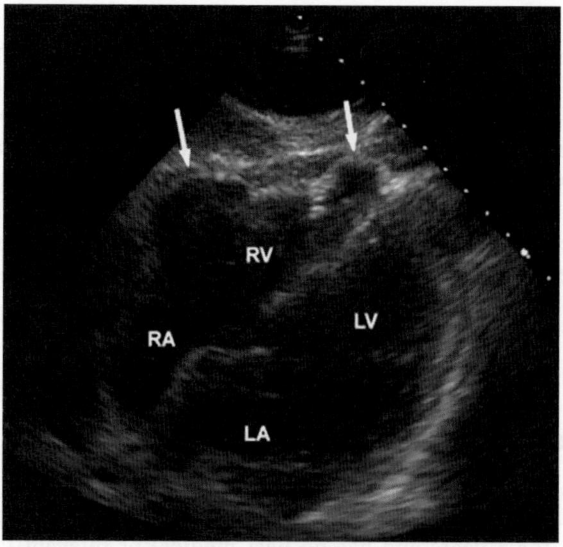

Fig. 3.3 Transthoracic echocardiogram. Subcostal view demonstrating two discrete aneurysmal outpouchings of the right ventricular free wall (*arrows*)

Table 3.2 Frequency of qualitative echocardiographic abnormalities in probands with arrhythmogenic right ventricular dysplasia/cardiomyopathy (n = 29)

	Number	Percent
RV global function		
Normal	11	38
Mildly reduced	8	28
Severely reduced	10	34
RV regional WMA	23	79
RVOT	13	45
Anteroseptal	16	55
Anterior	20	70
Apex	21	72
Septal	16	55
Inferior basal	17	59
Inferior apical	15	52
Hyperreflective moderator band	9	31
Excessive/abnormal trabeculations	15	54
Sacculations	5	17

RV right ventricle, *WMA* wall motion abnormality, *RVOT* right ventricular outflow tract
From [54]

diagnosed with ARVD/C [54]. All subjects had normal LV size and function. The most frequent RV morphologic abnormalities were trabecular derangement, hyper-reflective moderator band, and RV sacculations (Table 3.2). The systolic and diastolic RV outflow (RVOT) and inflow tract dimensions were significantly increased, while global RV function was impaired in 66% of subjects. An RVOT long-axis dimension of >30 mm had the highest sensitivity and specificity for the diagnosis of ARVD (89 and 86%, respectively). Of note, RVOT tachycardia, a more benign and treatable condition, has also been associated with evidence of RVOT tract dilation [55].

The detection of subtle changes in RV function not apparent with conventional two-dimensional TTE is paramount in the assessment of suspected ARVD/C. This is especially important in individuals with Naxos disease (plakoglobin mutation) in whom the phenotype does not appear until adolescence and in some athletes who may have very mild or unapparent structural abnormalities but are still at risk for malignant arrhythmia [48, 56]. Changes in RV function by quantitative tissue Doppler and strain TTE in patients with known ARVD/C but otherwise normally appearing RVs have been described [57]. Peak RV systolic velocity (S'), early diastolic velocity (E'), displacement, strain (ε), and strain rate were all significantly lower in patients with ARVD/C than in controls (Table 3.3). Peak RV systolic velocity <7.5 cm/s and peak RV strain <18% best identified patients with ARVD/C. Imaging patients with suspected ARVD/C with three-dimensional TTE has been shown to be feasible and provides an accurate assessment of RV structure and function [58, 59]. Intracardiac echocardiography (ICE) of the right ventricle during electrophysiological interventions has demonstrated reliability and superiority in comparison to

Table 3.3 Tissue Doppler and strain echocardiography measurements in patients with ARVD/C

	Mean ±SD	Sensitivity (%)	Specificity (%)
RV systolic velocity (*S*′, cm/s)	6.4 ± 2.2	67	89
Early diastolic velocity (*E*, cm/s)	−6.7 ± 2.7		
RV displacement (mm)	13.7 ± 5.8	77	71
Strain (ε, %)	−10 ± 6	73	87
Strain rate (s^{-1})	−1 ± 0.7	50	96

Adapted from [57]

RV angiography [60]. Despite the previously summarized advances in the use of TTE for the diagnosis of ARVD, technical challenges of RV imaging by ultrasound may limit the yield of this test. Further, TTE has been suggested to lack optimal sensitivity and specificity for the detection of ARVD/C related structural or functional abnormalities [61–63].

MRI uses nonionizing radiofrequency stimulation to perform noninvasive multiplanar imaging and allows for accurate morphological and functional evaluation of the RV without any geometric assumptions [64–66]. Further, detection of intramyocardial fat and fibrosis is possible due to the ability of MRI to perform tissue characterization [61, 64, 67–72]. Recently, the group of Tandri et al. sought to define the prevalence, sensitivity, and specificity of quantitative MRI findings in 40 probands newly diagnosed with ARVD/C [73]. Intramyocardial RV fat infiltration was observed in 60% of subjects and was most commonly located in the basal RV free wall (Figs. 3.4 and 3.5). Qualitative global RV dysfunction was reported in 24 (60%) patients and was severe in ten patients (25%). A significant association between the area of fat infiltration and the area of regional dysfunction was observed. Aneurysmal dilation of the RV wall was most notable in the RV apex, RVOT, and in the RV basal and mid-free walls.

Contrary to prior reports, the study by Tandri et al. suggests that RV fat infiltration is seldom the only MRI abnormality in individuals with ARVD/C [69, 74, 75]. Further, this study found that RV fat infiltration had poor sensitivity for the diagnosis of ARVD/C compared to regional RV dysfunction (Fig. 3.6). Notably, significant fatty infiltration of the RV occurs in more than 50% of normal elderly people [76, 77]. Quantitative, instead of qualitative, estimates of RV function, as well as routine quantification of RV volumes, improved the sensitivity and specificity of ARVD/C diagnosis [78]. RVOT area by MRI was less predictive of ARVD/C compared with global RV volumes. Finally, MRI can also be used to assess both systolic and diastolic function in great detail. Several studies have addressed the presence of RV diastolic dysfunction as an early marker of disease, even when systolic function is still preserved [64, 79]. Kayser et al. showed that diastolic function of the right ventricle was significantly altered in 15 patients with nonischemic tachyarrhythmias of RV origin (five of whom had a clinical diagnosis of ARVD/C), even though systolic function was normal [80].

Although MRI has assumed a prominent role in the assessment of individuals with suspected ARVD/C, access to medical facilities with the required equipment and expertise may limit its widespread applicability. On the other hand, CT is a

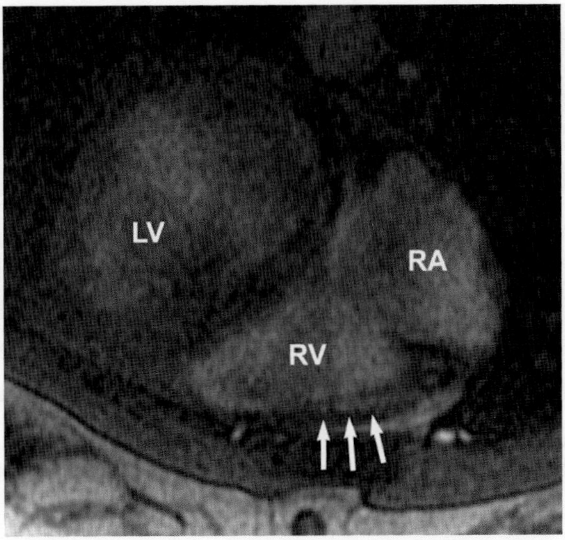

Fig. 3.4 Magnetic resonance imaging. Spoiled gradient echo sequence with the patient in prone position demonstrating hyperintense signal, consistent with fatty infiltration (*white arrows*), within the anterior free wall of the right ventricle

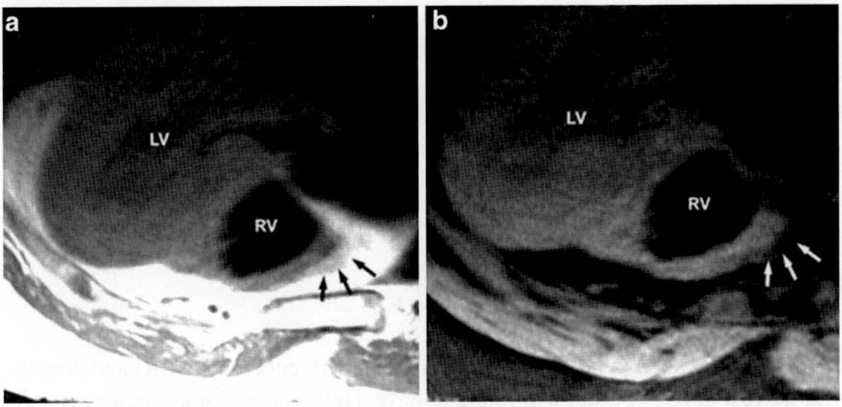

Fig. 3.5 Magnetic resonance imaging. Oblique axial high-resolution T1-weighted conventional spin echo sequence demonstrating the presence of intramyocardial fatty changes (*black arrows*) in basal portion of the anterior free wall of the right ventricle (Panel (**a**)). Panel (**b**) demonstrates signal voiding (*white arrows*) at the base of the RV anterior free wall after effective fat suppression, confirming the presence of intramyocardial fatty infiltration

more available imaging modality, and its role in the diagnosis of ARVD/C is being investigated. Dery et al. have used CT to demonstrate a dilated and hypokinetic right ventricle in a patient with ARVD/C [81]. Improved image resolution as well as decreased scan time has led to recent studies exploring the use of

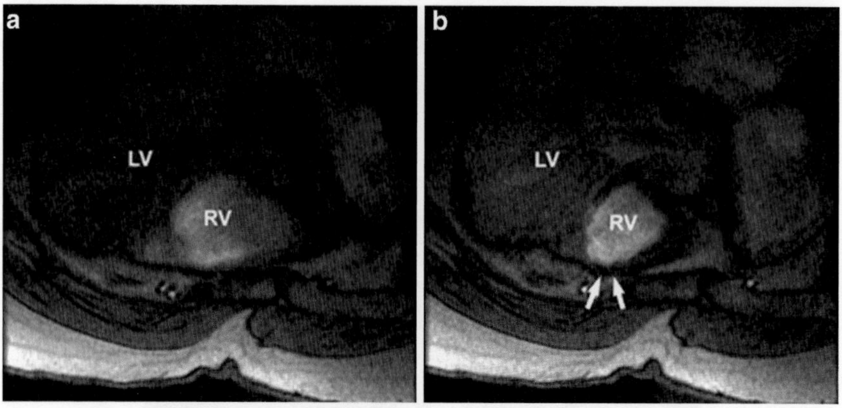

Fig. 3.6 Magnetic resonance imaging. Oblique axial spoiled gradient echo sequence in diastole (Panel (**a**)) and systole (Panel (**b**)) demonstrating dyskinesis of the distal portion of the RV anterior free wall

multidetector computed tomography (MDCT) as an alternative to MRI for the diagnosis of ARVD/C, especially in patients with contraindications to MRI [82–84]. In a study by Bomma et al., 31 patients underwent MDCT scanning for the evaluation of known or suspected ARVD/C [82]. Increased RV trabeculation, intramyocardial fat, and scalloping of myocardium were significantly associated with the final diagnosis of ARVD/C. RV volumes, RV inlet dimensions, and RVOT tract surface area were increased in patients with ARVD/C compared with patients who did not meet Task Force criteria for ARVD/C. Further study is required to determine the relative merits of CT for the evaluation of individuals with suspected ARVD/C.

Summary

In the preceding case presentation, the athlete underwent cardiac MRI and, together with the rest of his workup, was found to have a number of features consistent with ARVD/C. A recommendation was made to prohibit him from further exercise training and he was referred for consideration of implantable defibrillator placement. A high level of clinical suspicion should be employed for an athlete who complains of unexplained palpitations, presyncope, syncope, or aborted sudden death. Multiple modalities are available to ensure a correct and accurate diagnosis. Echocardiography remains the modality of choice initially to identify structural or functional abnormalities. Accurate and rapid imaging techniques such as MDCT are certainly gaining popularity and reliability. At this point, MRI remains the gold standard for the diagnosis of RV structural and functional abnormalities typical of ARVD/C.

References

1. Maron BJ, Pelliccia A. The heart of trained athletes: cardiac remodeling and the risks of sports, including sudden death. Circulation. 2006;114:1633–1644.
2. Morganroth J, Maron BJ, Henry WL, Epstein SE. Comparative left ventricular dimensions in trained athletes. Ann Intern Med. 1975;82:521–524.
3. Pelliccia A, Culasso F, Di Paolo FM, Maron BJ. Physiologic left ventricular cavity dilatation in elite athletes. Ann Intern Med. 1999;130:23–31.
4. Abernethy WB, Choo JK, Hutter AM Jr. Echocardiographic characteristics of professional football players. J Am Coll Cardiol. 2003;41:280–284.
5. Scharhag J, Schneider G, Urhausen A, Rochette V, Kramann B, Kindermann W. Athlete's heart: right and left ventricular mass and function in male endurance athletes and untrained individuals determined by magnetic resonance imaging. J Am Coll Cardiol. 2002;40:1856–1863.
6. Van Camp SP, Bloor CM, Mueller FO, Cantu RC, Olson HG. Nontraumatic sports death in high school and college athletes. Med Sci Sports Exerc. 1995;27:641–647.
7. Maron BJ, Shirani J, Poliac LC, Mathenge R, Roberts WC, Mueller FO. Sudden death in young competitive athletes. Clinical, demographic, and pathological profiles. JAMA. 1996;276:199–204.
8. Savage DD, Seides SF, Clark CE, Henry WL, Maron BJ, Robinson FC, Epstein SE. Electrocardiographic findings in patients with obstructive and nonobstructive hypertrophic cardiomyopathy. Circulation. 1978;58:402–408.
9. Maron BJ, Mathenge R, Casey SA, Poliac LC, Longe TF. Clinical profile of hypertrophic cardiomyopathy identified de novo in rural communities. J Am Coll Cardiol. 1999;33:1590–1595.
10. Pelliccia A, Maron BJ, Culasso F, Di Paolo FM, Spataro A, Biffi A, Caselli G, Piovano P. Clinical significance of abnormal electrocardiographic patterns in trained athletes. Circulation. 2000;102:278–284.
11. Kinoshita N, Nimura Y, Okamoto M, Miyatake K, Nagata S, Sakakibara H. Mitral regurgitation in hypertrophic cardiomyopathy. Non-invasive study by two dimensional Doppler echocardiography. Br Heart J. 1983;49:574–583.
12. Maron BJ, Gardin JM, Flack JM, Gidding SS, Kurosaki TT, Bild DE. Prevalence of hypertrophic cardiomyopathy in a general population of young adults. Echocardiographic analysis of 4111 subjects in the CARDIA study. Coronary artery risk development in (young) adults. Circulation. 1995;92:785–789.
13. Klues HG, Schiffers A, Maron BJ. Phenotypic spectrum and patterns of left ventricular hypertrophy in hypertrophic cardiomyopathy: morphologic observations and significance as assessed by two-dimensional echocardiography in 600 patients. J Am Coll Cardiol. 1995;26:1699–1708.
14. Spirito P, Bellone P, Harris KM, Bernabo P, Bruzzi P, Maron BJ. Magnitude of left ventricular hypertrophy and risk of sudden death in hypertrophic cardiomyopathy. N Engl J Med. 2000;342:1778–1785.
15. Elliott PM, Gimeno Blanes JR, Mahon NG, Poloniecki JD, McKenna WJ. Relation between severity of left-ventricular hypertrophy and prognosis in patients with hypertrophic cardiomyopathy. Lancet. 2001;357:420–424.
16. Pelliccia A, Maron BJ, Spataro A, Proschan MA, Spirito P. The upper limit of physiologic cardiac hypertrophy in highly trained elite athletes. N Engl J Med. 1991;324:295–301.
17. Sharma S, Maron BJ, Whyte G, Firoozi S, Elliott PM, McKenna WJ. Physiologic limits of left ventricular hypertrophy in elite junior athletes: relevance to differential diagnosis of athlete's heart and hypertrophic cardiomyopathy. J Am Coll Cardiol. 2002;40:1431–1436.
18. McMahon CJ, Nagueh SF, Pignatelli RH, Denfield SW, Dreyer WJ, Price JF, Clunie S, Bezold LI, Hays AL, Towbin JA, Eidem BW. Characterization of left ventricular diastolic function by tissue Doppler imaging and clinical status in children with hypertrophic cardiomyopathy. Circulation. 2004;109:1756–1762.

19. Cardim N, Oliveira AG, Longo S, Ferreira T, Pereira A, Reis RP, Correia JM. Doppler tissue imaging: regional myocardial function in hypertrophic cardiomyopathy and in athlete's heart. J Am Soc Echocardiogr. 2003;16:223–232.
20. Matsumura Y, Elliott PM, Virdee MS, Sorajja P, Doi Y, McKenna WJ. Left ventricular diastolic function assessed using Doppler tissue imaging in patients with hypertrophic cardiomyopathy: relation to symptoms and exercise capacity. Heart. 2002;87:247–251.
21. Zoncu S, Pelliccia A, Mercuro G. Assessment of regional systolic and diastolic wall motion velocities in highly trained athletes by pulsed wave Doppler tissue imaging. J Am Soc Echocardiogr. 2002;15:900–905.
22. Caso P, Galderisi M, Cicala S, Cioppa C, D'Andrea A, Lagioia G, Liccardo B, Martiniello AR, Mininni N. Association between myocardial right ventricular relaxation time and pulmonary arterial pressure in chronic obstructive lung disease: analysis by pulsed Doppler tissue imaging. J Am Soc Echocardiogr. 2001;14:970–977.
23. Serri K, Reant P, Lafitte M, Berhouet M, Le Bouffos V, Roudaut R, Lafitte S. Global and regional myocardial function quantification by two-dimensional strain: application in hypertrophic cardiomyopathy. J Am Coll Cardiol. 2006;47:1175–1181.
24. Neilan TG, Ton-Nu TT, Jassal DS, Popovic ZB, Douglas PS, Halpern EF, Marshall JE, Thomas JD, Picard MH, Yoerger DM, Wood MJ. Myocardial adaptation to short-term high-intensity exercise in highly trained athletes. J Am Soc Echocardiogr. 2006;19:1280–1285.
25. Saghir M, Areces M, Makan M. Strain rate imaging differentiates hypertensive cardiac hypertrophy from physiologic cardiac hypertrophy (athlete's heart). J Am Soc Echocardiogr. 2007;20:151–157.
26. Rickers C, Wilke NM, Jerosch-Herold M, Casey SA, Panse P, Panse N, Weil J, Zenovich AG, Maron BJ. Utility of cardiac magnetic resonance imaging in the diagnosis of hypertrophic cardiomyopathy. Circulation. 2005;112:855–861.
27. Maron BJ, Epstein SE, Roberts WC. Causes of sudden death in competitive athletes. J Am Coll Cardiol. 1986;7:204–214.
28. Corrado D, Thiene G, Nava A, Rossi L, Pennelli N. Sudden death in young competitive athletes: clinicopathologic correlations in 22 cases. Am J Med. 1990;89:588–596.
29. Frescura C, Basso C, Thiene G, Corrado D, Pennelli T, Angelini A, Daliento L. Anomalous origin of coronary arteries and risk of sudden death: a study based on an autopsy population of congenital heart disease. Hum Pathol. 1998;29:689–695.
30. Basso C, Maron BJ, Corrado D, Thiene G. Clinical profile of congenital coronary artery anomalies with origin from the wrong aortic sinus leading to sudden death in young competitive athletes. J Am Coll Cardiol. 2000;35:1493–1501.
31. Cheitlin MD, De Castro CM, McAllister HA. Sudden death as a complication of anomalous left coronary origin from the anterior sinus of valsalva, a not-so-minor congenital anomaly. Circulation. 1974;50:780–787.
32. Benson PA. Anomalous aortic origin of coronary artery with sudden death: case report and review. Am Heart J. 1970;79:254–257.
33. Taylor AJ, Rogan KM, Virmani R. Sudden cardiac death associated with isolated congenital coronary artery anomalies. J Am Coll Cardiol. 1992;20:640–647.
34. Roberts WC, Shirani J. The four subtypes of anomalous origin of the left main coronary artery from the right aortic sinus (or from the right coronary artery). Am J Cardiol. 1992;70:119–121.
35. Pelliccia A, Spataro A, Maron BJ. Prospective echocardiographic screening for coronary artery anomalies in 1,360 elite competitive athletes. Am J Cardiol. 1993;72:978–979.
36. Zeppilli P, dello Russo A, Santini C, Palmieri V, Natale L, Giordano A, Frustaci A. In vivo detection of coronary artery anomalies in asymptomatic athletes by echocardiographic screening. Chest. 1998;114:89–93.
37. Fernandes F, Alam M, Smith S, Khaja F. The role of transesophageal echocardiography in identifying anomalous coronary arteries. Circulation. 1993;88:2532–2540.
38. Dawn B, Talley JD, Prince CR, Hoque A, Morris GT, Xenopoulos NP, Stoddard MF. Two-dimensional and Doppler transesophageal echocardiographic delineation and flow characterization of anomalous coronary arteries in adults. J Am Soc Echocardiogr. 2003;16:1274–1286.

39. Datta J, White CS, Gilkeson RC, Meyer CA, Kansal S, Jani ML, Arildsen RC, Read K. Anomalous coronary arteries in adults: depiction at multi-detector row CT angiography. Radiology. 2005;235:812–818.
40. van Ooijen PM, Dorgelo J, Zijlstra F, Oudkerk M. Detection, visualization and evaluation of anomalous coronary anatomy on 16-slice multidetector-row CT. Eur Radiol. 2004;14:2163–2171.
41. Schmid M, Achenbach S, Ludwig J, Baum U, Anders K, Pohle K, Daniel WG, Ropers D. Visualization of coronary artery anomalies by contrast-enhanced multi-detector row spiral computed tomography. Int J Cardiol. 2006;111:430–435.
42. Memisoglu E, Ropers D, Hobikoglu G, Tepe MS, Labovitz AJ. Usefulness of electron beam computed tomography for diagnosis of an anomalous origin of a coronary artery from the opposite sinus. Am J Cardiol. 2005;96:1452–1455.
43. Ropers D, Moshage W, Daniel WG, Jessl J, Gottwik M, Achenbach S. Visualization of coronary artery anomalies and their anatomic course by contrast-enhanced electron beam tomography and three-dimensional reconstruction. Am J Cardiol. 2001;87:193–197.
44. McConnell MV, Ganz P, Selwyn AP, Li W, Edelman RR, Manning WJ. Identification of anomalous coronary arteries and their anatomic course by magnetic resonance coronary angiography. Circulation. 1995;92:3158–3162.
45. Casolo G, Del Meglio J, Rega L, Manta R, Margheri M, Villari N, Gensini G. Detection and assessment of coronary artery anomalies by three-dimensional magnetic resonance coronary angiography. Int J Cardiol. 2005;103:317–322.
46. Bunce NH, Lorenz CH, Keegan J, Lesser J, Reyes EM, Firmin DN, Pennell DJ. Coronary artery anomalies: assessment with free-breathing three-dimensional coronary MR angiography. Radiology. 2003;227:201–208.
47. Furlanello F, Bertoldi A, Dallago M, Furlanello C, Fernando F, Inama G, Pappone C, Chierchia S. Cardiac arrest and sudden death in competitive athletes with arrhythmogenic right ventricular dysplasia. Pacing Clin Electrophysiol. 1998;21:331–335.
48. Thiene G, Nava A, Corrado D, Rossi L, Pennelli N. Right ventricular cardiomyopathy and sudden death in young people. N Engl J Med. 1988;318:129–133.
49. Basso C, Thiene G, Corrado D, Angelini A, Nava A, Valente M. Arrhythmogenic right ventricular cardiomyopathy. Dysplasia, dystrophy, or myocarditis? Circulation. 1996;94:983–991.
50. Corrado D, Fontaine G, Marcus FI, McKenna WJ, Nava A, Thiene G, Wichter T. Arrhythmogenic right ventricular dysplasia/cardiomyopathy: need for an international registry. European Society of Cardiology and the Scientific Council on Cardiomyopathies of the World Heart Federation. J Cardiovasc Electrophysiol. 2000;11:827–832.
51. Metzger JT, de Chillou C, Cheriex E, Rodriguez LM, Smeets JL, Wellens HJ. Value of the 12-lead electrocardiogram in arrhythmogenic right ventricular dysplasia, and absence of correlation with echocardiographic findings. Am J Cardiol. 1993;72:964–967.
52. Pinamonti B, Sinagra G, Camerini F. Clinical relevance of right ventricular dysplasia/cardiomyopathy. Heart. 2000;83:9–11.
53. McKenna WJ, Thiene G, Nava A, Fontaliran F, Blomstrom-Lundqvist C, Fontaine G, Camerini F. Diagnosis of arrhythmogenic right ventricular dysplasia/cardiomyopathy. Task Force of the Working Group Myocardial and Pericardial Disease of the European Society of Cardiology and of the Scientific Council on Cardiomyopathies of the International Society and Federation of Cardiology. Br Heart J. 1994;71:215–218.
54. Yoerger DM, Marcus F, Sherrill D, Calkins H, Towbin JA, Zareba W, Picard MH. Echocardiographic findings in patients meeting task force criteria for arrhythmogenic right ventricular dysplasia: new insights from the multidisciplinary study of right ventricular dysplasia. J Am Coll Cardiol. 2005;45:860–865.
55. Carlson MD, White RD, Trohman RG, Adler LP, Biblo LA, Merkatz KA, Waldo AL. Right ventricular outflow tract ventricular tachycardia: detection of previously unrecognized anatomic abnormalities using cine magnetic resonance imaging. J Am Coll Cardiol. 1994;24:720 –727.
56. Protonotarios NI, Tsatsopoulou AA, Gatzoulis KA. Arrhythmogenic right ventricular cardiomyopathy caused by a deletion in plakoglobin (Naxos disease). Card Electrophysiol Rev. 2002;6:72–80.

57. Prakasa KR, Wang J, Tandri H, Dalal D, Bomma C, Chojnowski R, James C, Tichnell C, Russell S, Judge D, Corretti M, Bluemke D, Calkins H, Abraham TP. Utility of tissue Doppler and strain echocardiography in arrhythmogenic right ventricular dysplasia/cardiomyopathy. Am J Cardiol. 2007;100:507–512.
58. Kjaergaard J, Hastrup Svendsen J, Sogaard P, Chen X, Bay Nielsen H, Køber L, Kjaer A, Hassager C. Advanced quantitative echocardiography in arrhythmogenic right ventricular cardiomyopathy. J Am Soc Echocardiogr. 2007;20:27–35.
59. Prakasa KR, Dalal D, Wang J, Bomma C, Tandri H, Dong J, James C, Tichnell C, Russell SD, Spevak P, Corretti M, Bluemke DA, Calkins H, Abraham TP. Feasibility and variability of three dimensional echocardiography in arrhythmogenic right ventricular dysplasia/cardiomyopathy. Am J Cardiol. 2006;97:703–709.
60. Peters S, Brattström A, Götting B, Trümmel M. Value of intracardiac ultrasound in the diagnosis of arrhythmogenic right ventricular dysplasia–cardiomyopathy. Int J Cardiol. 2002;83:111–117.
61. White RD, Trohman RG, Flamm SD, VanDyke CW, Optican RJ, Sterba R, Obuchowski NA, Carlson MD, Tchou PJ. Right ventricular arrhythmia in the absence of arrhythmogenic dysplasia: MR imaging of myocardial abnormalities. Radiology. 1998;207:743–751.
62. Marcus FI, Fontaine GH, Guiraudon G, Frank R, Laurenceau JL, Malergue C, Grosgogeat Y. Right ventricular dysplasia: a report of 24 adult cases. Circulation. 1982;65:384–398.
63. Mehta D, Odawara H, Ward DE, McKenna WJ, Davies MJ, Camm AJ. Echocardiographic and histologic evaluation of the right ventricle in ventricular tachycardias of left bundle branch block morphology without overt cardiac abnormality. Am J Cardiol. 1989;63:939–944.
64. Auffermann W, Wichter T, Breithardt G, Joachimsen K, Peters PE. Arrhythmogenic right ventricular disease: MR imaging vs angiography. AJR Am J Roentgenol. 1993;161:549–555.
65. van der Wall EE, Kayser HW, Bootsma MM, de Roos A, Schalij MJ. Arrhythmogenic right ventricular dysplasia: MRI findings. Herz. 2000;25:356–364.
66. Corrado D, Basso C, Thiene G. Arrhythmogenic right ventricular cardiomyopathy: diagnosis, prognosis, and treatment. Heart. 2000;83:588–595.
67. Ricci C, Longo R, Pagnan L, Dalla Palma L, Pinamonti B, Camerini F, Bussani R, Silvestri F. Magnetic resonance imaging in right ventricular dysplasia. Am J Cardiol. 1992;70:1589–1595.
68. Midiri M, Finazzo M, Brancato M, Hoffmann E, Indovina G, Maria MD, Lagalla R. Arrhythmogenic right ventricular dysplasia: MR features. Eur Radiol. 1997;7:307–312.
69. Tandri H, Calkins H, Nasir K, Bomma C, Castillo E, Rutberg J, Tichnell C, Lima JA, Bluemke DA. Magnetic resonance imaging findings in patients meeting task force criteria for arrhythmogenic right ventricular dysplasia. J Cardiovasc Electrophysiol. 2003;14:476–482.
70. Tandri H, Saranathan M, Rodriguez ER, Martinez C, Bomma C, Nasir K, Rosen B, Lima JA, Calkins H, Bluemke DA. Noninvasive detection of myocardial fibrosis in arrhythmogenic right ventricular cardiomyopathy using delayed-enhancement magnetic resonance imaging. J Am Coll Cardiol. 2005;45:98–103.
71. Blake LM, Scheinman MM, Higgins CB. MR features of arrhythmogenic right ventricular dysplasia. AJR Am J Roentgenol. 1994;162:809–812.
72. Markowitz SM, Litvak BL, Ramirez de Arellano EA, Markisz JA, Stein KM, Lerman BB. Adenosine-sensitive ventricular tachycardia: right ventricular abnormalities delineated by magnetic resonance imaging. Circulation. 1997;96:1192–1200.
73. Tandri H, Macedo R, Calkins H, Marcus F, Cannom D, Scheinman M, Daubert J, Estes Iii M, Wilber D, Talajic M, Duff H, Krahn A, Sweeney M, Garan H, Bluemke DA. Role of magnetic resonance imaging in arrhythmogenic right ventricular dysplasia: insights from the North American arrhythmogenic right ventricular dysplasia (ARVD/C) study. American Heart Journal. 2008;155:147–153.
74. Molinari G, Sardanelli F, Gaita F, Ottonello C, Richiardi E, Parodi RC, Masperone MA, Caponnetto S. Right ventricular dysplasia as a generalized cardiomyopathy? Findings on magnetic resonance imaging. Eur Heart J. 1995;16:1619–1624.
75. Dumousset E, Alfidja A, Lamaison D, Ponsonnaille J, Ravel A, Garcier JM, Boyer L. MRI and arrhythmogenic right ventricular dysplasia (ARVD). Retrospective evaluation of 50 patients. J Radiol. 2004;85:313–320.

76. Burke AP, Farb A, Tashko G, Virmani R. Arrhythmogenic right ventricular cardiomyopathy and fatty replacement of the right ventricular myocardium: are they different diseases? Circulation. 1998;97:1571–1580.
77. Fontaliran F, Fontaine G, Fillette F, Aouate P, Chomette G, Grosgogeat Y. Nosologic frontiers of arrhythmogenic dysplasia. Quantitative variations of normal adipose tissue of the right heart ventricle. Arch Mal Coeur Vaiss. 1991;84:33–38.
78. Tandri H, Castillo E, Ferrari VA, Nasir K, Dalal D, Bomma C, Calkins H, Bluemke DA. Magnetic resonance imaging of arrhythmogenic right ventricular dysplasia: sensitivity, specificity, and observer variability of fat detection versus functional analysis of the right ventricle. J Am Coll Cardiol. 2006;48:2277–2284.
79. Appleton CP, Hatle LK, Popp RL. Relation of transmitral flow velocity patterns to left ventricular diastolic function: new insights from a combined hemodynamic and Doppler echocardiographic study. J Am Coll Cardiol. 1988;12:426–440.
80. Kayser HW, Schalij MJ, van der Wall EE, Stoel BC, de Roos A. Biventricular function in patients with nonischemic right ventricle tachyarrhythmias assessed with MR imaging. AJR Am J Roentgenol. 1997;169:995–999.
81. Dery R, Lipton MJ, Garrett JS, Abbott J, Higgins CB, Schienman MM. Cine-computed tomography of arrhythmogenic right ventricular dysplasia. J Comput Assist Tomogr. 1986;10:120–123.
82. Bomma C, Dalal D, Tandri H, Prakasa K, Nasir K, Roguin A, Piccini J, Dong J, Mahadevappa M, Tichnell C, James C, Lima JAC, Fishman E, Calkins H, Bluemke DA. Evolving role of multidetector computed tomography in evaluation of arrhythmogenic right ventricular dysplasia/cardiomyopathy. Am J Cardiol. 2007;100:99–105.
83. Kantarci M, Bayraktutan U, Sevimli S, Bayram E, Durur I. Multidetector computed tomography findings of arrhythmogenic right ventricular dysplasia: a case report. Heart Surg Forum. 2008;11:E56–E58.
84. Wu Y-W, Tadamura E, Kanao S, Yamamuro M, Nishiyama K, Kimura T, Kita T, Togashi K. Structural and functional assessment of arrhythmogenic right ventricular dysplasia/cardiomyopathy by multi-slice computed tomography: comparison with cardiovascular magnetic resonance. Int J Cardiol. 2007;115:e118–e121.

Chapter 4
Exercise Training and Prescription

Steven J. Keteyian and John R. Schairer

The task of prescribing exercise in competitive athletes and in patients with cardiovascular disease (CVD) is more similar than one might think, which makes life a bit easier when faced with patients with CVD who also choose to participate in vigorous, competitive sports. Regardless of whether you are prescribing exercise for the athlete, or the patient-athlete, there are two basic tenets that apply to everyone when establishing an exercise program. These are *specificity of training* (e.g., mode of training) and *progressive overload* (i.e., intensity, duration, and frequency of training).

Before discussing each of these tenets in detail, it is necessary to first briefly review several of the major components or types of physical fitness. These are aerobic power, anaerobic power, anaerobic endurance or capacity, muscular strength, and muscular endurance.

Aerobic Power

The determination of peak aerobic capacity or oxygen uptake (VO_2) can be easily accomplished during a maximal exercise test using a bike or treadmill and an automated gas collection/analysis system. And although this information is important relative to either categorizing one's fitness level or assessing change in exercise capacity due to training, one can also derive from such testing heart rate or pace at ventilatory threshold, which can be quite useful when developing an exercise prescription.

Figure 4.1 depicts the measurment of peak VO_2 using open circuit, indirect spirometry. Since testing mode or type of exercise can influence results among highly trained athletes, it is appropriate to test the athlete using the mode that best simulates her or his activity – the principle of specificity of testing [1]. Therefore,

S.J. Keteyian (✉)
Division of Cardiovascular Medicine, Department of Internal Medicine, Henry Ford Hospital, Detroit, MI, USA

C.E. Lawless (ed.), *Sports Cardiology Essentials: Evaluation, Management and Case Studies*, DOI 10.1007/978-0-387-92775-6_4,

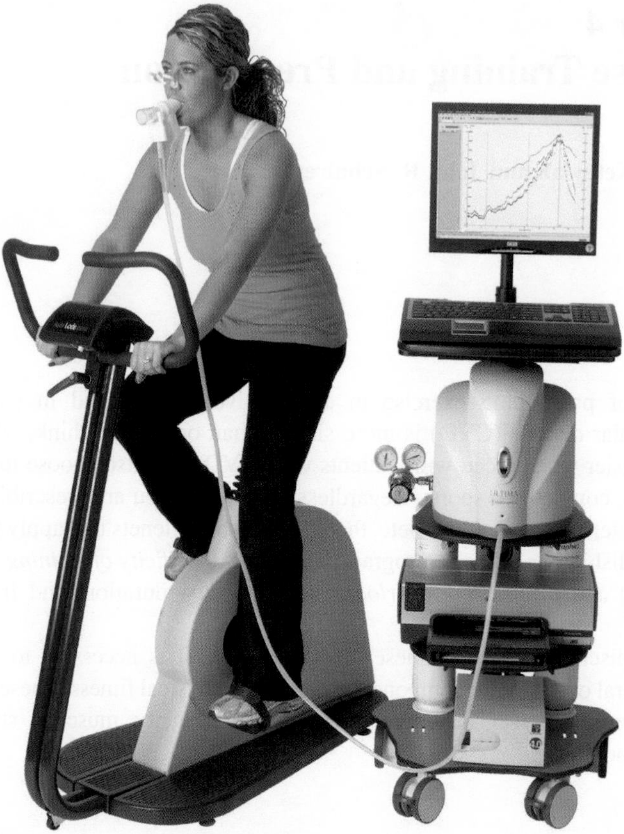

Fig. 4.1 Example of equipment needed to conduct a cardiopulmonary exercise test to measure peak oxygen uptake and other gas exchange parameters

elite competitive cyclists should be tested on a cycle ergometer, swimmers in a swim flume, and runners on a treadmill. Among healthy untrained and less competitive individuals, treadmill testing usually results in a higher peak VO_2, by about 5–15%, when compared to testing performed using other ergometers.

Typically, peak VO_2 is reported in $mL \cdot kg^{-1} \cdot min^{-1}$ and, assuming normal pulmonary function and the absence of clinically meaningful anemia or a skeletal muscle disorder, it reflects the ability of the body to transport (cardiac output) and utilize oxygen (i.e., arterial-mixed venous O_2 difference). A simple rearrangement of the Fick equation provides a nice illustration of this concept:

$$VO_2 = Q \times \text{a-v}O_2\text{diff},$$

where VO_2 is the oxygen consumption ($L \cdot min^{-1}$), Q is the cardiac output ($L \cdot min^{-1}$), and a-vO_2 diff is the arterial-mixed venous O_2 difference ($mL \cdot L^{-1}$).

At peak exercise, cardiac output may reach 22–25 $L \cdot min^{-1}$ in the nonathlete and exceed 35 $L \cdot min^{-1}$ in the athlete. In general, this difference in the ability to maximally transport O_2 to the metabolically more active tissues is due to a greater stroke volume during exercise in the athlete versus the nonathlete (~170 $mL \cdot beat^{-1}$ versus ~120 $mL \cdot beat^{-1}$, respectively). In contrast, peak heart rate is influenced little by exercise training, and peak a-vO_2 diff is only slightly greater in the athlete (~15.5 mL of $O_2 \cdot 100$ mL of $blood^{-1}$) versus the nonathlete (~13.8 mL of $O_2 \cdot 100$ mL of $blood^{-1}$).

Anaerobic Power and Capacity

Whereas the ability of skeletal muscle to generate adenosine triphosphate (ATP) over a long period of time relates to the capabilities of the aerobic metabolic pathways (i.e., Kreb's cycle, oxidative phosphorylation, and beta-oxidation), a person's ability to generate ATP during sudden, short duration and all-out tasks is related to the amount and rate of ATP produced via anaerobic pathways [i.e., phosphocreatine (PC) system and anaerobic glycolysis]. The preferred test used today to assess anaerobic power is the Wingatė anaerobic test [2], which involves pedaling a cycle ergometer for 30 s using maximal effort against a fixed braking force that is set at two to four times a previously determined maximum. Peak power is determined in watts or horsepower, usually attained in the first 5 s of the test.

Muscle Strength and Endurance

Measures of muscle strength and endurance have long been performed, and established norms exist for boys and girls, men, and women and athletes and nonathletes. A convenient and common method used today to assess muscle performance, more so for muscle strength than muscle endurance, is the one repetition maximum (1 RM). Using either free weights or fixed bar resistance machines, isotonic or concentric muscle strength is measured as the maximum amount of weight that can be lifted during one repetition – thus 1 RM. Prior work, expressed as percentiles, is available to help categorize an athlete's 1 RM upper body strength (bench press) and leg strength (leg press) [3]. When a 1 RM is not advised or available for whatever reason, equations to predict 1 RM exist for leg press and chest press using submaximal effort [4].

Over the past 30 years the use of isokinetic or other accommodating resistance devices had flourished because of their ability to quantify muscle power, force, or torque across a wide range of fixed joint movement speeds – from 0 to 300° per second. With this methodology the tester can identify points of high and low force output that may occur throughout a limb's measured range of motion. Such information is generally advantageous for clinical evaluation and research aimed at monitoring training progress or rehabilitation.

Additionally, with isokinetic devices muscle endurance can be assessed using a testing approach that provides a *fatigue index*. This variable represents the loss of maximally generated force at a given joint movement speed and over a given period of time (e.g., 20–30 s). Generally, the smaller the drop in mean force when comparing the first five repetitions in a test to the last five, the greater the level of muscle endurance. When using muscle endurance testing to help guide readiness for return to play in competitive athletes, a common goal is the restoration to less than 10% any differences in fatigue index (loss of power) that exist when comparing one limb to the other.

Prescribing Exercise

As mentioned earlier, improving an athlete's ability or capacity to perform a certain task or event involves working specific muscles or organ systems at a progressively increased resistance. Thus, the two key training principles of *specificity of training* and *progressive overload*.

Specificity of Training

To develop or improve the predominate energy or organ system(s) needed to perform a sport you must first identify its associated performance time. For example, near-world caliber time for the men's 5,000-m ice speed skate is approximately 6 min and 30 s. Similarly, a near record time for the men's 3,000 m run sits just above 7 min. Although these two forms of locomotion are substantially different, skating versus running, they both have similar performance times. As a result, the energy contributions from the muscle's energy systems are similar as well. Specifically, for both events approximately 35–40% of training time should be spent developing the anaerobic glycolysis system, with the balance spent training the aerobic metabolic pathways.

Contrast the above example to shorter duration events such as the 100 m dash; the 25 m swim; or the shuffle, jump, and block maneuver in volleyball – all of which predominately rely on the ATP-PC and glycolysis systems for energy production. Obviously, substantially less training time should be spent on aerobic training in these athletes and more on high-intensity, short-duration drills. Finally, the 3,200 m distance runner should spend 4 or 5 days each week training the cardiorespiratory system and aerobic metabolic pathways, and 1 or 2 days developing anaerobic glycolysis. To summarize, the energy sources for a given activity are time- and intensity-dependent.

In addition to the above, it is important to also point out that the ability to *repeatedly* perform anaerobic activities relies on an efficient aerobic system. This means that even the striker in soccer, center forward in ice hockey, or running back in football, all of whom should spend a great deal of their training time developing the ATP-PC and anaerobic glycolysis systems of the legs must also spend some time training the aerobic system. The reason for this is that it is the aerobic metabolic pathways that are responsible to restore muscle PC stores – in between bouts of repetitive exercise. The more efficient the aerobic system, the quicker is one's recovery between anaerobic bouts.

There is one final point concerning specificity of training. The more and more proficient an athlete becomes within a certain sport, the greater the need to focus training time on sport-specific tasks and drills. In other words, elite runners should run, volleyball players should play volleyball, and tennis players should play tennis. Although there is benefit gained by having volleyball players do sprints or tennis players do repetitive jumps because both activities rely on the ATP-PC system and anaerobic glycolysis, this is not an optimal training model for the elite competitive athlete. Among these individuals conditioning exercises and skill development drills should mimic the athlete's sport. Training in this manner allows the athlete to not only develop the metabolic pathway(s) for their sport but the necessary neuromuscular patterns as well.

Progressive Overload

Although the concept of overload training also applies to resistance training or weight lifting, we begin our discussion by first focusing on whole body anaerobic and aerobic training programs. To accomplish this it is necessary to introduce intensity, duration, and frequency of training. Ultimately, these concepts are used to provide a sufficient "overload" stimulus upon the energy pathways, in hopes that corresponding adaptations lead to improved athletic performance.

Intensity

Of the above three factors, intensity is clearly the most important. The three methods that are typically used to guide intensity are blood lactate level, heart rate, and training velocity or training pace.

Blood lactate is an important biomarker indicating whether the athlete is predominately stressing the muscle's aerobic systems, anaerobic glycolysis, or both. Measuring this blood chemistry during exercise requires specialized equipment, but fingerstick methodology makes it relatively easy – often measured poolside among swimmers. Blood lactate increases with increases in exercise pace or power output, from around 1 $mmol \cdot L^{-1}$ to values that may exceed 12 $mmol \cdot L^{-1}$ during exhaustive work. Note, however, that at or around 4 $mmol \cdot L^{-1}$ there is a definitive break in the curve that is referred to as lactate threshold (LT). It is at this point that lactate production, predominately from anaerobic glycolysis in the more quickly recruited type II muscle fibers, exceeds the ability of the liver, muscle, and kidney to clear lactate from the blood [5]. In practice, one common approach is to identify the heart rate at which LT occurs and be sure a predominate amount of training occurs at a

Table 4.1 Examples of computing exercise training intensity in younger and older untrained individuals using the Heart Rate Reserve (HRR) Method

	Measured peak heart rate (beats min^{-1})	Resting heart rate (beats min^{-1})	Exercise training heart rate range (beats min^{-1})	
			Lower limit	Upper limit
60-year-old	168	70	119	148
20-year-old	198	60	129	170

Heart rate reserve is computed as: (peak HR – resting HR) × 0.50 + resting HR = lower limit; (peak HR – resting HR) × 0.8 + resting HR = upper limit

heart rate that is 5% or more above the heart rate at LT in athletes predominately involved in more anaerobic type activities or two to four beats below the heart rate at LT among athletes competing in a more aerobic-type activity.

Since the relationship between heart rate and exercise intensity (i.e., power output or peak VO_2) is generally quite linear in healthy athletes, one can also train at the heart rate that elicits the necessary overload stimulus on the muscles and organ systems involved. The most common formula used when determining training intensity using heart rate alone is the heart rate reserve (HRR) method.

Table 4.1 depicts examples using the heart rate reserve method for younger and older individuals. Typically, for the health and general fitness needs of apparently healthy nonathletes, training intensities set at 50–80% of heart rate reserve are sufficient to produce the metabolic and organ system overload stimulus needed to improve aerobic performance. For athletes involved in competitive aerobic or anaerobic sports, heart rate during exercise may be maintained at 85% or more of heart rate reserve. The use of the heart rate reserve method to guide exercise intensity remains safe and applicable, regardless of whether the athlete is taking a beta-adrenergic blocking agent.

Frequency and Duration

Duration can refer to both the length of a single training bout (number of minutes or hours) or how long the athlete has been training overall (months vs. years). Generally, the more frequent the program (5 days per week vs. 2 days per week) and the longer the overall program, the greater will be the increase in fitness or performance.

The recommended frequency for most endurance athletes is, at minimum, 5 days per week. However, many train seven or more times in a week. Obviously, the latter may require more than one work out in a day, which is quite common in swimmers and track athletes.

Concerning training, if one maintains the same intensity of training, duration and frequency of training can, to a certain extent, be traded off. For example, if training 1 week needs to be decreased from 6 to 4 days in a week, then the total duration

Table 4.2 General training guidelines for aerobic and anaerobic sports

Training factor	Aerobic sport	Anaerobic sport
Intensity	75–85% of HRR or just below (or at) HR at lactate threshold	HR 5–15% above HR at lactate threshold
Frequency	4–6 days/week	3–4 days/week
Sessions/day	1 (maybe 2)	1 (maybe 2)
Duration	≥8 weeks	≥10–12 weeks
Duration/session		
ATP/PC system	–	Repeated work bouts of 25 s or less
Anaerobic glycolysis	–	Repeated work bouts of 3–4 min or less
Aerobic	20–25 min fast work bouts with 5 min of slow work in between or a slow, continuous bout for 30–60 min or more	

HR heart rate; *HRR* heart rate reserve

(minutes) for that week should be increased to ensure that the overload stimulus that is applied is similar to that of a 6 days per week workout regimen.

Table 4.2 shows a typical training program for both aerobic and anaerobic athletes. Notice that the frequency of anaerobic training occurs fewer times each week. This is because of the marked strain or overload that high-intensity training provides on the metabolic systems. Adequate time must be given for recovery and adaptation.

Resistance Training

All of the above discussion concerning specificity of training and progressive overload has been focused on activities that involve the entire body during an anaerobic or aerobic activity. Common among athletes, however, is the use of weight training or resistance training to improve athletic performance [4, 5]. Clearly, it is well documented that resistance training-induced increases in muscle strength (due to improved neuromuscular coordination and increased cross-sectional muscle size) lead to improvements in athletic performance. The difference here is that resistance training does so by focusing on a single muscle or muscle group. As a result, the concepts of intensity, duration, and frequency of activity take on slightly different meanings.

There are a couple of important points to consider when discussing/recommending resistance training to athletes. First, specificity of weight training in athletes means that the training exercises or lifts you recommend must be relevant to the energy source and movement pattern of the event. Second, maximal strength gains are best achieved by an overload program that incorporates higher intensities (more weight) with more sets and fewer repetitions. Interestingly, maximal gains in endurance are also derived from this same type of program. Therefore, since most competitive athletes require optimal gains in both muscle strength and endurance to best perform, a high-weight, low-repetition concentric or isotonic program is usually recommended – e.g., four sets of six to eight repetitions at ≥85% of 1 RM. Obviously, any recommendations made for resistance training must consider individual safety and population-specific issues. It is often prudent to use a lower weight, fewer set, and higher repetition training model for older people and those with clinically manifest disease – e.g., two sets of 12 repetitions at 50–75% of 1 RM.

Types of Training Programs

Interval Training

Just as the name implies, interval training requires the completion of a series of repeated exercise bouts, alternated with periods of relief. The work interval is that period where exercise intensity or pace is high, such as completing a 100 m swim in no more than 3 s above an athlete's best time from a moving start.

The relief interval is the time in between work intervals and there are two types. The first is called rest-relief, which means it contains very light work. The second is a work-relief interval and it may include mild or moderate work.

If the specific metabolic system you are trying to enhance is the ATP-PC system, then a rest-relief interval is used to allow the aerobic metabolic pathways to more quickly replenish muscle ATP-PC stores during recovery. If, however, you strive to improve anaerobic glycolysis in order to improve performance during either a longer duration anaerobic event or an aerobic event, then a work-relief interval is used. This approach is effective as it partially blocks the complete restoration of the ATP-PC system during the relief phase. As a consequence, anaerobic glycolysis is forced to provide more energy during the subsequent work bout.

A final point about interval training. It is important to determine the correct ratio between work and relief. Generally, the shorter the duration of the sport the greater the number of workout sets, the greater the number of repetitions, and the greater the duration or time of the relief interval. For example, the 25 m swimmer might do three sets of eight repetitions with a work to relief (rest-relief) ratio of 1:3. Compare this to the 800-m runner who might do two sets of three repetitions, with a work to relief (work-relief) ratio of 1 to 1.

Fartlek

A Swedish word meaning *speed play*, fartlek training is felt to be the precursor to interval training. It usually involves alternating a slow exercise pace with a faster pace. Often used by distance swimmers, runners, cross-country skiers and cyclists, fartlek training should be employed no more than once a week. In this method, the duration of the faster and slower paced periods is not prespecified, and all exercise is performed continuously. Most often used among aerobic athletes to improve aerobic metabolic pathways, there is some improvement in anaerobic glycolysis as well. The net effect is an improvement in race pace.

Tempos

In this method of endurance training exercise intensity is set at heart rate at LT or race pace, with the plan to continue to exercise for 20–60 min. Occasionally, the intensity can be increased if the duration is shortened to just 10–15 min or so. Sometime called aerobic intervals, the main objective of tempos is to improve tolerance to racing at LT. Among athletes who have plateaued relative to increasing peak VO_2, tempos can improve race performance with little increase in peak VO_2 [5].

The Patient-Athlete

So far we have discussed the general principles associated with prescribing exercise in healthy athletes. The remainder of this chapter will address the unique challenges of prescribing exercise in patient-athletes with various types of cardiovascular disease, specifically those participating in vigorous and competitive sport activity. In this section we assume that the athlete has already undergone screening, has been correctly diagnosed, and now stands before you asking for guidance on participation in a sport that is classified as vigorous and/or competitive.

Just as not all heart disease is the same, not all competitive sports require the same level of exertion. Therefore, special modifications in the exercise prescription are needed. Table 4.3 lists those forms of heart disease for which the athlete should never participate in vigorous competitive sports and thus will not be discussed in this chapter. Participation in athletics should not be considered an all-or-none process. If it is determined that an athlete should not participate in vigorous level sports, the benefits of regular exercise for prolonging life, treating risk factors, delaying the onset of coronary artery disease and certain cancers, and improving quality of life should not be forgotten. An exercise prescription can still be written that takes into account both the patient's heart disease and important need to maintain an active and healthy lifestyle. To paraphrase George Sheehan, a writer, physician, and athlete "We are all athletes, some of us are just training more regularly."

The 36th Bethesda Conference developed prudent consensus recommendations regarding the eligibility of the trained athlete with heart disease to participate in vigorous and/or competitive sports [6]. The competitive athlete by definition is one who trains at high levels of intensity and then competes, usually against another athlete or athletes, at maximal or near maximal work rates. Writing an exercise prescription for a competitive athlete must take into account the unique variables associated with the type of heart disease present (Table 4.4). Although it is usually easy to advise an athlete to monitor and maintain a certain level of intensity during training, the clinician must assume that the athlete will be achieving maximum or

Table 4.3 Patient athletes who should not participate in vigorous sports

- Symptomatic athletes (see Table 4.5)
- Athletes with evidence of hemodynamic compromise (see Table 4.5)
- Hypertrophic cardiomyopathy
- Marfan's syndrome
- Bicuspid aortic valve with aortic dilatation > 40 mmHg
- Moderate or severe stenotic or regurgitant valvular heart disease
- Moderate or severe multivalvular heart disease
- Prosthetic heart valves
- Acute myocarditis or pericarditis
- Congenital heart disease with cyanosis or RV dysfunction
- Anomalous coronary artery coming from the opposite cusp
- Coarctation, corrected coarctation
- Congenitally corrected transposition of the great arteries
- Arrhythmogenic right ventricular cardiomyopathy
- Ventricular tachycardia with structural heart disease
- Long QT syndrome, short QT syndrome, Brugada's syndrome, and catecholaminergic polymorphic ventricular tachycardia
- Patient-athletes with a device should not participate in contact sports
- Prior embolic event
- Patients-athletes on coumadin should not participate in contact sports

Table 4.4 Approach to patient-athlete with cardiovascular disease

- Identify unique physiology of the heart disease present
- Assume a maximal or near maximal effort during competition
- Athletes do not always know when they are exceeding safe limits
- Identify medications they are taking and determine what influence they may have on the exercise response
- Identify if the athlete has had surgical correction
- Does the athlete have a pacemaker or automatic implantable cardioverter/defibrillator (AICD)?
- Does the athlete have symptoms or signs of hemodynamic compromise?

near-maximum intensity during competition. Finally, athletes can undergo surgical procedures or have devices inserted as treatment for their underlying heart disease, any of which may alter the exercise prescription.

Once the diagnosis of heart disease is made, the next step is to understand the severity of the condition. The cornerstone of the evaluation of the severity of the heart condition is whether the patient-athlete is having symptoms of chest pain, shortness of breath, worsening exercise tolerance, or syncope. With athletes this can be especially problematic because the athlete may not feel it is in his or her best interest to admit to symptoms that may result in their physician recommending they no longer participate in vigorous or competitive sports. Generally, athletes with symptomatic heart disease should avoid vigorous competitive sports. Other testing modalities can be used to quantify the severity of the heart disease, including echocardiography with Doppler, stress testing, and Holter monitoring. Rarely is cardiac catheterization necessary. Exercise testing is especially helpful in that it allows the clinician to assess the athlete's cardiovascular responses during exertion. If exercise testing is performed, the protocol can be modified to simulate the activity of the sport (i.e., if the athlete is a sprinter the stress test should begin abruptly and at a higher work rate to achieve maximum effort in a shorter duration). Conversely, if the athlete is an endurance athlete the exercise test could take place over a longer period of time than the traditional exercise test. Athletes whose heart disease is severe enough to cause hemodynamic compromise should not participate in vigorous or competitive sports (Table 4.5).

Since the intensity of exertion may vary with the type of sport itself as well as the level of competition, not all competitive athletes are involved in sports that are considered vigorous. The Bethesda conference devised a "Classification of Sports" based on peak static and dynamic components achieved during competition [7]. The static component is defined as the estimated percentage of maximal voluntary contraction (MVC), while the dynamic component is defined as the percentage of maximal VO_2. Also included in the classification is a designation for those sports where there is danger of bodily contact and increased risk if syncope occurs. In this chapter, we are concerned primarily with those sports with a high static component (> 50% of MVC; i.e., resistance training) or a high dynamic component (>70% peak VO_2; i.e., soccer) or both – sports we would classify as vigorous.

There are two populations of athletes that are at risk for sudden cardiac death and cardiac events [8]: those athletes less than 35 years old who are more likely to have structural heart disease and those athletes over the age 35 years old who are more likely to have coronary artery disease. Not only is this distinction important to help us in the screening of athletes and to understand the cause of sudden cardiac death in athletes, it also is important because athletes who have coronary artery disease generally derive a protective benefit from future cardiac events through moderate exercise. Conversely athletes with structural heart disease do not receive this benefit. It is not known, however, if participation in vigorous vs. moderate sports or exercise by athletes with coronary artery disease may diminish some of the protective benefits of exercise. Vigorous activity has been defined as an absolute exercise work rate of at least 6 metabolic equivalents (METs), which is equal to a VO_2 of approximately 21 $mL{\cdot}kg^{-1}{\cdot}min^{-1}$ and occurs at a level of exertion equivalent to jogging [9]. However, among the unfit and the elderly a similar level of physical stress may be placed on the cardiovascular system at work rates <6 METs. The remainder of this chapter will discuss unique aspects of prescribing exercise in

Table 4.5 Signs and symptoms of hemodynamic compromise

- Symptoms of chest pain, shortness of breath, change in exercise tolerance, or syncope
- LV enlargement with >6.0 cm end-diastolic dimension
- LV impairment with EF <50%
- Aortic root dilation >4.5 cm
- Pulmonary hypertension with systolic pressure >50 mmHg during exercise
- Resting sinus tachycardia or an exaggerated exercise tachycardia
- Exercise hypotension

patients with various forms of heart disease who elect to participate in vigorous and/or competitive sports.

Hypertrophic Cardiomyopathy

The complexity of the decision to allow the patient-athlete to participate in vigorous sports is no better observed than in athletes with hypertrophic cardiomyopathy (HCM). HCM is described in more detail in Chapter 13. Suffice it to say, however, the Bethesda Conference recommended that athletes with HCM should limit themselves to low-intensity activities only. However, there 12 mutant genes with 400 specific mutations implicated in the pathogenesis of HCM. Some patients have the genotype of HCM but not the phenotype. It is anticipated that at least some of these genotypically positive, phenotypically negative athletes will eventually develop the echocardiographic features of HCM. These athletes can participate in competitive vigorous sports, but they should be monitored with serial echocardiography, Holter monitors, ECGs, stress tests, or cardiac magnetic resonance every 12–18 months. Once they begin to manifest signs of HCM their participation in competitive sports should cease. For those patients with HCM and an implantable cardiac defibrillator (ICD) inserted to prevent sudden cardiac death (SCD) they should not be cleared to participate in competitive sports because there is no evidence that ICD's prevent SCD during vigorous exercise.

Mitral Valve Prolapse and Myocarditis

Athletes with mitral valve prolapse, i.e., myxomatous degeneration, who are asymptomatic and have no signs of hemodynamic compromise (Table 4.5) or family history of MVP-related sudden death are at very low risk for SCD. Therefore, these athletes can participate in all vigorous competitive sports using the methods for prescribing exercise presented at the beginning of this chapter. Athletes with MVP and signs of hemodynamic compromise can participate in low-intensity competitive sports only. Athletes with myocarditis who are asymptomatic, without signs of hemodynamic compromise and whose ECG is normal or only showing mild nonspecific ST-T wave changes can participate in all competitive vigorous sports after a 6-month convalescent period.

Valvular Heart Disease

Valvular heart disease is discussed in more detail in Chapter 17. Athletes with normal hearts will often have regurgitant murmurs that are considered physiologic. These athletes have no restrictions and can participate in all sports and at all levels of intensity. Murmurs due to abnormal valve function are considered pathologic and require further diagnosis and quantification before recommendations regarding participation in competitive sports can be made. Athletes with valvular disease who are symptomatic or have signs of hemodynamic compromise (Table 4.5) have more advanced disease and are candidates for valve repair or replacement and should not participate in vigorous sports. Little is known about the effects of vigorous exercise on the progression of the valvular disease or the progression of left ventricular dysfunction.

Athletes with mild valvular heart disease who are asymptomatic and have no signs of hemodynamic compromise can participate in vigorous sports, using the methods for prescribing exercise outlined at the beginning of the chapter. Mild valvular heart disease such as mitral stenosis and aortic stenosis is defined as a valve area > 1.5 cm^2. Mild aortic and mitral regurgitation is defined by jets < 30 mL in volume or a jet width at just below the valve (Vena contracta) that is <3 mm or occupying less than 20% of the cavity area [10, 11].

Athletes with moderate regurgitant lesions should avoid training regimens and competitive sports that are considered to have a high (>50% MVC) static component [6]. If they have a mechanical valve or atrial fibrillation and one taking war farin, they should avoid contact sports. For athletes with regurgitant lesions or prosthetic valves, observing the athlete during an exercise test performed to the level of exertion simulating the type of physical activity that occurs during competition can often provide insight to how well the heart will tolerate the physical activity.

Congenital Heart Disease

As stated earlier, if the athlete is symptomatic or has signs of hemodynamic compromise he should not participate in vigorous sports. If the athlete has an uncomplicated form of congenital heart disease such as a shunt at the level of the atrium, ventricle, or pulmonary artery they can compete in training and sports of all duration, frequency, and intensities. If the shunt is large enough that it needs to be repaired, the athlete should wait until 3 months after the lesion has been repaired before resuming vigorous training or competition.

Patients with pulmonary stenosis can participate in vigorous competitive sports if the gradient across the valve is <40 mmHg. If the gradient is >40 mmHg they should not participate in competitive vigorous sports. If they have undergone treatment and the gradient is <40 mmHg they can resume competitive sports a minimum of 2 weeks after balloon valvuloplasty and 3 months after surgery.

Athletes with tetralogy of fallot or transposition of the great vessels who underwent corrective surgery as a child and now have no residual signs of hemodynamic compromise can undergo vigorous resistance training or cardiorespiratory training and competition without restriction. Ebstein's anomaly, if mild; anomalous coronary arteries after correction; and Kawaski's disease after regression of ectasia or aneurysms can participate in all levels of competitive sports. Exercise testing is recommended before participating in competitive sports to rule out exercise-induced ischemia or ventricular arrhythmias. CT angiography and MR angiography of the coronary arteries may be helpful to evaluate the coronary artery anatomy in some patients.

Arrhythmias are covered extensively in other chapters.

Cardiac Transplantation

While patients with nonischemic and ischemic cardiomyopathies with abnormal LV function should never participate in vigorous training or competition, there are accounts of athletes who have undergone heart transplantation and participated in endurance training and marathon running [12, 13]. One such patient organized a charity to promote organ donation and organ transplantation awareness. To promote his charity he has completed nine marathons. Additionally, the World Transplant Games allow cardiac transplant patients to compete regularly. Ruddy et al. [14] reported on a team of 14 cardiac transplant patients who participate yearly in a 600 km relay race for four consecutive years. All authors report an improvement in treadmill duration, peak VO_2, and peak power output with vigorous training.

The training program after heart transplantation typically includes both a resistance and aerobic component [15]. The training program begins with an exercise test to determine the level of fitness. Because heart rate response to exercise is an inaccurate way to estimate peak VO_2 in transplant patients, especially within the first year after surgery, peak VO_2 is often measured directly. Instead, exercise intensity is often set at a training work rate equivalent to 60–70% of peak VO_2 or a perceived exertion on the Borg scale of 12–14. The Toronto/Harefield program [16] began by having the patient walk 1.6 km 5 days weekly at a pace of 11–14 $min \cdot km^{-1}$. The distance is increased by 1.6 km every 2 weeks until by the 6th week the patient is walking 4.8 km 5 days weekly. The time is quickened by 1 min until the 4.8 km is performed in 45 min. Once this level is reached, 50-m bouts of a slow jog are introduced until the 4.8 km is covered in 36 min. If the patient plateaus at a particular stage, he is then encouraged to maintain that pace but increase the exercise session to 30–60 min. Although resistance training is quite helpful for the heart transplant patient, there are no reports addressing the safety of competitive lifting in these patients.

The development of coronary artery disease (CAD) is one of the complications of heart transplant. CAD does not typically cause chest pain or ST depression during a stress test. The symptoms of dyspnea, light headedness, syncope, or arrhythmias secondary to ischemia may be the only signs of CAD, so the athlete needs to be monitored closely for and instructed to look for these symptoms.

Elderly

With aging there is a decline in fitness, as measured by peak VO_2 of about 1% per year, so that by age 55 peak VO_2 has decreased by 30% when compared to values reported for people in their mid-twenties. In cross-sectional and longitudinal studies involving elite master's athletes, peak VO_2 begins at a higher level and declines at a lesser rate so that loss of fitness is only 15% after 30 years [17]. Clearly a lifetime of exercise can help offset some of the effects of aging. Also the type of sport an athlete chooses to engage in changes with age. Young athletes are generally involved in team sports while the older athlete is more likely to choose an individual sport such as long-distance running or cycling.

The elderly are not only undertaking exercise at increasing numbers to maintain fitness but are also competitively involved in sports, as is evidenced by the formation of competitive events such as master's level programs and the Senior Olympics. The elderly athlete can be divided into three categories. One category is the healthy elderly adult who has not exercised in the past, is free of heart disease, and is contemplating starting an exercise program. The second category is the elderly athlete, a person who has been exercising regularly throughout his life and is still competing in a sport. And the final category is the elderly adult who has had a cardiac event and wants to start or continue exercising, perhaps competitively to a level that was enjoyed prior to their cardiac event.

In the healthy elderly adult, habitual vigorous physical activity has a protective effect, reducing the likelihood of developing coronary artery disease and the incidence of cardiac events during exercise in athletes both with and without coronary artery disease [18]. In patients who have already had a myocardial infarction or undergone coronary revascularization, cardiac rehabilitation reduces the risk of recurrent events and cardiac death by 23% over 3 years [18].

Once the elderly athlete has been screened by his physician, usually with a stress test, and determined to be either free of heart disease or to have stable coronary artery disease, there is no reason vigorous exercise cannot be prescribed. Although all athletes involved in vigorous activity are at a very slight increased risk for SCD during the physical activity or immediately afterward, their overall risk for SCD when compared to the sedentary individual is lower. A very important variable associated with any person's risk of SCD during exercise is their current exercise habit. Those individuals who exercise on a regular basis have a lower likelihood of SCD during exercise. In fact, the Onset Study estimated that the risk of acute myocardial infarction during or immediately after vigorous exertion was 50 times greater in the least active vs. the most active cohort [19]. Those athletes who have the highest intensity and frequency of activity are at the lowest risk for SCD either at rest or during exercise [17,19]. It is important then that these elder-athletes begin exercise training at a low intensity, gradually increasing first duration then frequency of effort, before increasing the intensity of their workout – all the time monitoring for symptoms that might suggest exercise-related ischemia. If the athlete does not have a history of heart disease, the exercise prescription is written using the standard guidelines.

For the elderly athlete who suffers a myocardial infarction or undergoes revascularization, cardiac rehabilitation should be the first step. Comprehensive cardiac rehabilitation programs offer education, an individualized exercise prescription, risk factor modification, surveillance, restoration of self-confidence, and counseling. Today cardiac rehabilitation is divided into inpatient, early outpatient, and maintenance programs. Following a cardiac event the patient enters a continuous program that evolves from being highly structured and monitored to an unmonitored maintenance program.

A summary of the guidelines for writing an exercise prescription for patients with coronary artery disease is as follows:

Frequency = most days of the week
Intensity = 60–80% of peak VO_2 or Heart Rate Reserve (see Table 4.1)
Time = at least 30 min

For the athlete some additional modifications must be taken into consideration. Note that exercise intensity is guided by heart rate response, usually based on peak heart rate during an exercise test. However, during prolonged submaximal exercise lasting over 30 min, stroke volume tends to decrease and heart rate proportionately increases to maintain cardiac output. This is referred to as cardiac or cardiovascular drift. Thus, at the end of an endurance event it is not uncommon to find near maximal heart rates [20].

Cardiac drift should be considered when writing an exercise prescription for the endurance athlete who has evidence of ischemia, such that additional modifications may need to be made to the exercise prescription if the athlete is participating in endurance events that exceed 30 min. Specifically, and regardless of duration, if exercise-induced ischemia is present, the exercise heart rate throughout training and competition should remain ten beats below the heart rate at which ischemia occurred (ischemic threshold).

Two cardiac rehabilitation programs have published their experience with returning the patients with cardiac disease to vigorous competitive sports such as marathon running. Gottheiner reported his experience [21] with vigorous endurance sports training for cardiac reconditioning and rehabilitation at the Centre for Sports Medicine in Tel-Aviv Israel. In that report, 3,000 patients [1,461 with ischemic heart disease, 629 with "other" heart disease (rheumatic, hypertensive, etc.), and 910 sedentary patients without heart disease] were enrolled in an exercise program that systematically increased exercise intensity until they were ultimately participating in vigorous sports training program. After testing for cardiovascular fitness and work tolerance, the participants were exposed to a several month-long preparatory period of mild warm-up and strength-building exercises. Within approximately 9 months they qualified for systematic training in rhythmic endurance and locomotive sports (hiking, swimming, cycling, rowing, running) and volley-ball. The program culminated in competitive team games. Of 1,103 trainees with ischemic heart disease who remained under observation for 5 years, a total of 49 deaths were reported; nine of the deaths were noncardiac (automobile accidents, cancer, and stroke). Only 3.6% of the patients with ischemic heart disease died from recurrent MI or other complications. In a survey of 390 postinfarction patients in Israel who did not receive sports training, the mortality rate over 4 years was 12%.

The second report from Kavanagh et al. [22] chronicles the training of eight postinfarction patients who run a marathon. All patients participated in a program of progressive endurance running to the point of participating in the Boston Marathon. They were trained to take their pulse and were advised to drop out if they noticed an excessive increase in their pulse rate, arrhythmia, or chest pain. Seven of the eight completed the race at an average speed of 5.4 mph, which corresponded to 81% of their peak VO_2. While it is not necessary to return to this level of physical activity these seven patients showed that with proper supervision and monitoring, this level of participation in competitive sports could be done safely.

Case Presentation 1

Medical History

Mr. GJ is a 39-year-old male who presented to the ER with chest pain that began while performing vigorous weight training at the gym. The chest pain was left sided, radiated to the left arm, and was rated 8/10 in intensity. The pain was associated with diaphoresis and light headedness. His past medical history included placement of a bare metal stent in his left anterior descending (LAD) artery 7 years earlier, gastroesophageal reflux disease, hypercholesterolemia, and a family history of coronary artery disease.

Examination

His blood pressure was 88/54 mmHg with a heart rate of 99 beats per minute. He appeared anxious. Auscultation of his lungs revealed them to be clear. Auscultation of his heart demonstrated a regular rhythm without murmurs or extra heart sounds. His peripheral pulses are diminished and his feet cool.

Testing

ECG done by EMS showed anterior wall ischemic changes, and he was given 81 mg ASA and transferred to the ER.

Diagnosis

1. Acute anterior wall myocardial infarction with early cardiogenic shock

Hospital Course

In the ER his chest pain continued and his ECG now showed ST elevation anteriorly. He was transferred to the cardiac catheterization laboratory for emergent percutaneous coronary intervention. The cardiac catheterization demonstrated

100% occlusion of stent previously placed in his LAD. There was also 50% stenosis of the right coronary artery. The LAD was opened using PCI. The patient's hospital course was otherwise uncomplicated. His echocardiogram showed a mildly dilated (59 mm) left ventricle with an ejection fraction of 25–30%. He had an anterior wall motion abnormality consistent with an LAD occlusion. His medications at the time of discharge included 325 mg ASA, 75 mg clopidigrel, 80 mg atorvastatin, 6.25 mg carvedilol twice daily, and lisinopril 10 mg daily.

Post Discharge Plan

Following discharge he was enrolled in cardiac rehabilitation. Because of his moderate LV impairment, he had an AICD implanted at 45 days. After completing cardiac rehabilitation, he returned to the office for follow-up and asks if he can resume his vigorous weight training program.

His most recent exercise stress echocardiogram demonstrated a resting EF of 35% and no evidence of ischemia by symptoms, ECG or exercise echocardiography. His peak VO_2 on cardiopulmonary stress testing was low at 22.1 $mL \cdot kg^{-1} \cdot min^{-1}$. Based on the recommendations of the 36th Bethesda Conference, this patient is considered to be at substantially increased risk for sudden cardiac death because of his hemodynamically significant stenosis (≥50%) of a major coronary artery and impaired LV function (EF≤50%). Therefore, he was advised not to resume his vigorous weight training program. An exercise prescription was written recommending 2 days per week of resistance training, at 60–80% of a one rep maximum for each of 10–12 exercises emphasizing the major muscle groups. We recommended that the weight be light enough, such that he can perform two sets of 12–15 repetitions. We, also, recommended cardiorespiratory training at 60–80% of heart rate reserve based on the patient's most recent stress test. Additionally, he was instructed to maintain his heart rate 15 beats below the threshold for discharge of his ICD. His exercise program should include sessions that last at least 30 min and occur on most days of the week.

Case Presentation 2

Medical History

A former college track athlete, Mr. C.M. is a 29-year-old Caucasian male who was first seen 18 months ago secondary to his interest to resume a competitive, vigorous running regimen. He did go on to resume a regular running program, tolerating it well and for the past 6 months has been competing in approximately one 10 K race per month. Race times are generally sub 38 min.

He is seen today asking for assistance with how best to safely increase training volume, in preparation for participation in his first marathon road race that is to be held in approximately 5 months. Running history for the past 3 months consists of steady state runs four to five times per week of 4–7 miles per run; 7:05 pace. The patient also tries to complete a longer run each weekend of 6–9 miles. Interval workouts one time per month, with no tempo or Fartlek training employed.

He denies any complaints of dyspnea, palpitations, chest pain, or syncope. He states that he has no history of diabetes or cardiac disease, but he does have mild hypertension that is treated with hydrochlorothiazide. He also has a history of mitral valve prolapse with moderate mitral regurgitation diagnosed by echocardiography. The echocardiogram demonstrates normal left ventricular size, normal EF, normal left atrial size, and normal pulmonary artery pressures. Blood lipids or glucose not measured in past 5 years. He has a positive history of intermittent cocaine use, as recently as 3 weeks ago. Alcohol is limited to less than 3 drinks per week, and he denies tobacco use. He has a very strong family history of heart disease, with his living father having suffered a myocardial infarction at the age of 47 years. His mother is alive and apparently healthy.

Examination

Examination today revealed a healthy appearing, well-developed, well-nourished male; BMI 20; seated heart rate regular at 48 and blood pressure right arm of 124/82. No carotid bruits; lungs clear; normal PMI; and normal S1 and S2, mid systolic click with a soft late systolic murmur that increases in duration with valsalva maneurer. No edema present and normal peripheral vascular exam. Skin, no rashes. Normal gait, joints are normal, good range of motion throughout. Nail on great toe of right foot is absent, with new growth evident.

Testing

Results from symptom-limited maximal cardiopulmonary exercise test performed today in the office are as follows:

1. Completed four stages and exercised for 14 min using standard Bruce protocol. Exercise limited by fatigue.
2. Resting ECG is normal with exercise there is no evidence of myocardial ischemia.
3. Appropriate heart rate response to exercise to a peak rate of 184 per min.
4. Appropriate blood pressure response to a peak value of 208/84.
5. No ectopy.

6. Excellent exercise capacity based on a measured peak VO_2 of 63.3 mL·kg^{-1} · min^{-1}; this equates to 121% of age predicted. Ventilatory-derived anaerobic threshold estimated using the v-slope method occurred at a VO_2 that was 79% of peak VO_2 and an exercise heart rate of 160 per min.

Diagnosis

1. Normal examination
2. Hypertension controlled by exercise and medical therapy
3. Mitral valve prolapse with moderate mitral regurgitation without signs of hemodynamic compromise
4. Substance above, with cocaine

Plan

1. Counseled about cardiovascular dangers/risks of cocaine use, with and without superimposed exercise, and recommended complete avoidance.
2. Continue exercise and hydrochlorothiazide daily for management of hypertension.
3. Given family history will order lipid profile, and fasting blood sugar.
4. Based on the recommendations of the 36th Bethesda Conference, the patient is at low risk for sudden cardiac death and can participate in all competitive sports.
5. Based on CPX test results and the patient's current training habits, suggested the following to better prepare him for marathon event.
   (a) Over the next 2 months, progressively modify current training regimen to achieve approximately 35–40 miles per week using the following:
      (i) Two days per week run 6–8 miles at a heart rate that is between 152 and 156 per min.
      (ii) One day per week run initially 9–13 miles at a heart rate that is between 152 and 156 per min. Within 2 months of race day these runs should begin to lengthen, such that 2–3 weeks before race day this one time per week longer run is 18–20 miles.
      (iii) One time per week conduct a Fartlek run, cover about 5 miles and at patient's discretion vary pace (for no pre-specified period of time) between slower (heart rate = 154–158 per min), moderate (heart rate = 156–160 per min), and tempo (heart rate = 158–162 per min) paces.
      (iv) One day per week (no more than 3 per month) run a tempo run for 3.5–4 miles at a heart rate of 158–162 per min. Instead of the tempo run, intervals can be conducted to improve leg speed also. This would include eight, 1,000 m runs (at tempo pace of heart rate = 159–162 per min), with 2.5–3 min of walking recovery in between each 1,000 m run.

(b) Rest, do not exercise 1 day per week.
(c) Progressively modify diet, such that 65–70% of calories are derived from carbohydrates, predominately complex carbohydrates. Maintain/adjust hydration commensurate with training volume and sweat loss to avoid dehydration.
(d) Using rest/reduced training/cross-training and ice, compression and elevation, initiate self-treatment of any developing muscle or joint problem. Any problem that does not measurably improve in 3 days using this approach should be evaluated.
(e) Pay close attention to integrity of footwear and replace as needed.

Summary

The death of an athlete during training or while participation in vigorous activity or sport is dramatic and captures our attention because these athletes often represent youth, peak health and are engaging in a behavior seen as one of the cornerstones of a healthy lifestyle. As the name implies, the event of sudden cardiac death occurs suddenly, most of the time without warning and usually irreversibly. These vibrant individuals are removed suddenly from our communities.

Programs based on symptoms, family history, and physical findings have been developed to identify these high-risk athletes. Some athletes will be disqualified from participating in vigorous training or competitive sports. Other athletes who are deemed able to compete in vigorous training and competition may require modifications in their exercise prescription for training, such as the avoidance of ischemia in athletes with coronary artery disease, avoidance of high static component sports if the athlete has a dilated aorta, or avoidance of contact sports if a pacemaker was inserted or coumadin is taken.

Once identified, recommendations regarding the type and nature of training and competition can be made for the athlete, so that they can train and compete safely.

References

1. Magel JR, Foglia GF, McArdle WD, et al. Specificity of swim training on maximum oxygen uptake. J Appl Physiol. 1975;38:151–155.
2. Bar-Or O. The Wingate anaerobic test: An update on methodology, reliability and validity. Sports Med. 1978;4:381–394.
3. American College of Sports Medicine. *Guidelines for Exercise Testing and Prescription*. 6th ed. Philadelphia: Lippincott Williams & Wilkins, 2000.
4. Robergs RA, Keteyian SJ. *Fundamentals of Exercise Physiology*. New York: McGraw Hill, 2003.
5. Foss ML, Keteyian SJ. *Fox's Physiological Basis for Exercise and Sport*. New York: McGraw Hill, 1998.
6. Maron BJ, Zipes DP. 36th Bethesda Conference: Eligibility recommendations for competitive athletes with cardiovascular abnormalities. J Am Coll Cardiol. 2005;45:1318–1375.

7. Mitchell JH, Haskell W, Snell P, Van Camp SP. Task Force 8: Sports classification. J Am Coll Cardiol. 2005;35:1364–1367.
8. Maron BJ, Roberts WC, McAllister HA, Rosing DR, Epstein SE. Sudden death in young athletes. Circulation. 1980;62:218–229.
9. Thompson PD, Franklin BA, Balady GJ, et al. Exercise and acute cardiovascular events: Placing the risks in perspective. Circulation. 2007;115:2358–2368.
10. Bonow RO, Cheitlin MD, Crawford MH, Douglas PS. Task Force 3: Valvular heart disease. J Am Coll Cardiol. 2005;45:1334–1340.
11. Bonow RO, Carabello BA, Chaterjee K, et al. ACC/AHA guidelines for the management of patients with valvular heart disease. J Am Coll Cardiol. 2006;48:e1–e148.
12. Kavanaugh T, Yacoub MH, Campbell R, Mertens D. Marathon running after cardiac transplantation: A case history. J Cardiopulm Rehabil. 1986;6:16–20.
13. Niset G, Poortmans JR. Metabolic implications during a 20 km run after heart transplantation. Int J Sports Med. 1985;6:340–343.
14. Ruddy R, Verdier JC, Duvallet A, et al. Chronotropic competence in endurance trained heart transplant recipients: Heart rate is not a limiting factor for exercise capacity. J Am Coll Cardiol. 1999;33:192–197.
15. Kavanaugh T. Exercise rehabilitation in cardiac transplantation patients: A comprehensive review. Eur Med Phys. 2005;41:67–74.
16. Kavanaugh T, Yacoub MH, Mertens D, Kennedy J, et al. Cardiorespiratory responses to exercise training after orthotopic cardiac transplantation. Circulation. 1988;77;162–171.
17. Yu S, Christopher CC, Yarnell JWG. Is vigorous physical activity contraindicated in subjects with coronary heart disease? Evidence from the Caerphilly study. Eur Heart J. 2008;29:602–608.
18. Taylor RS, Brown A, Ebrahim S, et al. Exercised-based cardiac rehabilitation for patients with coronary heart disease: Systematic review and meta-analysis of randomized controlled trials. Am J Med. 2004;116:682–692.
19. Mittleman MA, Maclure M, Tofler GH. Triggering of acute myocardial infarction by heavy physical exertion: Protection against triggering by regular exertion: Determinants of Myocardial Infarction Onset Study Investigators. N Engl J Med. 1993;329:1677–1683.
20. Coyle EF, Gonzalez-Alonso J. Cardiovascular drift during prolonged exercise: New perspectives. Exerc Sport Sci Rev. 2001;29:86–92.
21. Gottheiner V. Long-range strenuous sports training for cardiac reconditioning and rehabilitation. Am J Cardiol. 1968;22:426–435.
22. Kavanagh T, Shepard RH, Pandit V. Marathon running after myocardial infarction. JAMA. 1974;229:1602–1605.

Chapter 5
Role of Genetic Testing for Sudden Death Predisposing Heart Conditions in Athletes[1]

Andrew P. Landstrom, David J. Tester, and Michael J. Ackerman

Introduction

Sudden death in a young competitive athlete occurs with a prevalence of approximately 1 per 100,000 athletes per year [2, 3]. Despite its rarity, the sudden death of an athlete is devastating to both the family and community. These tragic events often garner widespread attention due to the sudden, unexpected, and seemly paradoxical nature of the death of a trained athlete in good health. This underscores the occult nature of the diseases responsible for such youthful deaths. While the causes of sudden unexpected death (SUD) in the young are diverse, approximately two-thirds are explained following a conventional autopsy while one-third are classified as autopsy-negative SUD [4, 5]. Chief among autopsy-positive SUD are the heritable cardiomyopathies, particularly hypertrophic cardiomyopathy (HCM) and arrhythmogenic right ventricular cardiomyopathy (ARVC). On the other hand, the cardiac channelopathies including long QT syndrome (LQTS) and catecholaminergic polymorphic ventricular tachycardia (CPVT) represent the most common cause(s) of autopsy-negative SUD [6, 7]. For the athlete, however, sudden cardiac death (SCD) stemming from a variety of cardiac conditions predominates and accounts for approximately 90% of "on-the-field" SUD among young athletes with the heritable cardiomyopathies (HCM and ARVC) responsible for nearly half of all such deaths [8].

[1] Dr. Ackerman is a consultant for Boston Scientific, Medtronic, PGxHealth, and St. Jude Medical, Inc. and chairs PGxHealth's Scientific Advisory Board with respect to their FAMILION™ genetic tests for heritable channelopathies and cardiomyopathies. There is a royalty relationship between PGxHealth and Mayo Clinic Health Solutions with respect to genetic testing for long QT syndrome and catecholaminergic polymorphic ventricular tachycardia.

M.J. Ackerman (✉)
Department of Molecular Pharmacology and Experimental Therapeutics, Mayo Clinic, Rochester, Minnesota, USA

Division of Cardiovascular Diseases, Department of Medicine, Mayo Clinic, Rochester, Minnesota, USA

Division of Pediatric Cardiology, Department of Pediatrics and Adolescent Medicine, Mayo Clinic, Rochester, Minnesota, USA

C.E. Lawless (ed.), *Sports Cardiology Essentials: Evaluation, Management and Case Studies*, DOI 10.1007/978-0-387-92775-6_5,

The last two decades have witnessed tremendous advances in the identification of the genetic perturbations responsible for the pathogenesis of these heritable cardiomyopathies and channelopathies. These mutations offer the unique possibility of identifying the genetic biomarker responsible for disease pathogenesis, even in ostensibly healthy individuals. Thus, clinical genetic testing can play a crucial role in the prevention of SCD in athletes and identification of individuals at risk of SCD with occult underlying disease. Further, in some SCD-associated diseases, genetic testing may directly influence therapeutic options and clinical management.

Hypertrophic Cardiomyopathy Case Vignette

JPA is a highly recruited 6′ 5″ high school basketball player. Although entirely asymptomatic, he has a positive family history of premature SCD secondary to HCM involving his paternal uncle and his older brother. His father has echocardiographic evidence for nonobstructive HCM but is asymptomatic. Since his brother's death 5 years ago, yearly echocardiograms have revealed a left ventricular wall thickness of 10–14 mm with normal diastolic function. Contrast-enhanced cardiac MRI was negative for late enhancement. Nevertheless, his cardiologist disqualified him from all competitive sports except class IA activities (i.e., billiards, bowling, cricket, curling, golf, and riflery) because of the positive family history and his "borderline" wall thickness (Fig. 5.1a). The family sought a second opinion. Evaluation was again unremarkable except for the upper limit of normal wall thickness. Genetic testing of the patient's father, which is positive in 35–65% of cases that meet a clinical diagnosis of HCM, revealed the well-established R92W missense mutation in cardiac troponin T (TNNT2-R92W). Postmortem genetic testing on archived autopsy samples confirmed this mutation in the basketball player's deceased uncle and brother. Mutation-specific confirmatory testing in the high school recruit was negative, and JPA returned to the basketball court.

Summary of Cardiomyopathy Genetic Testing

Hypertrophic Cardiomyopathy

The most common cause of SCD among athletes is HCM, which is characterized as asymmetrical left ventricular hypertrophy in the absence of a clinically identifiable cause such as hypertension. Affecting 1 in 500 people, HCM is one of the most prevalent, heritable cardiovascular diseases and is underscored by both marked genetic heterogeneity and phenotypic heterogeneity in degree of hypertrophy (none to extreme), fibrosis and myocyte disarray (none to extreme), left ventricular outflow tract obstruction (none to severe), morphological subtype (reverse curve-, sigmoidal-, and apical-HCM, for example), symptoms (none to debilitating symptoms refractory to pharmacotherapy), and sudden death susceptibility (asymptomatic longevity to premature sudden death prior to first sports participation evaluation).

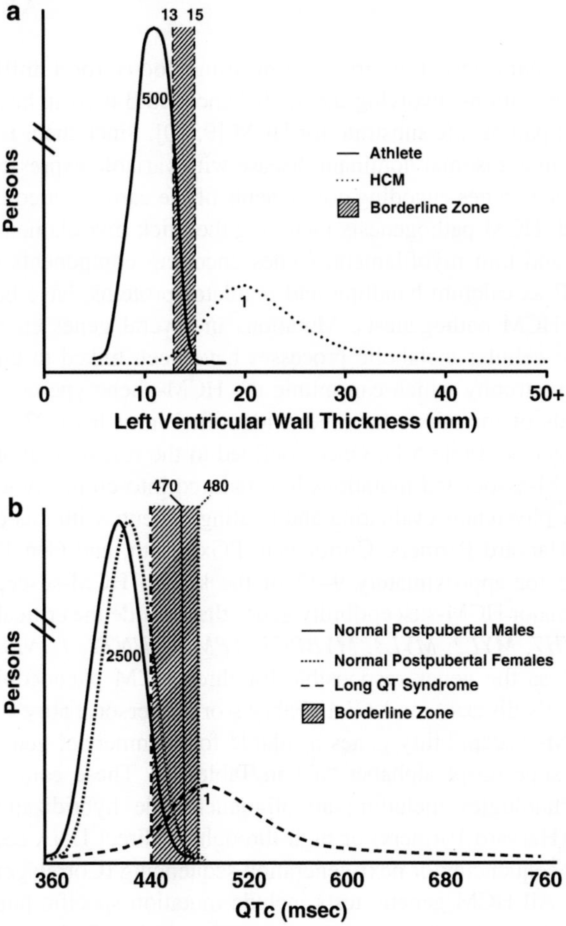

Fig. 5.1 "Borderline" and SCD-predisposing cardiomyopathies/channelopathies. (**a**) Graphical depiction of the overlap zone for left ventricular wall thickness between otherwise healthy athletes and patients with HCM. Note the average left ventricular wall thickness among patients with genetically proven HCM is about 22 mm. An estimated 20–30% of HCM is nonpenetrant, hence the completely normal septal wall thickness measurements. In contrast, a small percentage of normal subjects will have a wall thickness of 13–15 mm, so-called "borderline" hypertrophy. If a diagnosis of HCM has been assigned *solely* because of a wall thickness measurement that resides in this overlap zone, genetic testing may be utilized to provide genetic evidence for HCM or if negative, consider reclassification of the patient as possibly normal. The "athlete" distribution *curve* was adapted from Abernethy et al. [44]. (**b**) Graphical depiction of the normal distribution of QTc values in health and the normal distribution among patients with genetically proven LQTS seen at Mayo Clinic. The *solid line* depicts the distribution of QTc measurements in healthy men, *short dashed line* in healthy women, and the *long dashed line* in LQTS. Note that the so-called "borderline" QTc designation is often applied when the QTc exceeds 440 ms whereas the ~99th percentile values are 470 and 480 ms in males and females, respectively, giving rise to the zone of "borderline QT prolongation" (*oblique lines*). In contrast, the average QTc in our LQTS clinic is about 480 ms and approximately 30–40% of patients with genetically proven LQTS have a QTc < 460 ms. Note also the relative amplitudes of the normal curves and the LQTS curve emphasizing the 1:2,500 estimated incidence of LQTS. Akin to HCM and "borderline" values, if an athlete has been disqualified based solely upon his/her residence in this *gray zone*, a repeat evaluation that may include genetic testing should be considered. The distribution *curves* were adapted from Taggart et al. [43]

Nearly 20 years ago, the first chromosome locus for familial HCM and subsequently mutations involving the *MYH7*-encoded β myosin heavy chain were elucidated as a pathogenic substrate for HCM [9, 10]. Since then, HCM is viewed principally as an autosomal dominant disease with variable expressivity and penetrance. Additional genes encoding components of the cardiac sarcomere have been associated with HCM pathogenesis including the thick myofilament, intermediate myofilament, and thin myofilament. Genes encoding components of the cardiac Z-disc, as well as calcium-handling and regulator proteins, have been associated recently with HCM pathogenesis. Mutations in several genes encoding proteins responsible for cellular metabolic processes have been linked to unexplained left ventricular hypertrophy which can mimic the HCM-phenotype or "phenocopies." In all, hundreds of mutations have been identified in at least 27 putative HCM-susceptibility genes (Table 5.1). Once confined to the research laboratory, genetic testing for HCM-associated mutations has matured into clinically available, diagnostic tests for physicians evaluating and treating patients with this disease.

Currently, Harvard Partners, Correlagen, PGxHealth, and GeneDx offer HCM genetic testing for approximately 9–17 of the known HCM-susceptibility genes including the major HCM-susceptibility genes that encode the critical cardiac myofilaments: *MYH7*, *MYL2*, *MYL3*, *MYBPC3*, *TPM1*, *TNNT2*, *TNNI3*, *TNNC1*, and *ACTC* as well as the genes responsible for three HCM phenocopies: *PRKAG2*, *LAMP2* (Danon's disease), and *GLA* (Fabry's or Anderson Fabry's cardiomyopathy). The HCM-susceptibility genes available for commercial genetic testing are indicated (by superscript alphabet "a") in Table 5.1. These companies utilize a variety of technologies including an oligonucleotide hybridization-based chip methodology (Harvard Partners) or high-throughput direct DNA sequencing with either dideoxy sequencing or next-generation sequencing (Correlagen, PGxHealth, and GeneDx). All HCM genetic tests include mutation-specific family confirmatory testing to determine the presence of a proband-identified mutation in family members. The index test ranges in price from about $3,500–$5,500 (USA), while the family specific test costs between $250 and $900 with insurance reimbursement being quite variable for HCM genetic testing presently.

Regardless of the applied technology, each platform has a diagnostic accuracy exceeding 99%. Although no laboratory has published the results of genotyping the major HCM-susceptibility genes among ostensibly healthy individuals to determine the so-called "background noise rate" of rare genetic variants, the "false-positive" rate is estimated to be quite low («5%). The yield of HCM genetic testing using these commercial tests has declined from its original estimates of 80–90%. Instead, the yield has ranged from 35 to 65% in several different, international research cohorts of unrelated patients who met the clinically accepted definition of HCM [11, 12]. *MYBPC3*-encoded myosin binding protein C and *MYH7*-encoded β myosin heavy chain are, by far, the most common HCM-associated genes with an estimated prevalence of 25–35% for each gene and account for the majority of positive genetic tests. Expansion of commercial testing to include all 27 currently known HCM-susceptibility genes would not enhance the overall yield significantly as the other genes are extremely rare causes of HCM.

Table 5.1 Molecular basis of cardiomyopathies

Gene	Locus	Protein	Frequency
Myofilament (sarcomeric) hypertrophic cardiomyopathy (HCM)			
Giant filament			
TTN	2q31	Titin	<1
Thick filament			
MYH6	14q11.2–q12	α-Myosin heavy chain	Rare
MYH7[a]	14q11.2–q12	β-Myosin heavy chain	25–35%
MYL2[a]	12q23–q24.3	Regulatory myosin light chain	Rare
MYL3[a]	3p21.2–p21.3	Essential myosin light chain	Rare
Intermediate filament			
MYBPC3[a]	11p11.2	Cardiac myosin-binding protein C	25–35%
Thin filament			
ACTC[a]	15q14	α-Cardiac actin	Rare
TNNC1[a]	3p21.1	Cardiac troponin C	Rare
TNNI3[a]	19p13.4	Cardiac troponin I	1–5%
TNNT2[a]	1q32	Cardiac troponin T	3–5%
TPM1[a]	15q22.1	α-Tropomyosin	1–5%
Z-disc HCM			
ACTN2	1q42–q43	α-Actinin 2	Rare
CSRP3	11p15.1	Muscle LIM protein	Rare
LBD3	10q22.2–q23.3	LIM binding domain 3	Rare
MYOZ2	4q26–q27	Myozenin 2	Rare
TCAP	17q12–q21.1	Telethonin	Rare
VCL	10q22.1–q23	Vinculin/metavinculin	Rare
Calcium-handling HCM			
JPH2	20q13.12	Junctophilin 2	Rare
PLN	6q22.1	Phospholamban	Rare
CALR3	19p13.11	Calreticulin 3	Rare
CASQ2	1p13.3–p11	Calsequestrin 2	Rare
Metabolic cardiac hypertrophy (HCM mimickers)			
FXN	9q13	Frataxin	Rare
GLA[a]	Xq22	α-Galactosidase A	Rare
LAMP2[a]	Xq24	Lysosome-associated membrane protein 2	Rare
PRKAG2[a]	7q35–q36.36	AMP-activated protein kinase	Rare
RAF1	3p25.2	RAF serine/threonine kinase	Rare
Arrhythmogenic right ventricular cardiomyopathy (ARVC)			
DSC2[a]	18q12	Desmocollin 2	Rare
DSG2[a]	18q12.1–q12.2	Desmoglein 2	10–15%
DSP[a]	6p24	Desmoplakin	10–20%
JUP	17q21	Plakoglobin	Rare
PKP2[a]	12p11	Plakophilin 2	10–40%
RYR2	1q42.1–q43	Ryanodine receptor 2	Rare
TGFB3	14q23–q24	Transforming growth factor-β3	Rare
TMEM43[a]	3p25	Transmembrane protein 43	Rare

[a] Genes available as a commercial genetic test

Instead, echocardiography may help in providing appropriate genetic counseling as to the a priori probability of a positive genetic test (i.e., echo-guided genetic testing). Analysis of the echocardiograms of nearly 400 unrelated patients demonstrated that sigmoidal-septal, in which the septal hypertrophy is greater near the left ventricular outlet (so-called subaortic basal bulge) giving the septum a sigmoidal shape, and reverse curve-septal, in which the hypertrophic septum bulges into the left ventricular cavity "reversing" its usual curvature, morphologies were the two most prevalent anatomical HCM subtypes (47 and 35%, respectively). Apical HCM, in which the hypertrophy is localized to the apex of the heart and left ventricular cavity, constituted 10% of the cohort. In patients demonstrating reverse curve-HCM, the yield of myofilament genetic testing was 80% while sigmoidal-HCM had a 10% yield [13]. In this respect, septal contour was the strongest predictor of a positive HCM genetic test, regardless of age, with an odds ratio of 21 ($p < 0.001$) when reverse curve morphology was present [13].

Unlike the channelopathies, LQTS in particular, where there are clear diagnostic, prognostic, and therapeutic implications with the clinical genetic test, HCM genetic testing contributes primarily as a diagnostic tool. While a negative genetic test is not sufficient to "rule out" HCM, a positive genetic test may help distinguish HCM from physiologic cardiac hypertrophy and the "athlete heart." Further, genetic testing may play a key role in distinguishing HCM from other HCM phenocopies such as Anderson–Fabry's, glycogen (*PRKAG2*) and lysosomal (*LAMP2*) storage, mitochondrial, Noonan and LEOPARD syndromes, for which there are definitive and alternative therapies distinct from HCM treatments.

Most importantly, however, genetic testing of the index case has the potential of providing the diagnostic gold standard for his/her offspring, siblings, parents, as well as more distant relatives. A positive genetic test would then enable systematic scrutiny of the index case's relatives to identify affected individuals who carry the biomarker independent of clinical phenotype. On the other hand, a negative genetic test, as depicted in the case vignette, would effectively "rule out" HCM in this family setting enabling the athlete to once again pursue his/her dreams and forego yearly echocardiographic examinations.

Arrhythmogenic Right Ventricular Cardiomyopathy

In addition to HCM, arrhythmogenic right ventricular cardiomyopathy/dysplasia (ARVC) is a notable cause of SCD in athletes due to fibro-fatty replacement of ventricular myocardium. Despite its name, ARVC can involve the left ventricle, in addition to the right, and is not necessarily arrhythmogenic [14]. The variable clinical course may include: (1) a subclinical phase with concealed structural abnormalities during which the affected individual may present with SCD as their sentinel manifestation of the disease, (2) an overt electrical disorder with palpitations and syncope due to tachyarrhythmias stemming from the right ventricle often triggered during exertion, and (3) severe right ventricular or biventricular failure requiring cardiac transplantation [15].

Studies have shown that up to 20% of youthful SCD may be attributed to ARVC, and the disease may be even more common in athletes who die suddenly. In one study comprising 100 ARVC patients from the Johns Hopkins ARVC registry, palpitations and syncope were common presenting symptoms (27 and 26%, respectively) and fatal ventricular arrhythmias were the first manifestation in 22% [16]. Of the 29 patients experiencing SCD, 18 (62%) were involved in a routine activity, 9 (31%) in active exercise, 1 (3.5%) was pregnant, and 1 (3.5%) was in bed at the time of death. Nearly 25% of these SCD victims had other symptoms prior to death and may have benefited from an earlier diagnosis and an implantable defibrillator [16].

About half of all ARVC is recognized as familial with an autosomal dominant inheritance and the now expected disclaimer of incomplete penetrance and variable expressivity. To date, mutations in five ARVC-susceptibility genes that encode essential desmosomal proteins have been identified [14]. Desmosomes, also known as macula adherens, are macromolecular cellular structures composed of plasma membrane proteins involved in linking intracellular keratin filaments into a cell-spanning network allowing for effective transmission of force across cells. Functional deficits in these proteins imparted by genetic mutations result in cardiocyte detachment and cell death while subsequent inflammation results in fibro-fatty remodeling. Three nondesmosomal proteins, and the genes which encode them, have been linked to ARVC pathogenesis through varying mechanisms. Overall, eight genes have been implicated as pathogenic determinants of ARVC (Table 5.1).

PKP2, *DSP*, and *DSG* harbor the majority of identified mutations accounting for approximately 40% of ARVC cases in studies from the Netherlands [17], Italy [18], and the USA [16]. *PKP2* represents the most common gene mutated in ARVC, with a prevalence ranging from 40% (identified as the sole cause of ARVC in the cohort) [16, 17] to approximately 10% [18]. Harvard Partners, PGxHealth, and GeneDX currently offer ARVC clinical genetic testing with an estimated yield of approximately 50%.

Long QT Syndrome Case Vignette

LLH is a Division I, female collegiate swimmer with a history of dizziness, presyncope, and two fainting episodes associated with the sight of blood but not during exercise (including swimming). A pre-sports participation electrocardiogram demonstrated a QTc of 480 ms (99.5th percentile for postpubertal women, Fig. 5.1b). Her family history was negative but surveillance ECGs on her first-degree relatives revealed that her asymptomatic mother's QTc was 470 ms. Her cardiologist concluded that she has long QT syndrome, disqualified her from swimming, and implanted an ICD. One year later, her ICD lead fractured resulting in inappropriate ICD shocks and significant psychological sequelae. She and her family sought a second opinion that was unremarkable except for a resting QTc of 480 ms. Her treadmill stress test demonstrated normal shortening of her QTc during exercise and recovery. Her epinephrine QT stress test failed to demonstrate paradoxical prolongation of her absolute QT interval characteristic for patients with type 1 LQTS. Genetic testing elucidated an LQT3-causing mutation. Following explantation of her defective ICD lead and given her asymptomatic state and LQT3 status, LLH returns to the sport she loves consistent with recommendation no. 2 of the Bethesda Conference guidelines (task force 7) for LQTS [19].

Summary of Channelopathy Genetic Testing

Long QT Syndrome

Congenital long QT syndrome (LQTS), with a prevalence as high as 1 in 2,500 persons, comprises a distinct group of cardiac channelopathies characterized by delayed cardiac repolarization and increased risk for syncope, seizures, and SCD. Individuals with LQTS may or may not manifest QT prolongation on a resting 12-lead surface electrocardiogram (ECG, Fig. 5.1b). For virtually every heart beat in a person's life, this repolarization abnormality is without direct consequence; however, should the affected individual be exposed to triggers such as physical exertion (swimming), emotion, auditory stimuli (alarm clocks, door bells, etc.), or during the postpartum period, the depolarization delay can electrically destabilize the heart leading to the potentially lethal dysrhythmia of *torsades de pointes*. While in most incidences, the heart's normal sinus rhythm spontaneously returns, resulting in syncope, 5% of untreated and unsuspecting LQTS individuals succumb to a fatal arrhythmia as their sentinel event. Upon additional evaluation, it is estimated that nearly half of the victims of a LQT-triggered sudden death had exhibited prior warning signs, such as exertional syncope or a family history of premature sudden death, that went unrecognized [20].

LQTS, previously known as Romano-Ward syndrome, is a genetically heterogeneous disorder most often inherited in an autosomal dominant manner. Rarely, LQTS presents as the recessive trait first described by Drs. Jervell and Lange-Nielsen and is characterized by a severe cardiac phenotype and sensorineural hearing loss. In addition, 5–10% of LQTS results from a spontaneous germline mutation. To date, hundreds of mutations have been identified in 12 LQTS-susceptibility genes with approximately 75% of clinically robust LQTS due to mutations in three genes: *KCNQ1*-encoded I_{Ks} potassium channel (Kv7.1, LQT1, loss-of-function), *KCNH2*-encoded I_{Kr} potassium channel (Kv11.1, LQT2, loss-of-function), and *SCN5A*-encoded I_{Na} sodium channel (NaV1.5, LQT3, gain-of-function) that are responsible for the orchestration of the cardiac action potential [21]. The remainder of genotype-positive LQTS stems from mutations in genes that encode either other cardiac channels and channel interacting proteins or structural membrane scaffolding proteins that modulate channel function (Table 5.2). These minor genes contribute <5% of LQTS. Thus, 20–25% of LQTS remains genetically elusive.

Since 2004, LQTS genetic testing of the three major LQTS-susceptibility genes: *KCNQ1*, *KCNH2*, and *SCN5A*, and two of the minor genes: *KCNE1* and *KCNE2*, has been a clinically available diagnostic test offered by PGxHealth (FAMILION™). The yield is approximately 75% [22]. Thus, akin to HCM genetic testing, a negative genetic test cannot categorically exclude LQTS as a stand-alone test. Like with HCM genetic testing, the diagnostic accuracy is >99.5%. Approximately 5% of healthy volunteers possess a rare missense mutation of uncertain functional/clinical significance when genotyped through these five LQTS-susceptibility genes and this potential for a "false positive" must be kept in sharp focus especially as the veracity of the evidence for a clinical diagnosis of LQTS softens [23, 24]. Similar to HCM genetic testing, the index case genetic testing for LQTS costs ~$5,400. In contrast to HCM genetic testing, LQTS genetic testing has been acknowledged already as a bonafide clinical test, rather than an "investigational test," having diagnostic, prognostic, and therapeutic implications. Consequently, the LQTS genetic test is reimbursed by many private health insurance companies, is a Medicare-covered test, and is a Medicaid-approved test in 37 states as of December 2008.

Much like septal morphology can be used to guide genetic testing in HCM, the emergence of phenotype–genotype associations has facilitated rapid mutational analysis of the LQTS-causing genes. Swimming and exertion-induced cardiac events strongly suggest mutations in *KCNQ1*, whereas auditory triggers and events occurring during the postpartum period should prompt suspicion for LQT2, and an event during sleep is associated with LQT3 [25–29]. Importantly, the underlying genetic basis heavily influences the response to standard LQTS pharmacotherapy (β blockers), where β blockers are extremely protective in LQT1 patients, moderately protective in LQT2, and may not provide sufficient protection for those with LQT3 [30].

Catecholaminergic Polymorphic Ventricular Tachycardia

Among the other channelopathies whose genetic substrates are summarized in Table 5.2, the channelopathy most relevant to the SCD of an athlete is catecholaminergic polymorphic ventricular tachycardia (CPVT), a heritable arrhythmia syndrome that classically manifests with exertion-induced syncope or sudden death [31, 32]. CPVT is associated with a normal resting ECG, with possible bradycardia and U waves, and is electrocardiographically suspected following either exercise or catecholamine-induced ventricular ectopy. Like LQTS, CPVT is generally associated with a structurally normal heart. However, CPVT is more lethal with a positive family history of juvenile (<40 years) SCD for more than 30% of CPVT individuals and up to 60% in families hosting mutations in *RYR2* [31].

CPVT stems from genetic mutations in genes encoding components of the macromolecular intracellular Ca^{2+} release channel complex within the sarcoplasmic reticulum (SR) of the cardiocyte. Mutations in the *RYR2*-encoded cardiac ryanodine receptor 2/calcium release channel (RyR2 or CRC, CPVT1) represent the most common genetic subtype of CPVT accounting for approximately 50–60% of cases [31]. Gain-of-function mutations in RyR2 lead to SR Ca^{2+} leakage resulting in excessive store Ca^{2+} release, particularly during sympathetic stimulation. Ultimately, this may precipitate Ca^{2+} overload, delayed depolarization, and ventricular arrhythmias [31]. A rare subtype of CPVT is mediated in an autosomal recessive manner with mutations in *CASQ2*-encoded calsequestrin 2 (CPVT2) [33].

RYR2 is one of the largest genes in the human genome containing 105 coding exons. In this regard, current CPVT genetic testing has focused on a targeted mutation analysis of *RYR2*. PGxHealth offers genetic testing of 38 *RYR2* exons (3, 8–15, 37, 41, 44–50, 83, and 87–105) with a purported yield of 50–55% of CPVT cases. Prevention Genetics analyzes 20 *RYR2* exons (8, 14, 15, 44, 45, 46, 47, 49, 50, 83,

Table 5.2 Molecular basis of cardiac channelopathies

Gene	Locus	Protein	Frequency
Long QT syndrome (LQTS)			
KCNQ1 (LQT1)[a]	11p15.5	Kv7.1	30–35%
KCNH2 (LQT2)[a]	7q35–36	Kv11.1	25–30%
SCN5A (LQT3)[a]	3p21–p24	NaV1.5	5–10%
ANKB	4q25–q27	Ankyrin B	Rare
AKAP9	7q21–q22	Yotiao	Rare
CACNA1C	12p13.3	L-type calcium channel	Rare
CAV3	3p25	Caveolin 3	Rare
KCNE1[a]	21q22.1	MinK	Rare
KCNE2[a]	21q22.1	MiRP1	Rare
KCNJ2	17q23	Kir2.1	Rare
KCNJ5	11q24	Kir3.4	Rare
SCN4B	11q23.3	Sodium channel β4 subunit	Rare
SNTA1	20q11.2	Syntrophin α1	Rare
Catecholaminergic polymorphic ventricular tachycardia (CPVT)			
RYR2 (CPVT1)[a]	1q42.1–q43	Ryanodine receptor 2	50–60%
CASQ2	1p13.3–p11	Calsequestrin 2	Rare
Brugada syndrome (BrS)			
SCN5A (BrS1)[a]	3p21–p24	NaV1.5	20–30%
CACNA1C	12p13.3	L-type calcium channel	~5–10%
CACNB2	10p12	L-type calcium channel β2 subunit	~5–10%
GPD1L	3p22.3	Glycerol-3-phosphate dehydrogenase 1-like	Rare
KCNE3	11q13.4	MiRP2	Unknown
SCN1B	19q13.1	Sodium channel β1 subunit	Unknown
Short QT syndrome (SQTS)			
KCNH2[a]	7q35–36	Kv11.1	Unknown
KCNJ2	17q23	Kir2.1	Unknown
KCNQ1[a]	11p15.5	Kv7.1	Unknown

[a]Genes available as a commercial genetic test

88, 90, 93, 95, 97, 100, 101, 102, 103, and 105). The false-positive potential is estimated to be low but results from genotyping a large cohort of healthy subjects have not been published so far.

Brugada Syndrome

Brugada syndrome (BrS) is another heritable arrhythmia syndrome associated with SCD characterized by an ECG pattern of coved type ST-segment elevation in the right V_1 through V_3 precordial leads and an increased risk for sudden death resulting from episodes of polymorphic ventricular tachyarrhythmias [34]. The penetrance and expressivity are highly variable, ranging from entirely asymptomatic individuals to SCD during the first year of life. Fever represents the most common precipitating factor for arrhythmic cardiac events, including syncope and SCD [35].

Approximately 20–25% of BrS stems from loss-of-function mutations in the *SCN5A*-encoded cardiac sodium channel (NaV1.5, BrS1). In addition to primary mutations of the sodium channel, mutations in genes (*GPD1L* [36] and *SCN1B* [37]) that modulate the sodium channel function have been associated with BrS. Recently, mutations involving the L-type calcium channel α (*CACNA1C*) and β (*CACNB2B*) subunits have been implicated in nearly 10% of BrS cases [38] while mutations in the putative β-subunit of the transient outward potassium channel (Ito, *KCNE3*) have been reported as a rare cause [39]. These are summarized in Table 5.2. To date, only PGxHealth offers genetic testing for only type 1 BrS analyzing all 27 translated exons of *SCN5A*.

Short QT Syndrome

Short QT syndrome (SQTS), a relatively new clinical syndrome first described in 2000, is associated with a short QT interval (<320 ms) on a 12-lead ECG, paroxysmal atrial fibrillation, syncope, and an increased risk for SCD [40]. Cardiac arrest has been the most common initial presentation among 29 patients with SQTS while nearly one-third presented with atrial fibrillation [41]. Symptoms such as syncope or cardiac arrest occurred most often during periods of rest/sleep. To date, gain-of-function mutations in the potassium channel encoding genes *KCNH2*, *KCNQ1*, and *KCNJ2* have been identified as pathogenic substrates for SQTS [42] (Table 5.2).

Indications for Genetic Testing in the Athlete

The "Borderline" Patient

Genetic testing plays a universal, yet variable, role in the diagnosis of SCD-associated cardiomyopathies and channelopathies. While wise clinical judgment remains paramount, genetic testing can offer evidence to support (move towards) or refute (move away from) a contemplated cardiomyopathic/channelopathic diagnosis which can be particularly important in questionable cases. For example, while a negative genetic test is not sufficient to "rule out" either HCM or LQTS all by its own, genetic testing might help distinguish borderline pathologic HCM from extreme physiologic hypertrophy/athlete heart (both between 13 and 15 mm septal thickness, Fig. 5.1a). Indeed, a positive *MYH7* or *MYBPC* genetic test in an athletic adolescent with borderline left ventricular hypertrophy would confirm the diagnosis of HCM while a negative test might provide an independent, objective data point to move away from this consideration especially if the sole determinant for considering HCM in the first place was a borderline wall thickness measurement. Further, genetic testing may play a key role in distinguishing HCM from treatable, metabolic diseases such as Fabry's disease. Correct diagnosis of these diseases would guide the use of definitive and alternative therapies, such as recombinant enzyme-replacement therapy in Fabry's disease.

Similar to "borderline hypertrophy," genetic testing may assist in the evaluation of the athlete who has been disqualified solely because of "borderline QT prolongation" (Fig. 5.1b). Recently, we demonstrated that 40% of unrelated patients coming to Mayo Clinic with the diagnosis of LQTS have left without the diagnosis, the vast majority being reclassified as otherwise normal with only neurocardiogenic presyncope/syncope [43]. Among this subset of diagnostic reversals, no LQTS-causative mutations have been identified so far providing an independent, objective piece of evidence falling more in line with our clinical judgment than the patient's originally rendered diagnosis.

"Gold Standard" Diagnostic Marker for the Asymptomatic Athlete Who Is Part of a Family with a Sudden Death Predisposing Heart Condition

One of the most important roles for genetic testing is potential identification of an at-risk, disease-conferring genetic biomarker in the index case which can be used as the diagnostic gold standard in the clinical evaluation of his/her offspring, siblings, parents, as well as more distant relatives. This is especially crucial in SCD-associated cardiomyopathies/channelopathies in which SCD can be the sentinel event. A positive genetic test would enable systematic scrutiny of the index case's athletic and nonathletic relatives to identify genetically affected individuals. In this way, the genetic testing of an HCM index case, for example, permits separation of family members into two management groups: (1) close surveillance of the genotype-positive, preclinical individual and (2) casual observation or dismissal of the genotype-negative/phenotype-negative relative (like case vignette no. 1) and his/her future progeny.

Finally, the results of familial genetic testing should be communicated to the affected individuals in the context of appropriate genetic counseling by either genetic counselors, cardiovascular geneticists, or genetic/molecular cardiologists. It is critical that the effect(s) of the genetic test on lifestyle, physical activities, insurance, and family planning be considered in the context of each individual. Thus, while genetic testing may play an important role in the evaluation of the athlete being investigated for a possible SCD-predisposing cardiomyopathy/channelopathy, the wise use and even wiser interpretation of such genetic testing is of paramount importance.

Glossary

Dideoxy DNA sequencing: To directly determine a DNA sequence, a primer binds to the region of interest on the sample DNA and initiates polymerization of DNA which is terminated in small amounts after each nucleotide addition. Each resulting oligonucleotide is labeled with a fluorescent tag identifying the sequence of the final nucleotide. The collection of fluorescent products is separated based on size, where the smallest fragment represents the first sequenced nucleotide, and the sequence is determined by the order of the nucleotide-specific fluorescent signals. Generally, this can yield a DNA sequence up to 800 nucleotides per reaction.

Exon — DNA sequence of a gene that is present in the mature mRNA after splicing removal of introns. Generally, the exonic DNA sequence ultimately codes for the corresponding amino acid sequence of the protein. There is exonic sequence at the termini of the mature mRNA of variable lengths which do not code for protein in this manner and remain untranslated (5′ and 3′ untranslated regions).

Gene — The basic hereditary unit of life which, in humans, is composed of a DNA sequence traditionally containing "coding" exonic sequence that is ultimately *transcribed* into mRNA and *translated* into protein as well as intervening "noncoding" intronic sequences which are removed during transcription and do not code for protein.

Genome — The hereditary information of an organism encoded by nucleic acid including all chromosomes. In humans, there are two complete homologous sets of DNA – one paternal and one maternal – and are thus considered diploid genomes.

Germline — The cells within an organism that pass genetic information to progeny. In humans, this refers to sperm and egg cells specifically.

Intron — A gene's DNA sequence that is removed during splicing of the mature mRNA and does not ultimately code for protein during translation.

Mutation — Changes in the DNA sequence of an organism. In humans, mutations can generally be described as synonymous (does not ultimately alter the coding protein sequence) or nonsynonymous (does ultimately alter the original coding sequence). Nonsynonymous mutations include missense (altering a single amino acid), nonsense (changes an amino acid to a stop codon which truncates the protein), and insertion/deletion (addition or subtraction of DNA which often shifts the open reading frame of the gene resulting in an altered, "frameshifted," protein sequence after that point and usually an early truncation of the protein). For the hypertrophic cardiomyopathy-associated missense mutation, TNNT2-R92W, for example, the DNA mutation has changed an arginine amino acid (R) to a tryptophan (W) at position 92 of the protein troponin T which is encoded by *TNNT2*.

Next-generation DNA sequencing	A conglomeration of recently developed DNA sequencing methodologies capable of sequencing over 20×10^9 nucleotides per reaction depending on the platform [1].
Oligonucleotide hybridization mutation detection	Sample (patient) DNA is fluorescently labeled and exposed to a microarray chip containing thousands of short sequences of DNA (oligonucleotides) corresponding to mutated sequences of the genes of interest. If a mutation is present in the patient, it will bind (hybridize) to the known oligonucleotide on the chip and deliver an identifiable fluorescent signal.

References

1. Morozova O, Marra MA. 2008. Applications of next-generation sequencing technologies in functional genomics. *Genomics*. 92(5):255–264.
2. Maron BJ, Gohman TE, Aeppli D. 1998. Prevalence of sudden cardiac death during competitive sports activities in Minnesota High School athletes. *J Am Coll Cardiol*. 32(7):1881–1884.
3. Corrado D, Basso C, Schiavon M, Thiene G. 2006. Does sports activity enhance the risk of sudden cardiac death? *J Cardiovasc Med*. 7(4):228–233.
4. Puranik R, Chow CK, Duflou JA, Kilborn MJ, McGuire MA. 2005. Sudden death in the young. *Heart Rhythm*. 2(12):1277–1282.
5. Ellsworth EG, Ackerman MJ. 2005. The changing face of sudden cardiac death in the young. *Heart Rhythm*. 2(12):1283–1285.
6. Tester DJ, Ackerman MJ. 2007. Postmortem long QT syndrome genetic testing for sudden unexplained death in the young. *J Am Coll Cardiol*. 49(2):240–246.
7. Tester DJ, Ackerman MJ. 2006. The role of molecular autopsy in unexplained sudden cardiac death. *Curr Opin Cardiol*. 21(3):166–172.
8. Maron BJ. 2003. Sudden death in young athletes. *N Engl J Med*. 349(11):1064–1075.
9. Jarcho JA, McKenna W, Pare JA, Solomon SD, Holcombe RF, Dickie S, Levi T, Donis-Keller H, Seidman JG, Seidman CE. 1989. Mapping a gene for familial hypertrophic cardiomyopathy to chromosome 14q1. *N Engl J Med*. 321(20):1372–1378.
10. Geisterfer-Lowrance AA, Kass S, Tanigawa G, Vosberg H, McKenna W, Seidman CE, Seidman JG. 1990. A molecular basis for familial hypertrophic cardiomyopathy: A beta cardiac myosin heavy chain gene missense mutation. *Cell*. 62:999–1006.
11. Marian AJ, Roberts R. 2001. The molecular genetic basis for hypertrophic cardiomyopathy. *J Mol Cell Cardiol*. 33:655–670.
12. Van Driest SL, Ommen SR, Tajik AJ, Gersh BJ, Ackerman MJ. 2005. Yield of genetic testing in hypertrophic cardiomyopathy. *Mayo Clin Proc*. 80(6):739–744.
13. Binder J, Ommen SR, Gersh BJ, Van Driest SL, Tajik AJ, Nishimura RA, Ackerman MJ. 2006. Echocardiography-guided genetic testing in hypertrophic cardiomyopathy: septal morphological features predict the presence of myofilament mutations. *Mayo Clin Proc*. 81(4):459–467.

14. Sen-Chowdhry S, Syrris P, McKenna WJ. 2007. Role of genetic analysis in the management of patients with arrhythmogenic right ventricular dysplasia/cardiomyopathy. *J Am Coll Cardiol*. 50(19):1813–1821.
15. Thiene G, Corrado D, Basso C. 2007. Arrhythmogenic right ventricular cardiomyopathy/dysplasia. *Orphanet J Rare Dis*. 2:45.
16. Dalal D, Molin LH, Piccini J, Tichnell C, James C, Bomma C, Prakasa K, Towbin JA, Marcus FI, Spevak PJ, Bluemke DA, Abraham T, Russell SD, Calkins H, Judge DP. 2006. Clinical features of arrhythmogenic right ventricular dysplasia/cardiomyopathy associated with mutations in plakophilin-2. *Circulation*. 113(13):1641–1649.
17. van Tintelen JP, Entius MM, Bhuiyan ZA, Jongbloed R, Wiesfeld ACP, Wilde AAM, van der Smagt J, Boven LG, Mannens MMAM, van Langen IM, Hofstra RMW, Otterspoor LC, Doevendans PAFM, Rodriguez L-M, van Gelder IC, Hauer RNW. 2006. Plakophilin-2 mutations are the major determinant of familial arrhythmogenic right ventricular dysplasia/cardiomyopathy. *Circulation*. 113(13):1650–1658.
18. Pilichou K, Nava A, Basso C, Beffagna G, Bauce B, Lorenzon A, Frigo G, Vettori A, Valente M, Towbin J, Thiene G, Danieli GA, Rampazzo A. 2006. Mutations in desmoglein-2 gene are associated with arrhythmogenic right ventricular cardiomyopathy. *Circulation*. 113(9):1171–1179.
19. Zipes DP, Ackerman MJ, Estes Iii NAM, Grant AO, Myerburg RJ, Van Hare G. 2005. Task Force 7: Arrhythmias. *J Am Coll Cardiol*. 45(8):1354–1363.
20. Tester DJ, Ackerman MJ. 2007. Postmortem long QT syndrome genetic testing for sudden unexplained death in the young. *J Am Coll Cardiol*. 49(2):240–246.
21. Tester DJ, Will ML, Haglund CM, Ackerman MJ. 2005. Compendium of cardiac channel mutations in 541 consecutive unrelated patients referred for long QT syndrome genetic testing. *Heart Rhythm*. 2:507–517.
22. Tester DJ, Will ML, Haglund CM, Ackerman MJ. 2006. Effect of clinical phenotype on yield of long QT syndrome genetic testing. *J Am Coll Cardiol*. 47(4):764–768.
23. Ackerman M, Tester D, Jones G, Will M, Burrow C, Curran M. 2003. Ethnic differences in cardiac potassium channel variants: implications for genetic susceptibility to sudden cardiac death and genetic testing for congenital long QT syndrome. *Mayo Clin Proc*. 78(12):1479–1487.
24. Ackerman MJ, Splawski I, Makielski JC, Tester DJ, Will ML, Timothy KW, Keating MT, Jones G, Chadha M, Burrow CR, Stephens JC, Xu C, Judson R, Curran ME. 2004. Spectrum and prevalence of cardiac sodium channel variants among black, white, Asian, and Hispanic individuals: Implications for arrhythmogenic susceptibility and Brugada/long QT syndrome genetic testing. *Heart Rhythm*. 1(5):600–607.
25. Ackerman MJ, Tester DJ, Porter CJ. 1999. Swimming, a gene-specific arrhythmogenic trigger for inherited long QT syndrome. *Mayo Clin Proc*. 74(11):1088–1094.
26. Wilde AA, Jongbloed RJ, Doevendans PA, Duren DR, Hauer RN, van Langen IM, van Tintelen JP, Smeets HJ, Meyer H, Geelen JL. 1999. Auditory stimuli as a trigger for arrhythmic events differentiate HERG- related (LQTS2) patients from KVLQT1-related patients (LQTS1). *J Am Coll Cardiol*. 33(2):327–332.
27. Moss AJ, Robinson JL, Gessman L, Gillespie R, Zareba W, Schwartz PJ, Vincent GM, Benhorin J, Heilbron EL, Towbin JA, Priori SG, Napolitano C, Zhang L, Medina A, Andrews ML, Timothy K. 1999. Comparison of clinical and genetic variables of cardiac events associated with loud noise versus swimming among subjects with the long QT syndrome. *Am J Cardiol*. 84(8):876–879.
28. Schwartz PJ, Priori SG, Spazzolini C, Moss AJ, Vincent GM, Napolitano C, et al. 2001. Genotype-phenotype correlation in the long-QT syndrome: gene-specific triggers for life-threatening arrhythmias. *Circulation*. 103:89–95.
29. Khositseth A, Tester DJ, Will ML, Bell CM, Ackerman MJ. 2004. Identification of a common genetic substrate underlying postpartum cardiac events in congenital long QT syndrome. *Heart Rhythm*. 1:60–64.
30. Khositseth A, Ackerman MJ. Clinical evaluation, risk stratification, and management of congenital long QT syndrome. In: Gussak I, Antzelevitch C, eds. *Contemporary Cardiology: Cardiac Repolarization: Bridging Basic and Clinical Science*. Totowa: Humana; 2003.

31. Priori SG, Napolitano C, Memmi M, Colombi B, Drago F, Gasparini M, DeSimone L, Coltorti F, Bloise R, Keegan R, Cruz Filho FE, Vignati G, Benatar A, DeLogu A. 2002. Clinical and molecular characterization of patients with catecholaminergic polymorphic ventricular tachycardia [see comment]. *Circulation.* 106(1):69–74.
32. Tester DJ, Kopplin LJ, Will ML, Ackerman MJ. 2005. Spectrum and prevalence of cardiac ryanodine receptor (RyR2) mutations in a cohort of unrelated patients referred explicitly for long QT syndrome genetic testing. *Heart Rhythm.* 2(10):1099–1105.
33. Eldar M, Pras E, Lahat H. 2003. A Missense mutation in the CASQ2 gene is associated with autosomal-recessive catecholamine-induced polymorphic ventricular tachycardia. *Trends Cardiovasc Med.* 13:148–151.
34. Chen PS, Priori SG. 2008. The Brugada syndrome. *J Am Coll Cardiol.* 51(12):1176–1180.
35. Probst V, Denjoy I, Meregalli PG, Amirault JC, Sacher F, Mansourati J, Babuty D, Villain E, Victor J, Schott JJ, Lupoglazoff JM, Mabo P, Veltmann C, Jesel L, Chevalier P, Clur SA, Haissaguerre M, Wolpert C, Le Marec H, Wilde AA. 2007. Clinical aspects and prognosis of Brugada syndrome in children. *Circulation.* 115(15):2042–2048.
36. London B, Michalec M, Mehdi H, Zhu X, Kerchner L, Sanyal S, Viswanathan PC, Pfahnl AE, Shang LL, Madhusudanan M, Baty CJ, Lagana S, Aleong R, Gutmann R, Ackerman MJ, McNamara DM, Weiss R, Dudley SC, Jr. 2007. Mutation in glycerol-3-phosphate dehydrogenase 1-like gene (GPD1-L) decreases cardiac Na+ current and causes inherited arrhythmias. *Circulation.* 116(20):2260–2268.
37. Watanabe H, Koopmann T, Le Scouarnec S, Yang T, Ingram C, Schott J, Demolombe S, Probst V, Anselme F, Escande D, Wiesfeld A, Pfeufer A, Kääb S, Wichmann H, Hasdemir C, Aizawa Y, Wilde A, Roden D, Bezzina C. 2008. Sodium channel beta1 subunit mutations associated with Brugada syndrome and cardiac conduction disease in humans. *J Clin Invest.* 118(6):2260–2268.
38. Antzelevitch C, Pollevick GD, Cordeiro JM, Casis O, Sanguinetti MC, Aizawa Y, Guerchicoff A, Pfeiffer R, Oliva A, Wollnik B, Gelber P, Bonaros EP, Jr., Burashnikov E, Wu Y, Sargent JD, Schickel S, Oberheiden R, Bhatia A, Hsu LF, Haissaguerre M, Schimpf R, Borggrefe M, Wolpert C. 2007. Loss-of-function mutations in the cardiac calcium channel underlie a new clinical entity characterized by ST-segment elevation, short QT intervals, and sudden cardiac death. *Circulation.* 115(4):442–449.
39. Delpon E, Cordeiro JM, Nunez L, Bloch Thomsen PE, Guerchicoff A, Pollevick GD, Wu Y, Kanters JK, Larsen CT, Burashnikov E, Christiansen M, Antzelevitch C. 2008. Functional effects of KCNE3 mutation and its role in the development of Brugada syndrome. *Circ Arrhythm Electrophysiol.* 1(3):209–218.
40. Gussak I, Brugada P, Brugada J, Wright RS, Kopecky SL, Chaitman BR, Bjerregaard P. 2000. Idiopathic short QT interval: a new clinical syndrome? *Cardiology.* 94(2):99–102.
41. Giustetto C, Di Monte F, Wolpert C, Borggrefe M, Schimpf R, Sbragia P, Leone G, Maury P, Anttonen O, Haissaguerre M, Gaita F. 2006. Short QT syndrome: clinical findings and diagnostic-therapeutic implications. *Eur Heart J.* 27(20):2440–2447.
42. Brugada R, Hong K, Dumaine R, Cordeiro J, Gaita F, Borggrefe M, Menendez TM, Brugada J, Pollevick GD, Wolpert C, Burashnikov E, Matsuo K, Wu YS, Guerchicoff A, Bianchi F, Giustetto C, Schimpf R, Brugada P, Antzelevitch C. 2004. Sudden death associated with short-QT syndrome linked mutations in HERG. *Circulation.* 109:30–35.
43. Taggart NW, Haglund MC, Tester DJ, Ackerman MJ. 2007. Diagnostic miscues in congenital long-QT syndrome. *Circulation.* 115(20):2613–2620.
44. Abernethy WB, III, Choo JK, Hutter AM, Jr. 2003. Echocardiographic characteristics of professional football players. *J Am Coll Cardiol.* 41(2):280–284.

Part II
The Athlete with Signs and Symptoms

Chapter 6
Shortness of Breath

Jonathan P. Parsons

Introduction

Exercise is rarely limited by pulmonary causes in healthy individuals. During exercise, large, steep rises in ventilatory demands are met efficiently by the respiratory system while maintaining a substantial breathing reserve. The respiratory system including the lungs and chest wall are often considered "overbuilt" in meeting the demands of exercise.

However, exercise tolerance and performance can indeed be limited by respiratory symptoms. One of the most common symptoms of individuals experiencing respiratory problems provoked by exercise is shortness of breath or dyspnea which is defined as discomfort associated with breathing. Dyspnea can be difficult to describe by people experiencing it. Often, phrases such as "shortness of breath," "chest tightness," and "can't seem to take a deep, satisfying breath" are used by patients experiencing dyspnea on exertion.

Variations of the case described at the outset of the chapter occur frequently. Complaints of respiratory symptoms during exercise are very common reasons for presentation to both primary care providers and to specialists. The differential diagnosis of shortness of breath in athletes can include several disorders including exercise-induced bronchospasm (EIB), vocal cord dysfunction, gastroesophageal reflux disease (GERD) and others. Proper evaluation of cases similar to the one presented in this chapter require comprehensive history and objective diagnostic testing to accurately make the correct diagnosis.

J.P. Parsons (✉)
OSU Asthma Center, The Ohio State University Medical Center, Columbus, OH, USA
e-mail: Jonathan.Parsons@osumc.edu

C.E. Lawless (ed.), *Sports Cardiology Essentials: Evaluation, Management and Case Studies*, DOI 10.1007/978-0-387-92775-6_6,

Common Causes of Shortness of Breath During Exercise

Case 1

A 16-year-old female high school athlete presents to a medical clinic complaining of breathing problems that occur frequently with exercise. She is on the varsity soccer team and notes that she occasionally has trouble keeping up with the other players during practice and games as a result of shortness of breath, cough, and fatigue. Her coach has been criticizing her frequently for what he construes as "poor effort." Her cough is episodic and is nonproductive. Her shortness of breath seems to occur after several minutes of exercise, and she states that she feels as if she cannot get a "deep breath in." She does not notice symptoms at other times of the day when she is not exercising. Her review of symptoms is otherwise unremarkable.

Her past medical history is only significant for a broken arm 2 years prior to her current presentation. She has no known history of asthma and does not have problems with perennial allergies. She takes nutritional supplements and denies any known drug allergies. She does not smoke, and her family medical history is unremarkable.

On physical exam, she is a healthy, age-appropriate female in no acute distress. The head and neck exam is benign without stridor. Lung exam reveals normal breath sounds without wheezing. Heart exam reveals a regular rhythm with no murmurs, gallops, or rubs. Abdominal exam is benign. The extremities are without cyanosis, clubbing, or edema. The neurologic exam is nonfocal.

Office-based spirometry and chest radiograph are normal. Eucapnic voluntary hyperventilation (EVH) testing is performed which demonstrates a 13% decline in the forced expiratory volume in one second (FEV_1) from baseline. Based on EVH test results, a diagnosis of EIB is made. The patient is instructed to use albuterol prophylactically 15–20 min prior to exercise. She returns 2 months later for follow up and reports that her symptoms are very much improved and her athletic performance has returned to peak levels since she began using her inhaler.

Exercise-Induced Bronchospasm

EIB is acute and reversible airway narrowing that occurs as a result of exercise. EIB can occur during exercise and also happens frequently after an exercise session is completed. The clinical manifestations of EIB are extremely variable and can range from mild impairment of athletic performance to severe bronchospasm and significant respiratory distress. Common symptoms of EIB include cough, wheezing, dyspnea, fatigue, and chest tightness.

EIB occurs commonly in people with and without chronic asthma. In people with a known history of asthma, exercise is one of the most common triggers of bronchospasm and affects 40–90% of asthmatics [1]. In the general population without asthma or atopy, the prevalence of EIB is approximately 10% [2]. The prevalence of EIB is even higher in athletes at both the competitive and elite/Olympic levels, as reported prevalence rates in these groups are as high as 50% [1, 3, 4].

It is important to recognize that the occurrence of bronchospasm during exercise does not mean that a person has chronic asthma. Many people with EIB do not have the typical features of chronic asthma (i.e. frequent daytime symptoms, nocturnal symptoms, or impaired lung function). Exercise may be the only stimulus that causes respiratory symptoms in this population. The important clinical implication of this observation is that the vast majority of people with EIB who do not have chronic asthma can be managed very effectively with prophylactic use of bronchodilators before exercise and rarely require asthma controller medications. In contrast, chronic asthmatics that experience EIB often require maintenance asthma regimens.

The exact cause of EIB is not completely understood, but the two prevailing theories are the thermal theory [5] and the osmotic theory [6]. The upper airway is responsible for warming air as it enters the lungs. During exercise, large volumes of cold air relative to body temperature enter the lungs. If the volume of air is large enough, the capacity of the upper airway to effectively heat the air can be overwhelmed. As the relatively cool air reaches the distal airways, vasoconstriction occurs initially. Subsequently, a reactive hyperemia of the lung vasculature occurs presumably in response to the vasoconstriction which results in increased hydrostatic pressure in the vasculature leading to airway edema and mechanical narrowing of the small airways. The thermal theory may help explain why people with EIB often have more significant symptoms during cold weather.

The osmotic theory hypothesizes that as people inhale large volumes of relatively dry air during exercise, there is water loss from the airway surfaces via evaporation. As a result, changes in the osmolarity of the epithelial cells lining the airways occur. It is postulated that dehydration of epithelial cells triggers the release of inflammatory mediators many of which cause bronchospasm [7, 8].

Several environmental factors may be important factors in the development of EIB. Exposure to chlorine in swimmers [9], chemicals and by-products released during ice-resurfacing in ice rinks [10], and environmental and industrial air pollution [11] have all been linked to increased prevalence rates of EIB.

The presence of EIB has been shown to be difficult to diagnose clinically as symptoms are nonspecific. Common symptoms of EIB include cough, wheezing, dyspnea, fatigue, and chest tightness. However, these symptoms could occur as a result of many medical problems other than EIB. A history of symptoms occurring in specific environments (i.e., ice rinks or swimming pools) may also suggest EIB. More subtle indicators may include poor performance for the level of conditioning in competitive athletes or avoidance of physical activity, which is commonly seen in younger children.

Healthcare providers and coaches also may not consider EIB as a possible explanation for respiratory symptoms occurring during exercise. Athletes are generally fit and healthy and the presence of a significant medical problem often is not considered. The athlete is often considered to be "out of shape" and vague symptoms are not interpreted as a possible manifestation of EIB. Athletes themselves are often "poor perceivers" of EIB and are commonly not aware that they may have a physical problem. Furthermore, if they do recognize that they have a medical problem, they often do not want to admit to health personnel that a problem exists due to fear of social stigma or losing playing time.

The timing of onset and resolution of symptoms is an important issue. Initially during exercise, many times there is a transient period of bronchodilation. Symptoms of EIB usually peak 5–10 min after exercise and can last for 30–60 min [12, 13]. In most patients with EIB, symptoms will resolve even without treatment after about 60 min (Fig. 6.1) [13]. Symptoms that have a more abrupt onset or resolution may suggest alternative diagnoses such as vocal cord dysfunction.

All athletes are potentially susceptible to experiencing EIB. However, specific populations that may be at higher risk for EIB include athletes involved in cold weather sports or sports requiring sustained periods of high ventilatory demand or "high-ventilation sports" (i.e., long-distance running, soccer) [14, 15].

The physical examination at rest in patients with suspected EIB is most often normal and is not predictive of whether the patient has EIB. In those with a previous history of asthma, wheezing, or a prolonged expiratory time may be elicited during the pulmonary examination. Occasionally, abnormal physical findings such as heart murmurs may be found on examination that lead the clinician to specific diagnoses other than EIB, but in most cases the physical examination is not revealing.

Despite the value of a comprehensive history of the patient with symptoms suggestive of EIB, the diagnosis of EIB based on self-reported symptoms alone has been shown to be inaccurate. One study found that screening history identified subjects with symptoms or a previous diagnosis suggestive of EIB in 40% of the participants, but only 13% of these persons actually had objectively documented EIB [16]. Similarly, another study demonstrated 36% of athletes who complained of respiratory symptoms during exercise were found to be EIB-negative after testing [3]. These studies demonstrate that empirically diagnosing and treating

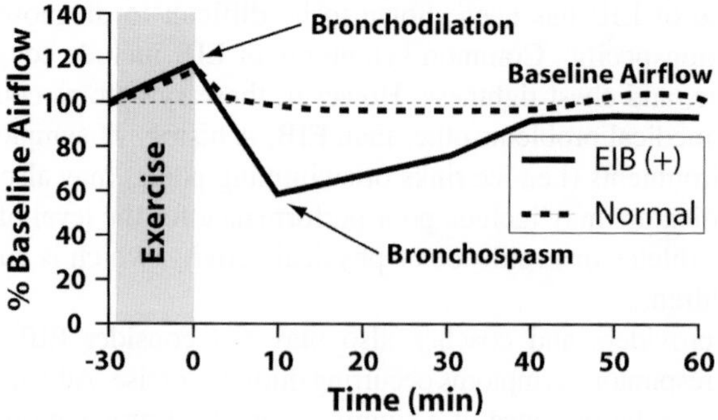

Fig. 6.1 Typical airflow changes in exercise-induced bronchospasm

symptomatic patients without objectively confirming a diagnosis of EIB leads to an inaccurate diagnosis in a significant proportion of cases.

The poor predictive value of the history and physical exam in the evaluation of EIB strongly suggests that clinicians should perform objective diagnostic testing when there is a suspicion of EIB. However, evidence has shown that many healthcare providers do not utilize objective testing when evaluating EIB despite the data that indicate that it is essential [17].

Objective testing should begin with spirometry before and after inhaled bronchodilator therapy, which will help identify athletes who may have chronic asthma at baseline. However, many people who experience EIB will have normal baseline lung function [18]. In these patients, spirometry alone is not adequate to diagnose EIB. Significant numbers of false-negatives may occur if adequate exercise and environmental stress is not provided in the evaluation for EIB. In patients being evaluated for EIB who have a normal physical examination and normal spirometry, bronchoprovocation testing is strongly recommended. A diagnostic algorithm for the initial work up of exercise-induced shortness of breath is shown in Fig. 6.2.

EVH testing is the modality recommended to document EIB in Olympians [19]. EVH involves hyperventilation of a gas mixture of 5% CO_2 and 21% O_2 at 85% of maximum voluntary ventilation (MVV) per minute (calculated as 30 times the baseline FEV_1 which approximates 85% MVV) and assessment of FEV_1 at specified intervals after the test. EVH has a high specificity for EIB [20], and has been shown to be more sensitive in some studies for detecting EIB than methacholine [21] or field or lab-based exercise testing [20, 22]. Alternatives to EVH testing include field- or lab-based exercise challenges. Methacholine challenge is a less preferred method for evaluation of suspected EIB as it is less specific than EVH or exercise. Mannitol inhalation is a recent promising method for diagnosing EIB [23] and may be approved for clinical use in the USA in the future.

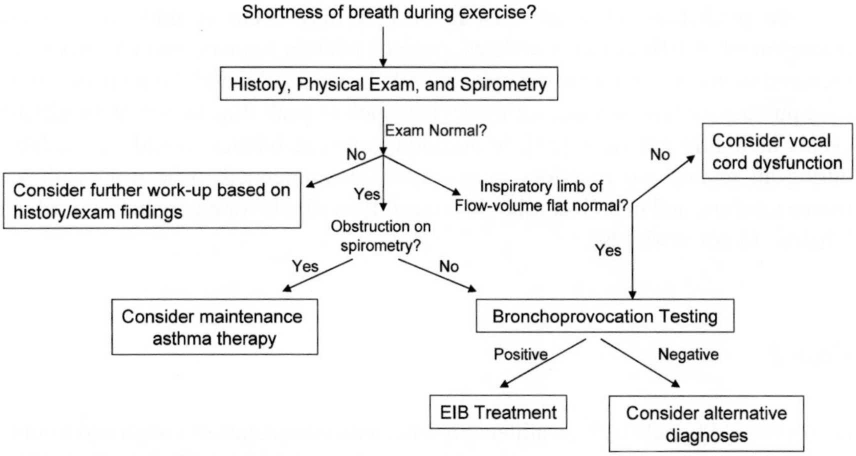

Fig. 6.2 Initial evaluation of exercise-induced shortness of breath

A positive bronchoprovocation test indicates the need for treatment for EIB. Interpretations of bronchoprovocation tests can vary, but a significant change (usually ≥10% decrease in FEV_1) between pre- and post-bronchoprovocation testing values is suggestive of EIB [24].

The most common therapeutic recommendation to minimize or prevent symptoms of EIB is the prophylactic use of short-acting bronchodilators such as albuterol shortly before exercise [25]. Treatment with two puffs of short-acting bronchodilator shortly before exercise (15 min) will provide peak bronchodilation in 15–60 min and protection from EIB for at least 3 h in most patients. Asthma controller medicines including inhaled corticosteroids, leukotriene modifiers, and long-acting bronchodilators have also been shown to be effective in attenuating or preventing EIB, however short-acting bronchodilators alone are effective in 80% of cases [26]. Athletes with chronic asthma should continue with prescribed controller therapy and should premedicate with albuterol prophylactically before exercise. Need for escalation of therapy to control presumed EIB in athletes without chronic asthma should raise questions to the clinician whether EIB is truly the source of the clinical presentation.

Many athletes find that a period of precompetition warm up reduces the symptoms of EIB that occur during their competitive activity. It has been shown by investigators that this phenomenon of the "refractory period" does occur in some athletes with asthma and that athletes can be refractory to an exercise task performed within 2 h of an exercise warm up [26].

There are other nonpharmacologic strategies that can be employed to help reduce the frequency and severity of symptoms of EIB. Breathing through the nose rather than the mouth and/or wearing a face-mask may also help prevent EIB by warming, filtering, and humidifying the air, when outdoor conditions are cold and dry and is especially valuable to elite and recreational athletes that exercise in the winter [27, 28]. In addition, people with knowledge of triggers (i.e., freshly cut grass) should attempt to avoid them if possible.

Since predicting when an episode of EIB may occur is impossible, acute management of EIB requires athletes, parents, athletic trainers, and coaches to be prepared to intervene if an acute episode of EIB occurs. All athletic trainers should have pulmonary function measuring devices such as peak flow meters at all athletic events including practices [29]. In addition, a rescue inhaler should be available during all games and practices. Spacers are recommended to be used with the rescue inhalers, and nebulizers should be readily available for emergencies in which inhalers do not work [29].

Case 2

A 20-year-old female college athlete presents with complaints of cough and trouble breathing that occurs with exercise. She is on the varsity basketball team and has had several episodes of acute onset of cough that occur both during games and practices. She has tried inhalers prophylactically without relief of symptoms. The coughing episodes often last 3–5 min and are associated with shortness of breath and tightness in her upper chest area. She has been particularly stressed emotionally recently as her final exam period is approaching, and her team has advanced to the semifinals of the conference tournament. Her past medical history is only significant for an appendectomy. She has no known history of asthma and does not have problems with perennial allergies. She takes no prescription medicine. She is a freshman in college and does not smoke. Her family medical history is unremarkable.

On physical exam, she is a healthy, age-appropriate female in no acute distress. The head and neck exam is benign without stridor. Lung exam reveals normal breath sounds without wheezing. Heart exam reveals a regular rhythm with no murmurs, gallops, or rubs. Abdominal exam is benign. The extremities are without cyanosis, clubbing, or edema. The neurologic exam is nonfocal.

Spirometry reveals no evidence of obstruction, but does show marked flattening of the inspiratory limb of her flow-volume loop, suggesting variable, extrathoracic airway obstruction and possibly vocal cord dysfunction (Fig. 6.3). Videolaryngostroboscopy testing subsequently confirms paradoxical vocal cord dysfunction. She undergoes several sessions of laryngeal control therapy with a certified speech pathologist. She returns to clinic after speech therapy reporting that her symptoms occur much less frequently, and when they do occur she is able to abort them effectively.

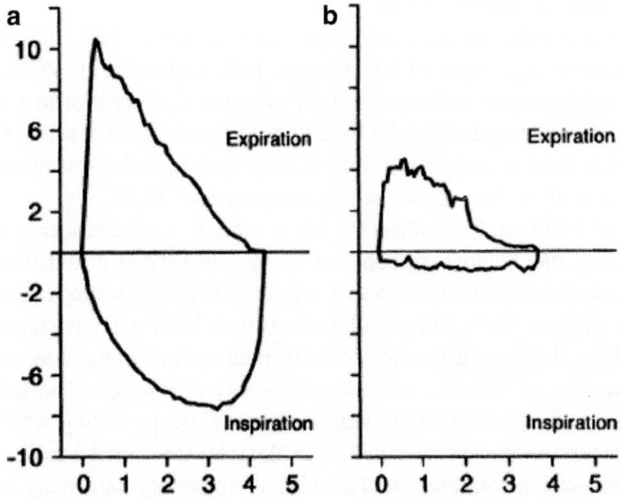

Fig. 6.3 Flow-volume loops showing a normal flow-volume loop (*left*) and variable extrathoracic airway obstruction which can be suggestive of vocal cord dysfunction (*right*)

Vocal Cord Dysfunction

Vocal cord dysfunction is upper airway obstruction caused by the paradoxical adduction or closure of the vocal cords. The abrupt, abnormal closure of the cords occurs predominately on inhalation. The clinical presentation of VCD is very similar to EIB and can range from mild dyspnea to acute, severe respiratory distress. Patients complain of sudden onset of difficulty breathing, usually on inhalation, tightness localized to the throat or neck, cough, and stridor. One of the most common triggers for episodes of VCD is exercise.

The epidemiology of VCD in athletes has not been well established. Rundell and Spiering [30] studied 370 elite athletes and found that 5% had inspiratory stridor suggestive of vocal-cord dysfunction. Interestingly, 53% of the athletes with vocal-cord dysfunction had EIB as well, indicating that vocal-cord dysfunction and EIB often occur concomitantly.

The etiology of VCD is largely unknown. Several theories have been proposed including upper airway hyperresponsiveness to stimuli such as GERD and/or postnasal drip. Other theories include autonomic dysfunction of the larynx or a primary psychiatric conversion disorder. However, the belief that psychologic dysfunction is an underlying feature of all VCD is not supported by the literature, which fails to document a greater incidence of psychologic dysfunction in patients with VCD than in the general population [31].

Because EIB and VCD have similar clinical presentations, VCD is very commonly mistaken for EIB. The literature has many case reports of VCD masquerading as uncontrolled asthma [32, 33]. Patients with VCD are frequently misdiagnosed as having EIB and do not respond to pharmacologic treatment for asthma. As a result, they are exposed to unnecessary medications and continue to be symptomatic despite treatment for presumed EIB.

Despite their similar presentations, there can be subtle clues elicited from the history that can be suggestive of VCD versus EIB. Patients with VCD commonly have a very sudden onset and resolution of symptoms in contrast to patients with EIB whose symptoms typically take time to both develop and resolve. Complaints of hoarse voice, stridor, inability to take a deep breath, and a sensation of persistently needing to clear their throat can be suggestive of VCD.

Diagnosis of VCD can be challenging. Many times it is not considered initially and is considered only after failure to respond to therapy aimed at presumed EIB occurs. This again emphasizes the critical importance of objective, diagnostic testing in the evaluation of dyspnea in athletes. Many, but not all, patients with VCD will have normal spirometry, but will have abnormal truncation of the inspiratory limb of the flow-volume loop, which is suggestive of variable, extrathoracic airway obstruction. The gold standard diagnostic test to document VCD is videolaryngostoboscopy testing which involves direct visualization of the vocal cords with flexible, transnasal laryngoscope after appropriate provocation with exercise. Paradoxical, inspiratory narrowing of the vocal cords during acute attacks is the most frequent finding (Fig. 6.4) [31].

Treatment of VCD in the acute setting includes reassurance and relaxation, removal from the offending agent, and in severe cases heliox (mixture of oxygen

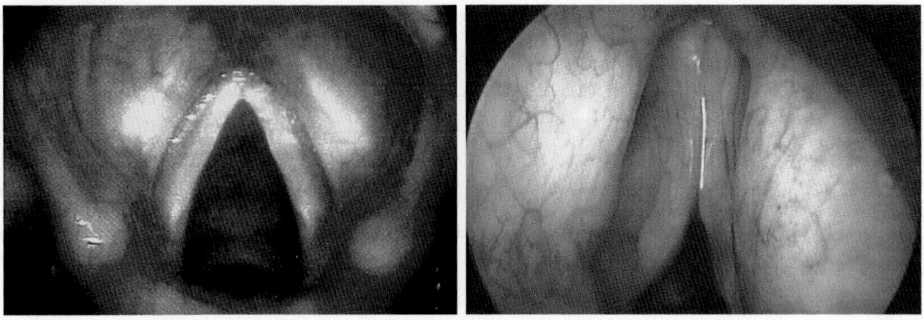

Fig. 6.4 Photograph of normal vocal cords (*left*) and during episode of vocal cord dysfunction (*right*)

and helium) and/or sedation. Heliox is less denser than air in our atmosphere, thus airway resistance is relatively reduced when inspiring heliox which facilitates movement of oxygen past areas of predominately upper airway obstruction. Many, if not most, attacks can be managed with reassurance alone. The primary component to the long-term management of VCD is speech therapy. Speech therapists provide respiratory techniques to abort attacks of VCD, patient education, and desensitization to specific irritants which can be extremely effective. Such therapy allows many athletes with VCD to exercise largely symptom free.

Gastroesophageal Reflux Disease

GERD is very common in the general population. Approximately 25–35% of the US population experiences GERD during their lifetime [34]. There is evidence that physical activity induces episodes of gastroesophageal reflux [35]. Mechanisms that may predispose to GERD during exercise include decreased gastrointestinal blood flow, alterations of hormone secretion, changes in the motor function of the esophagus and the stomach, and increased abdominal pressure with concomitant decrease in intrathoracic pressure [36]. Uncontrolled GERD can also lead to upper airway edema that can present in a similar fashion to vocal cord dysfunction. In one study, 19 of 22 patients with VCD had evidence of uncontrolled GERD leading to laryngeal edema [37]. Treatment of GERD includes appropriate timing of meals to avoid physical activity soon after eating and often requires pharmacologic therapy, typically with proton-pump inhibitors.

Less Common Causes of Dyspnea During Exercise

There are many other conditions that can cause shortness of breath but are much less common. Cardiac conditions such as cardiomyopathy, arrhythmia, and valvular heart disease can cause shortness of breath during exercise. Athletes with palpitations, dizziness, syncope, or significant exertional chest pain or those with significant cardiac findings on physical examination (i.e., murmurs) require evaluation for potential cardiac sources of their symptoms. Pneumothorax, pleural effusion, and chronic lung diseases such as interstitial lung disease or chronic obstructive pulmonary disease are conditions that certainly can cause shortness of breath, but would rarely be found in populations of competitive athletes. Congenital anomalies such as tracheomalacia, laryngomalacia, and vascular rings can also cause dyspnea during exercise; however these are very commonly observed in early childhood.

Exercise-induced urticaria/anaphylaxis is another rare condition that can lead to dyspnea. Patients with exercise-induced urticaria, complain of exercise-induced cutaneous warmth, pruritis, and erythema. If symptoms progress to dyspnea, wheezing, dizziness, or syncope, then the diagnosis becomes exercise-induced anaphylaxis. The mechanism of exercise-induced urticaria/anaphylaxis appears to be mast-cell mediated to a significant degree as increased levels of histamine, tryptase, and leukotrienes are demonstrated [38].

Conclusion

Despite the brilliant efficiency with which the respiratory system functions, there are a multitude of medical conditions that can lead to shortness of breath. Physicians, coaches, parents, and athletic trainers must have a high index of suspicion when healthy athletes complain of difficulty in breathing during exercise. While EIB and vocal cord dysfunction are two common diagnoses in athletes that present with shortness of breath, it is imperative that a comprehensive history is obtained and confirmatory diagnostic testing is performed when these diagnoses are suspected. The consequences of misdiagnosis or failure to diagnose entirely can result in impairment of performance and can be detrimental to health.

References

1. Rundell KW, Jenkinson DM. Exercise-induced bronchospasm in the elite athlete. Sports Med 2002; 32:583–600
2. Gotshall RW. Exercise-induced bronchoconstriction. Drugs 2002; 62:1725–1739
3. Parsons JP, Kaeding C, Phillips G, et al. Prevalence of exercise-induced bronchospasm in a cohort of varsity college athletes. Med Sci Sports Exerc 2007; 39:1487–1492
4. Parsons JP, Mastronarde JG. Exercise-induced bronchoconstriction in athletes. Chest 2005; 128:3966–3974
5. McFadden ER, Jr., Lenner KA, Strohl KP. Postexertional airway rewarming and thermally induced asthma. New insights into pathophysiology and possible pathogenesis. J Clin Invest 1986; 78:18–25
6. Anderson SD, Daviskas E. The mechanism of exercise-induced asthma is. J Allergy Clin Immunol 2000; 106:453–459

7. Finnerty JP, Holgate ST. Evidence for the roles of histamine and prostaglandins as mediators in exercise-induced asthma: the inhibitory effect of terfenadine and flurbiprofen alone and in combination. Eur Respir J 1990; 3:540–547
8. Hallstrand TS, Moody MW, Wurfel MM, et al. Inflammatory basis of exercise-induced bronchoconstriction. Am J Respir Crit Care Med 2005; 172:679–686
9. Helenius I, Haahtela T. Allergy and asthma in elite summer sport athletes. J Allergy Clin Immunol 2000; 106:444–452
10. Brauer M, Spengler JD. Nitrogen dioxide exposures inside ice skating rinks. Am J Public Health 1994; 84:429–433
11. Peden DB. Air pollutants, exercise, and risk of developing asthma in children. Clin J Sport Med 2003; 13:62–63
12. Brudno DS, Wagner JM, Rupp NT. Length of postexercise assessment in the determination of exercise-induced bronchospasm. Ann Allergy 1994; 73:227–231
13. Godfrey S. Clinical variables of exercise-induced bronchospasm. In: Dempsey J, ed. Muscular exercise and the lung. Madison: The University of Wisconsin Press, 1977; 247–288
14. Holzer K, Brukner P. Screening of athletes for exercise-induced bronchoconstriction. Clin J Sport Med 2004; 14:134–138
15. Wilber RL, Rundell KW, Szmedra L, et al. Incidence of exercise-induced bronchospasm in Olympic winter sport athletes. Med Sci Sports Exerc 2000; 32:732–737
16. Hallstrand TS, Curtis JR, Koepsell TD, et al. Effectiveness of screening examinations to detect unrecognized exercise-induced bronchoconstriction. J Pediatr 2002; 141:343–348
17. Parsons JP, O'Brien JM, Lucarelli MR, et al. Differences in the evaluation and management of exercise-induced bronchospasm between family physicians and pulmonologists. J Asthma 2006; 43:379–384
18. Rundell KW, Wilber RL, Szmedra L, et al. Exercise-induced asthma screening of elite athletes: field versus laboratory exercise challenge. Med Sci Sports Exerc 2000; 32:309–316
19. Anderson SD, Fitch K, Perry CP, et al. Responses to bronchial challenge submitted for approval to use inhaled beta2-agonists before an event at the 2002 Winter Olympics. J Allergy Clin Immunol 2003; 111:45–50
20. Eliasson AH, Phillips YY, Rajagopal KR, et al. Sensitivity and specificity of bronchial provocation testing. An evaluation of four techniques in exercise-induced bronchospasm. Chest 1992; 102:347–355
21. Holzer K, Anderson SD, Douglass J. Exercise in elite summer athletes: Challenges for diagnosis. J Allergy Clin Immunol 2002; 110:374–380
22. Rundell KW, Anderson SD, Spiering BA, et al. Field exercise vs laboratory eucapnic voluntary hyperventilation to identify airway hyperresponsiveness in elite cold weather athletes. Chest 2004; 125:909–915
23. Holzer K, Anderson SD, Chan HK, et al. Mannitol as a challenge test to identify exercise-induced bronchoconstriction in elite athletes. Am J Respir Crit Care Med 2003; 167:534–537
24. Anderson SD, Argyros GJ, Magnussen H, et al. Provocation by eucapnic voluntary hyperpnoea to identify exercise induced bronchoconstriction. Br J Sports Med 2001; 35:344–347
25. National Heart Lung and Blood Institute Expert Panel Report 3. Guidelines for the diagnosis and management of asthma. Bethesda, 2007
26. McKenzie DC, McLuckie SL, Stirling DR. The protective effects of continuous and interval exercise in athletes with exercise-induced asthma. Med Sci Sports Exerc 1994; 26:951–956
27. Shturman-Ellstein RZR, Buckley JM, Souhrada JF. The beneficial effect of nasal breathing on exercise-induced bronchoconstriction. Am Rev Respir Dis 1978; 118:65–73
28. Schacter E. The protective effects of a cold weather mask on EIA. Ann Allergy 1982:12–16
29. Miller MG, Weiler JM, Baker R, et al. National athletic trainers' association position statement: management of asthma in athletes. J Athl Train 2005; 40:224–245
30. Rundell KW, Spiering BA. Inspiratory stridor in elite athletes. Chest 2003; 123:468–474
31. Hicks M, Brugman SM, Katial R. Vocal cord dysfunction/paradoxical vocal fold motion. Prim Care 2008; 35:81–103, vii

32. McFadden ER, Jr., Zawadski DK. Vocal cord dysfunction masquerading as exercise-induced asthma. a physiologic cause for "choking" during athletic activities. Am J Respir Crit Care Med 1996; 153:942–947
33. Torrego Fernandez A, Santos Perez S, Brea Folco J, et al. Dysfunction of the vocal cords simulating exercise-induced asthma. Arch Bronconeumol 2000; 36:533–535
34. Eisen GM, Sandler RS, Murray S, et al. The relationship between gastroesophageal reflux disease and its complications with Barrett's esophagus. Am J Gastroenterol 1997; 92:27–31
35. Pandolfino JE, Bianchi LK, Lee TJ, et al. Esophagogastric junction morphology predicts susceptibility to exercise-induced reflux. Am J Gastroenterol 2004; 99:1430–1436
36. Jozkow P, Wasko-Czopnik D, Medras M, et al. Gastroesophageal reflux disease and physical activity. Sports Med 2006; 36:385–391
37. Powell DM, Karanfilov BI, Beechler KB, et al. Paradoxical vocal cord dysfunction in juveniles. Arch Otolaryngol Head Neck Surg 2000; 126:29–34
38. Truwit J. Pulmonary disorders and exercise. Clin Sports Med 2003; 22:161–180

Chapter 7
Chest Pain in the Athlete: Differential Diagnosis, Evaluation, and Treatment

John M. MacKnight and Dilaawar J. Mistry

Chest pain remains one of the most concerning complaints among athletes and active individuals. Fortunately, the vast majority of chest pain in this group is benign, noncardiac, and rarely associated with catastrophic manifestations such as sudden death [1, 2] A thorough assessment requires a full understanding of the differential of chest pain, a detailed history designed to elicit the nuances of each general category of chest pain, a directed physical examination, and prudent choices of ancillary testing as clinically warranted. This chapter will address the thoughtful evaluation of the symptomatic athlete with chest pain. Its primary focus will be on the differential diagnosis and management of noncardiac causes as the remainder of the text deals with the cardiac etiologies in great depth.

Chest pain is experienced by 25% of the US population [3] and is the chief complaint in 1–2% of outpatient encounters [4] and millions of physician visits in the USA each year [5]. Among athletes, epidemiologic studies vary considerably on etiology of chest pain. The overall incidence of cardiac chest pain in athletes under 35 years of age is less than 5% [6, 7] In this age group, gastroesophageal reflux is the most common cause of chest pain, followed by exercise-induced bronchospasm (see Table 7.1).

In pediatric athletes, idiopathic chest pain is most common, accounting for up to 40% of cases [8–10], while musculoskeletal causes account for at least 20% and panic disorder/hyperventilation account for another 10–20% [11]. As the population ages, cardiac etiologies account for an increasing percentage of chest pain presentations in athletes and active patients.

In the evaluation of chest pain, the care provider must first focus on excluding cardiac and life-threatening noncardiac conditions (see Table 7.2). It is particularly important to assess for cardiac etiologies when the chest pain complaint is associated with syncope or pre-syncope [12]. If this initial evaluation is negative, a broader search for the chest pain etiology should then be undertaken. With increasing age, coronary artery disease, valvular heart disease,

J.M. MacKnight (✉)
Clinical Internal Medicine and Orthopaedic Surgery, University of Virginia Sports Medicine, University of Virginia Health System, Charlottesville, VA, USA
e-mail: JM9M@hscmail.mcc.virginia.edu

C.E. Lawless (ed.), *Sports Cardiology Essentials: Evaluation, Management and Case Studies*, DOI 10.1007/978-0-387-92775-6_7,

Table 7.1 Differential diagnosis of chest pain in athletes

Cardiac/vascular
Hypertrophic cardiomyopathy
Dilated cardiomyopathy
Myocarditis
Aortic stenosis
Anomalous coronary artery
Coronary artery disease
Arrhythmogenic right ventricular dysplasia/cardiomyopathy
Brugada syndrome
Mitral valve prolapse
Atrial and ventricular tachyarrhythmias
Wolff-Parkinson-White syndrome
Congenital long QT syndrome
Aortic dissection
Non-cardiac
Musculoskeletal
Chest wall pain
Traumatic rib fracture
Rib stress fracture
Sternoclavicular sprain/dislocation
"Stitch"
Costochondritis
Tietze's syndrome
Slipping rib syndrome
Precordial catch syndrome
Cervical disk disease, "cervical angina"
Pulmonary
Exercise-induced bronchospasm (EIB)
Pneumothorax
Pulmonary contusion
Pneumomediastinum
Pulmonary embolus
Pneumonia
Pleurisy
Hyperventilation
Gastrointestinal
Gastroesophageal reflux disease (GERD)
Esophageal dysphagia
Psychiatric
Anxiety
Depression
Panic disorder
Somatization
Substance abuse
Stimulants
Psychostimulants
Cocaine
Alcohol

Table 7.2 Chest pain evaluation algorithm

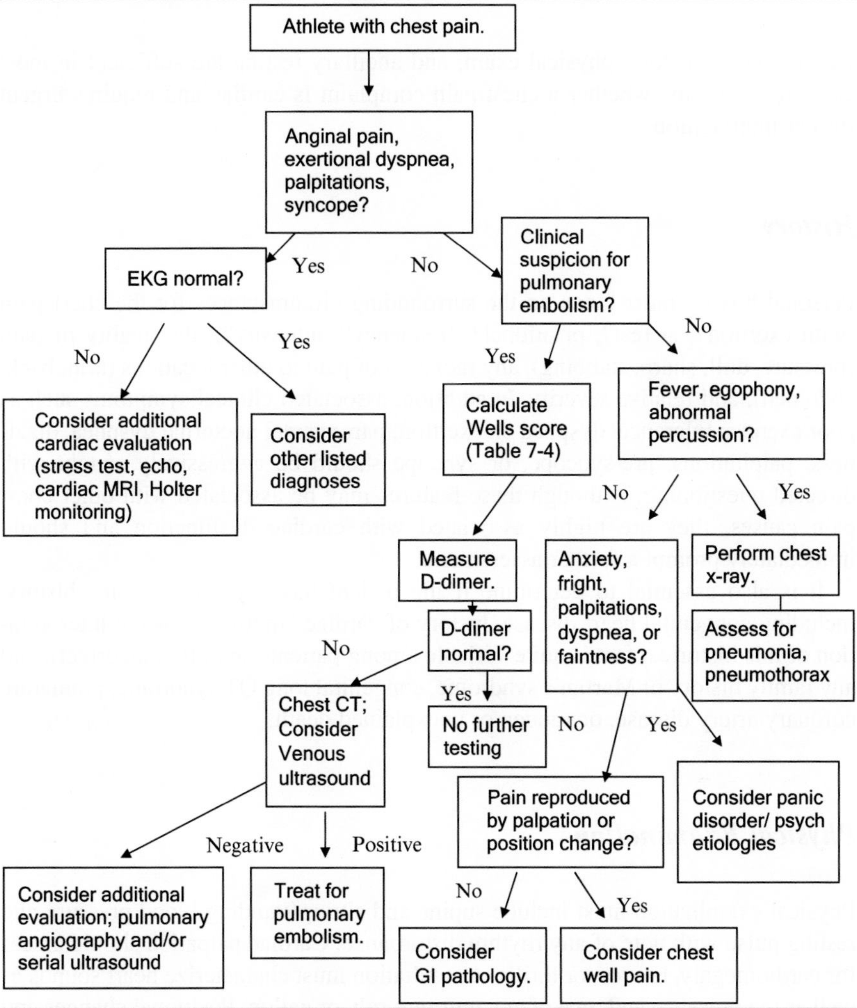

Adapted from Cayley, W., Diagnosing the cause of chest pain. Am Fam Physician, 2005.72.p.2012-21

thromboembolism, and gastrointestinal (GI) disorders become more common and should be actively sought. There is also a large overlap in the possible causes of noncardiac pain, with over one half of patients having two or more GI, respiratory, or psychiatric abnormalities [13]. This highlights the potential difficulty in diagnosing a discrete "cause" in noncardiac chest pain patients [14].

Cardiac Chest Pain

Key pieces of history, physical exam, and ancillary testing are sufficient in most cases to determine whether a chest pain complaint is cardiac and requires urgent further intervention.

History

Personal history must focus on the surrounding circumstances for the chest pain (with exertion?, at rest?, positional?, frequency?, intensity?), the quality of pain (pressure, dull, sharp, stabbing), any radiation of pain to other locations (arm, back, abdomen), and relative severity. In addition, associated clinical symptoms such as poor exercise tolerance, dyspnea on exertion, paroxysmal nocturnal dyspnea, dizziness, palpitations, pre-syncope, or syncope should be aggressively sought with directed questioning. Although these features may be associated with other chest pain causes, they are highly associated with cardiac dysfunction and should immediately prompt a further assessment.

It is also essential to determine if the patient has any prior cardiac history, including congenital heart disease, history of cardiac "murmur" (as the interpretation of this historical fact is quite variable among patients and often incorrect), and any family history of Marfan's syndrome, congenital long QT syndrome, premature coronary artery disease, or sudden or unexplained death.

Physical Examination

Physical examination must include supine and sitting/standing blood pressure and resting pulse with note of any rhythm disturbance. Cardiac palpation should assess for cardiomegaly, heaves, or thrills. Auscultation must characterize heart sounds as well as the presence and type of any murmur, rub, or gallop. Positional changes and the use of the Valsalva maneuver during auscultation are also critical techniques; these are discussed in detail elsewhere in the text. Peripheral pulse quality must also be assessed.

Finally, a resting ECG should be obtained on any athlete with a chest pain complaint. Although the initial history and physical may indicate the likelihood of a noncardiac source, an ECG should nonetheless be obtained to screen for cardiac pathology. The practitioner must consider, however, that the diagnostic accuracy and positive or negative predictive value of an ECG varies considerably for different cardiac conditions. Lawless and Best reported wide variations in ECG sensitivity for cardiac conditions commonly associated with sudden cardiac death ranging from <10 to 100% with virtually uniform poor specificity [15]. Therefore, even a "normal" ECG should be interpreted with caution when trying to exclude a cardiac cause of chest pain.

Based on the outcome of this focused cardiac assessment, additional studies may be undertaken including echocardiography, cardiac MRI, stress testing, and electrophysiologic testing as clinically warranted. Cardiac conditions classically associated with chest pain include hypertrophic cardiomyopathy, idiopathic dilated cardiomyopathy, myocarditis, coronary artery disease, anomalous coronary arteries, arrhythmogenic right ventricular dysplasia/cardiomyopathy, Brugada syndrome, congenital long QT syndrome, aortic stenosis, mitral valve prolapse, and aortic dissection in association with Marfan's syndrome (see below). These conditions are addressed in great detail throughout the remainder of the text.

Aortic Dissection

A special note should be made regarding aortic dissection. This rare but life-threatening cause of chest pain can present in a myriad of ways, making rapid diagnosis a challenge. Dissections may be associated with severe "ripping" chest pain or pain may be migratory involving anterior and posterior chest, neck, jaw, shoulder, upper and lower back, abdomen, or extremities. Patients may demonstrate a widened pulse pressure and new diastolic aortic murmur. Due to involvement of neighboring vascular or neurologic structures, aortic dissections may also cause altered mental status, dysesthesias, weakness, paralysis, or Horner's syndrome. Common associated conditions include congenital bicuspid aortic valve, Marfan's or Ehlers-Danlos syndrome, cocaine abuse [16], and weightlifting [17].

If aortic dissection is a consideration, techniques such as transesophageal echocardiography, CT, MRI, or angiography not only assist with the diagnosis but also help localize the dissection in preparation for emergent surgical repair.

Noncardiac Causes of Chest Pain

Musculoskeletal Etiologies of Chest Pain

Once cardiac chest pain has been reasonably excluded, other more common etiologies need to be explored. Musculoskeletal chest pain again generally accounts for at least 20% of chest pain presentations [18].

Chest Wall Pain

Blunt chest trauma or repetitive loading from activities such as weightlifting or rowing are responsible for most chest wall pain. Pain arises from significant muscle inflammation, muscle strain, spasm, and bone contusions. Most of these injuries are associated with a discrete activity or incident which is elicited by a comprehensive history. Patients typically complain of localized soreness and stiffness which is provoked by activity or positional change. Physical exam will generally reveal focal, palpable tenderness over the injured bone or soft tissue although some chest wall injuries, particularly those associated with overuse, may be difficult to reproduce. Management is symptomatic and conservative.

Traumatic Rib Fracture

The majority of these injuries are associated with direct, blunt chest trauma. Most rib fractures are not clinically significant beyond the acute pain and dysfunction that they create. However, displaced, penetrating injuries may cause pneumothorax, hemothorax, or splenic or liver lacerations. Direct blows to the chest most commonly create fractures at the posterior angle of the fourth through ninth ribs, their inherent weakest point. Fractures to the first and second ribs result from high velocity trauma and may be associated with injury to underlying neurovascular structures. The tenth through 12th ribs are more mobile and less apt to be injured.

Most athletes note a single, traumatic blow to the chest with the acute onset of sharp, stabbing pain locally at the fracture site. Pain is reproduced with deep inspiration, cough, or palpation. Patients demonstrate splinting on the side of injury and are generally unwilling to take a deep breath. Other clinical findings include bony crepitus, ecchymosis, and muscle spasm. Plain radiography has little influence on management as rib fractures are often difficult to distinguish even on rib-detailed X-rays; nonetheless, X-rays should be considered to rule out underlying complications (Fig. 7.1). Concern for organ injury as a result of a penetrating rib injury warrants CT imaging of chest or abdomen. Management of uncomplicated rib fractures is conservative.

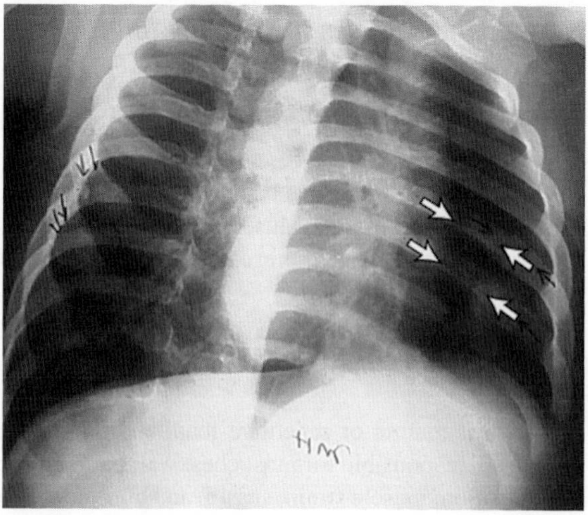

Fig. 7.1 Plain radiograph, displaced rib fracture

Rib Stress Fractures

These injuries result from repetitive stress to the ribs as is seen commonly in rowers, weightlifters, tennis players, beginner/amateur golfers, and throwers [19–26]. Stress fractures most commonly involve the first rib as the repetitive pull of the anterior scalene muscle produces bending forces at the subclavian sulcus, the most common site of fracture [27]. Contributing factors include lack of strength or flexibility, errors in technique, and equipment changes. Stress injuries to lower ribs generally occur at the posterolateral angle, where combined contraction of the serratus anterior and external oblique muscles generate a downward bending force [24].

Fractures of floating ribs are caused by avulsion of the attachments of external oblique muscles [28] due to opposing forces generated by latissimus dorsi and external oblique muscles [29, 30]. Plain radiographs may reveal a stress fracture (Fig. 7.2), but nuclear imaging via bone scan (Fig. 7.3) may be necessary for the diagnosis. Management includes relative rest and technique modification.

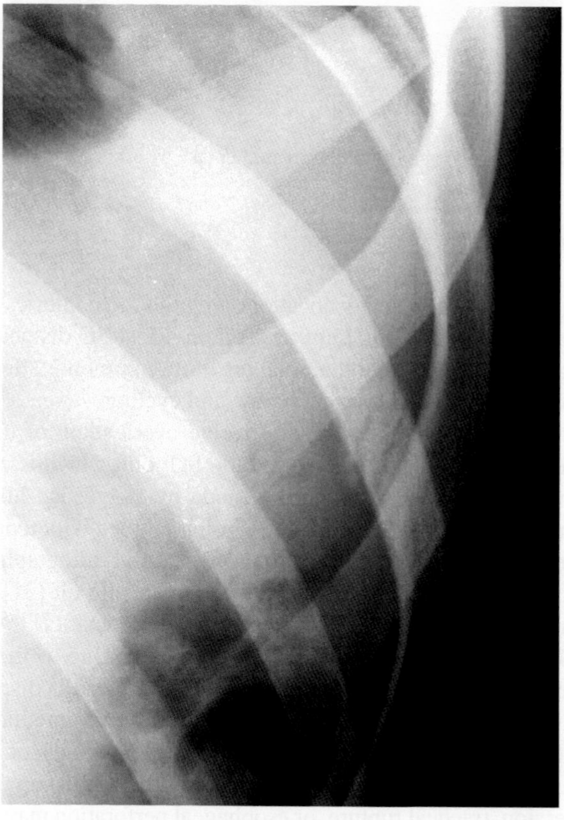

Fig. 7.2 Plain radiograph, callus formation in association with rib stress fracture

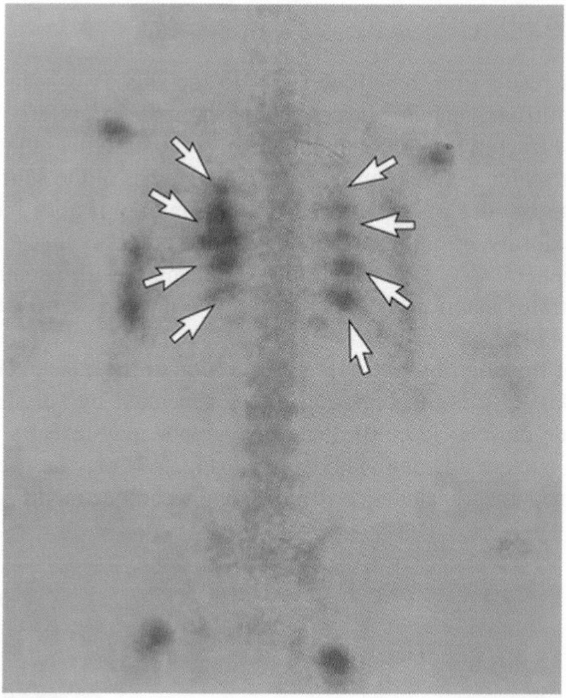

Fig. 7.3 Nuclear bone scan demonstrating increased uptake associated with rib stress fractures

Sternoclavicular Injury

Sternoclavicular (SC) sprains and dislocations are high force injuries resulting from levering or direct force to the SC joint or clavicle. Most SC dislocations occur in patients younger than 25, with football players most commonly affected [30]. The injury is also well described in hockey, rugby, and cycling.

Most SC dislocations are anterior and involve overloading of the anterior SC ligament. Patients complain of focal pain at the SC joint which is exacerbated by arm movement. The diagnosis is typically made by suggestive history of direct blow or levering trauma to the clavicle or SC joint coupled with tenderness, crepitus, and discernible clavicular dislocation on exam. Radiographic assessment includes chest radiography taken with a 40 degree cephalic tilt [31]. Management of uncomplicated anterior SC injuries is generally symptomatic.

Posterior SC dislocations deserve special attention. Due to the potential for compression of mediastinal structures as the clavicular head is displaced posteriorly, these injuries are a medical emergency and require immediate recognition and management. Clinically, these patients may present with dysphagia, dyspnea, venous congestion in the neck, and hoarseness [30]. Mediastinal hemorrhage, venous compression, tracheal rupture, or esophageal perforation may all complicate posterior SC dislocations [32, 33].

Counter-traction reduction maneuvers should be attempted on the field or in the athletic training room in the interest of obtaining the most rapid decompression of posterior soft tissue structures; reduction under general anesthesia may be required. Posterior injuries or SC injuries of unclear extent should undergo CT scanning for definitive identification [34] (Fig. 7.4).

"Stitch"

This common, cramping pain is typically experienced by less-trained individuals during vigorous, extended exercise. Pain is pleuritic and usually located over the lower left chest wall although it can occur on the right. Etiology is controversial but likely results from spasm or strain of musculoskeletal structures supporting the diaphragm. This is a benign, self-limited condition and may be managed via upper torso stretching and enhanced training status.

Costochondritis

A painful disorder of the rib/cartilage junction of the costo-sternal joints, costochondritis arises from overuse/overload of the chest wall during weightlifting or repeated chest compressing motions. The second to fifth costal cartilages [35, 36] are most commonly affected, and symptoms are generally unilateral, exacerbated by breathing, and may radiate to the back and abdomen.

Exam reveals localized costochondral tenderness without notable swelling, heat, or erythema. Pain is exacerbated by arm adduction on the affected side with rotation

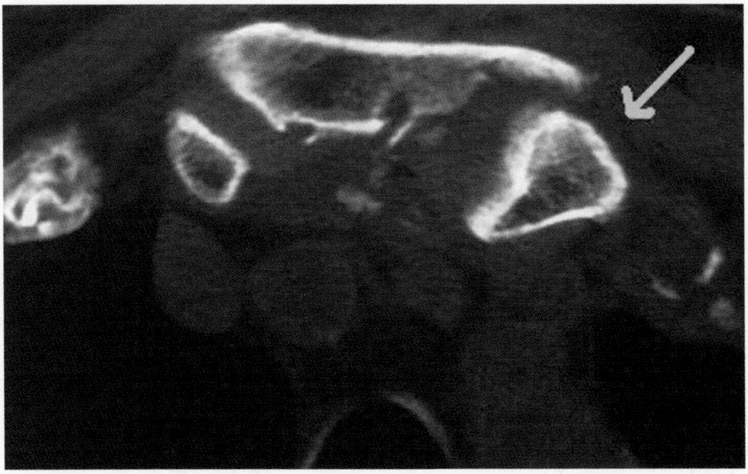

Fig. 7.4 Computed tomography (CT) scan, posterior sternoclavicular dislocation

of the head to the ipsilateral side. Management includes rest, technique modification, local modalities, and nonsteroidal antiinflammatories (NSAIDs).

Tietze's Syndrome

In contrast to costochondritis, Tietze's syndrome is an inflammatory, nontraumatic disorder manifest by painful nonsuppurative swelling of the second and third cartilaginous articulations of the anterior chest wall [35, 37]. Joint swelling distinguishes this condition from costochondritis. The exact etiology is unknown, but the inflammatory nature of the disorder is supported by elevated erythrocyte sedimentation rate and morning stiffness [38]. Management mimics that of costochondritis.

Slipping Rib Syndrome

An unusual chest pain etiology primarily in adolescent runners [39] and swimmers, slipping rib syndrome, results from laxity of the medial fibrous attachments of the lower ribs, allowing the affected cartilage to slip superiorly and impinge on the intercostal nerve above [40]. Pain may be reported in the inferior costal areas of the chest or upper abdomen, and a "slipping" or "popping" sensation may be experienced. Diagnosis is confirmed with the "hooking maneuver," where curved fingers pull the affected rib margin anteriorly to reproduce a popping sensation and/or pain. Management is conservative.

Precordial Catch Syndrome

Also known as "Texidor's twinge," precordial catch is described as a sharp, well-localized pain which occurs episodically at rest but may occur with mild to moderate exercise as well. Typically, pain lasts only seconds to minutes, is exacerbated by deep inspiration, and is often relieved by sitting upright. Etiology is unknown but may arise from the pleura. There is no specific management.

Cervical Disk Disease/"Cervical Angina"

Cervical disk disease can be a cause of referred chest pain [41, 42]. Compression of cervical roots C6 and C7 is the most common source of pain, mediated via medial and lateral pectoral nerves. Pain may be reproduced via cervical manipulation or the Spurling's maneuver with head rotation to the affected side of the chest. Routine MRI examination may be insufficient for the functional assessment of cervical angina; discography and/or selective nerve root infiltration should be considered. Management focuses on decompression of the affected nerve roots via traction and rehabilitative exercise with surgery for refractory cases.

Pulmonary Chest Pain

Asthma/Exercise-Induced Bronchospasm

The most common cause of exercise-related chest pain is exercise-induced bronchospasm (EIB) [43]. High rates of incidence for chest pain in association with EIB have been reported in pediatric patients [44, 45]; almost 75% of healthy children who presented with chest pain were diagnosed with EIB after provocative exercise testing in one study [45].

Airway hyper-reactivity, bronchospasm, and wheezing occur via one or more postulated environmental mechanisms and result in progressive airway narrowing in addition to mucus hypersecretion. Clinical features include burning substernal chest pain, chest tightness, wheezing, dry cough, shortness of breath, and increased sputum production. Patients often complain of difficulty with inspiration and a hyper-expanded, "full" chest because of air-trapping and inefficient exhalation. EIB is commonly associated with endurance activities with symptoms presenting several minutes into exercise or during recovery. EIB is also common in allergic/atopic individuals and amongst those in cold environment sports (figure skating, ice hockey) [46].

As many other conditions may mimic the "wheezing" of asthma (Table 7.3), it is essential to obtain a definitive diagnosis via spirometry [47]. In athletes, provocative testing via methacholine challenge, eucapneic voluntary hyperpnea, mannitol, or hypertonic saline may be required to discern a decline in pulmonary function with exercise.

Management varies from inhaled pre-exercise β2 agonist therapy (albuterol) to long-acting β2 agonist therapy (salmeterol) with or without inhaled corticosteroids (e.g., fluticasone, betamethasone), and oral leukotriene antagonists (e.g., montelukast). See Chapter 6 for detailed discussion of EIB.

Table 7.3 Nonasthmatic conditions which may be associated with a complaint of "wheezing"

Allergic rhinitis
Laryngotracheobronchitis
Foreign body
Vocal cord dysfunction (VCD)
Laryngeal webs, tracheal stenosis, enlarged lymph nodes, tumors
Cystic fibrosis
Tuberculosis
Bronchiectasis
Bronchopulmonary dysplasia
Congestive heart failure
α-1 antitrypsin deficiency
Bronchiolitis obliterans organizing pneumonia (BOOP)
Aspiration
GERD
Laryngeal reflux disease

Pneumothorax

Pneumothoraces arise from a tear in the protective pleural surfaces of the lung. Air entering the chest cavity decreases intrathoracic negative pressure resulting in relative collapse of the lung. Tall, thin athletes are predisposed to spontaneous pneumothoraces, most commonly seen in males aged 20–40 [48]; their primary mechanism is postulated to be rupture of pleural blebs or bullae. Other important associated clinical features include positive family history, smoking, and substance abuse. On the playing field, rib fractures and direct or compressive blows to the chest may all predispose to pneumothorax. Pneumothoraces are one of a small number of potential on-field emergencies, and they should always be considered high in the differential of any athlete presenting with new onset chest pain, even without trauma.

Chest pain affects 80–90% of patients with a pneumothorax, making it the most common clinical feature. In addition, shortness of breath, occasional hacking cough, hypotension, and tachycardia [49] may be observed as well. Physical exam reveals decreased or absent breath sounds in the affected lung field with associated hyperresonance to percussion. Progressive accumulation of air and positive pressure within the chest may create a *tension pneumothorax* which may be life threatening as it shifts mediastinal structures and compromises venous return to the heart. These athletes present as critically ill with cyanosis, tachypnea, and impending circulatory collapse.

Chest X-ray is the initial diagnostic study (Figs. 7.5 and 7.6). If a standard AP chest X-ray fails to demonstrate a pneumothorax in a patient with high clinical

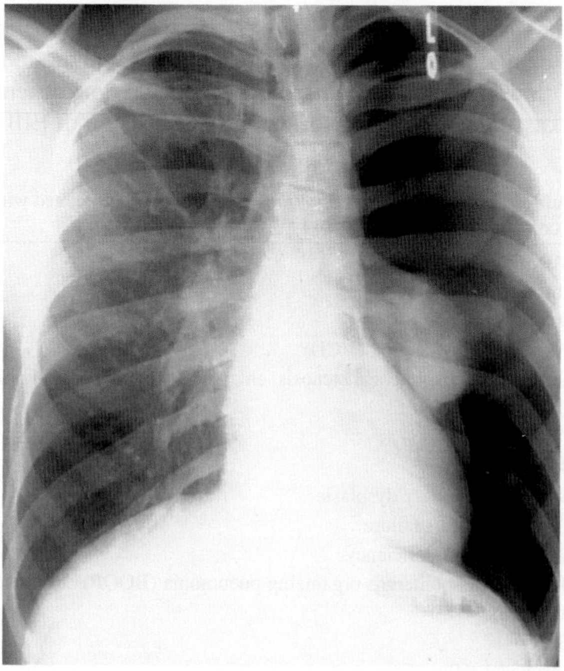

Fig. 7.5 Plain radiograph, pneumothorax

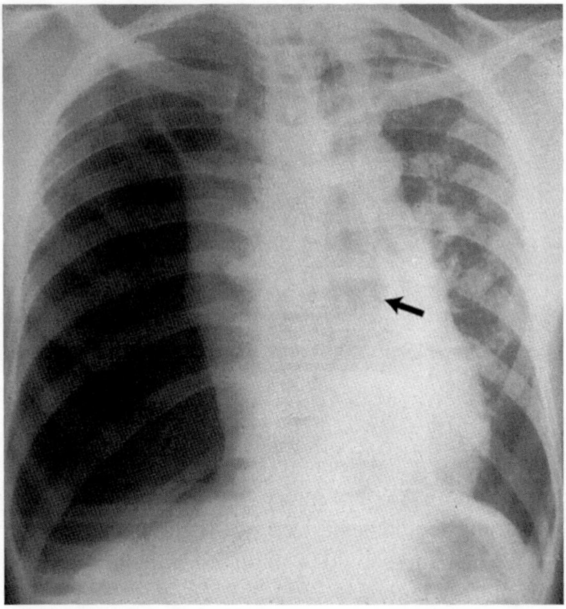

Fig. 7.6 Plain radiograph, tension pneumothorax Note mediastinal shift to left (arrow) away from the pneumothorax on the right

suspicion, an expiratory film should be considered as this will decrease the relative lung volumes and may accentuate the presence of a pneumothorax, if present. Any further investigation is best accomplished with a chest CT scan.

Small pneumothoraces (15–25% collapse) may be safely monitored via serial X-rays if the patient is clinically stable with no evidence of cardiopulmonary compromise. Moderate/large progressive, or bilateral pneumothoraces should be treated with chest tube decompression [50, 51]. Tension pneumothoraces require immediate needle decompression and emergent transport for definitive management. Recurrence rate for spontaneous pneumothorax is 20–50%, with increased risk associated with each subsequent recurrent event [48].

Pulmonary Contusion

Deep bruising of the lung parenchyma may result from high velocity blunt trauma as seen in bicycle racing or motor sports. The initial lung injury may progress to alveolar edema, hemorrhage, and significant respiratory compromise.

Onset of symptoms is insidious and includes dyspnea, tachypnea, cyanosis, and tachycardia; approximately 50% of patients will develop hemoptysis [51]. Exam may reveal rales or diminished breath sounds in the area of injury. Interestingly, the most severe pulmonary contusions are often found without concomitant rib fracture as the lack of dissipation of force when the rib does not break applies a more severe blow to the underlying lung [51].

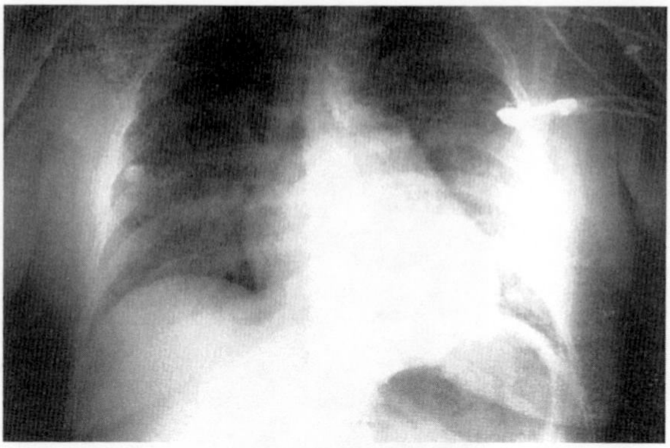

Fig. 7.7 Plain radiograph, patchy infiltrates associated with pulmonary contusion

Radiographic findings include patchy irregular alveolar infiltrates which are generally discernible within 4–6 h of injury (Fig. 7.7). When the diagnosis remains in question, CT scanning should be utilized as it is particularly effective at detecting early lung injury [52]. Patients should be observed in the hospital setting to monitor for progressive respiratory failure.

Pneumomediastinum

Most commonly associated with weightlifting, flying, or diving [53], a pneumomediastinum (PM) arises from injury to the alveolar space or to the communicating bronchial tree with resultant free air in the mediastinum. Chest pain is typically retrosternal, worsened by inspiration, and present in 50–90% of cases. Pain may radiate to the shoulders or back and may mimic myocardial infarction or pericarditis. Exam may reveal palpable subcutaneous crepitus. Auscultation may reveal precordial systolic crepitations and diminution of heart sounds, the "Hamman sign". Pneumothorax may be a concomitant finding and should be clinically suspected in individuals with respiratory distress, asymmetry of breath sounds, or hypoxemia.

Chest X-ray will usually demonstrate air in the mediastinum. Typical features of PM seen on chest radiography are caused by air outlining anatomic structures, producing such findings as the "double bronchial wall sign" (Fig. 7.8).

PM is rarely clinically significant. Management is conservative as spontaneous resolution is the rule, and treatment is directed toward comorbidities, particularly pneumothoraces or musculoskeletal injuries. There are no reported cases of athletes requiring intervention for PM.

Pulmonary Embolus

Pulmonary embolus (PE) as a potentially life-threatening complication of deep venous thrombosis (DVT) occurs uncommonly in athletes [54–58]. Nonetheless,

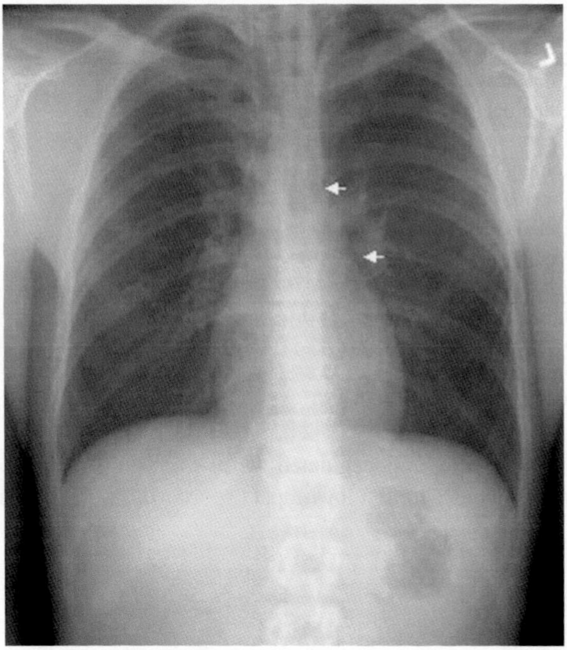

Fig. 7.8 Plain radiograph, pneumomediastinum; note the "double bronchial wall sign"

risks for thromboembolic disease in athletes are common. Venous stasis with immobilization from injury or recent surgery, venous trauma, hypercoagulability from dehydration [59], genetic clotting syndromes (Factor V Leiden mutation, Prothrombin/Factor II mutation, Protein S and Protein C deficiencies) or oral contraceptive use may predispose athletes to DVT and PE.

Presentations vary considerably in intensity and are often subtle. No symptom or physical finding has a high positive predictive value for the diagnosis of PE in either children or adults [55]. Chest pain is typically pleuritic and is associated with dyspnea, tachycardia, and hemoptysis. Physical exam may reveal an uncomfortable, tachypneic patient with tachycardia, fever, focal rales, and increased S2 heart sound, although the exam is notoriously benign in many cases. The classic electrocardiogram reveals sinus tachycardia and an S wave in Lead I, Q wave in Lead III, and T wave inversion in Lead III.

Diagnosis generally is made via clinical suspicion, ELISA D-dimer assay, and CT pulmonary arteriogram. The Wells scoring system [60] (Table 7.4) is a validated tool for determining low, moderate, or high clinical suspicion for PE. Low clinical suspicion for PE (Wells score < 2) and a normal quantitative ELISA D-dimer assay have a negative predictive value for PE of greater than 99.5% [60–62]. Although largely replaced by noninvasive CT scanning, selective pulmonary angiography is still considered the gold standard for diagnosis of PE. Lower extremity ultrasound may also support the likelihood of PE if a DVT is found.

Table 7.4 Wells prediction rule for pulmonary embolus

Clinical feature	Points
Clinical symptoms of DVT	3
Other diagnosis less likely than PE	3
Heart rate greater than 100 beats per minute	1.5
Immobilization or surgery within past 4 weeks	1.5
Previous DVT or PE	1.5
Hemoptysis	1
Malignancy	1
Total points	

Probability of Pulmonary Embolus
- >6 points: high risk (78.4%)
- 2–6 points: mod. risk (27.8%)
- <2 points: low risk (3.4%)

Pulmonary emboli are anticoagulated with warfarin for 6 months. Athletic participation may be considered in low impact sports with minimal risk for contact.

Pneumonia

Pneumonia is an uncommon cause of chest pain in athletes. Typically resulting from viral, atypical bacterial (e.g., mycoplasma), or community-acquired bacterial (e.g., *Streptococcus pneumoniae*, *Haemophilus influenzae*) pathogens, pneumonia may produce chest pain primarily as a function of pleural inflammation.

Clinically, patients may present with a broad constellation of symptoms including fever, chills, rigors, cough which may be variably productive of purulent sputum, malaise, pleuritic chest pain, and shortness of breath [63]. Physical exam may reveal inspiratory rales on auscultation, dullness to percussion, and egophony. Chest radiographs classically demonstrate focal areas of lobar consolidation or diffuse interstitial infiltrates, but may be normal (Fig. 7.9) Atypical pneumonias often demonstrate bilateral patchy infiltrates which appear more impressive than the clinical presentation of the patient. The Diehr diagnostic rule [64] (Table 7.5) can be a helpful adjunct in the evaluation of any patient with chest pain, cough, and fever. Management is either supportive or with broad-spectrum antibiotics depending on the causative organism.

Pleurisy

Inflammation of the pleura with resultant chest pain may arise from a variety of conditions. In the athlete population, the majority of pleuritic pain results from viral respiratory conditions due to adenovirus, Coxsackie, cytomegalovirus, Epstein-Barr virus, influenza, mumps, parainfluenza, and respiratory syncytial virus. Pneumonia may also produce pleuritic pain either by direct involvement of the pleura or via parapneumonic effusion. PE commonly presents with pleuritic pain and is the most frequently observed life-threatening cause of pleuritic chest pain.

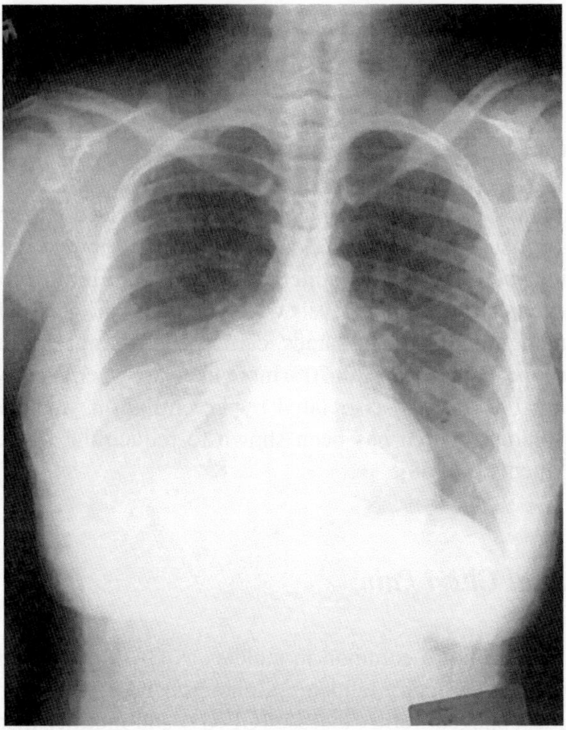

Fig. 7.9 Plain radiograph, lobar/segmental pneumonia consistent with community-acquired pneumonia

Table 7.5 Diehr diagnostic rule for pneumonia

Clinical features	Points
Rhinorrhea	−2
Sore throat	−1
Myalgia	1
Night sweats	1
Sputum all day	1
RR > 25	2
Temp > 100°F	2
Probability of pneumonia	
−3 pts	0.0%
−2	0.7%
−1	1.6%
0	2.2%
1	8.8%
2	10.3%
3	25.0%
≥ 4	29.4%

Management is condition-specific, and primary attention should be paid to the accurate diagnosis of the underlying cause.

Hyperventilation

Hyperventilation as a cause of chest pain is generally divided into sport-associated stress/anxiety or a sudden frightening or painful event (blow to the face or body, particularly with a ball) [65] during athletic participation. Elevated respiratory rates cause a decrease in carbon dioxide levels which produces the classic features of this condition including numb lips and hands, carpo-pedal spasm, dizziness/lightheadedness, and syncope. Females are 30–70% more likely to experience hyperventilation than males [66]. For anxiety-associated hyperventilation, management centers on behavioral therapy which has been shown to reduce the frequency of chest pain in these patients [67, 68].

Gastrointestinal Chest Pain

GI causes of chest pain are common in athletes as GI symptoms are reported by 20–50% of high performance athletes. Amongst those, esophageal disorders, including gastroesophageal reflux disease (GERD) and motility disorders, as well as dysphagia account for over 30% of cases of noncardiac chest pain [69]. Athletes are particularly predisposed because of slowed gastric emptying, prolonged exercise, postprandial state, lower esophageal sphincter (LES) relaxation, dehydration, protein supplementation, increased intra-abdominal pressure, NSAIDs, and sports drink use [70].

Gastroesophageal Reflux Disease

Esophageal reflux is the most common GI cause of chest pain. Symptomatic reflux of gastric contents into the esophagus is encountered in approximately 60% of athletes. Occurring more frequently during exercise [71, 72] the highest incidence is seen in runners [73] and weightlifters. GERD results from regurgitation of gastric contents and acid from the stomach into the esophagus due to failure of protective muscular actions of the esophagus [74]. Suggested mechanisms include gastric dysmotility [75], increased LES relaxation [76], enhanced pressure gradient between the stomach and esophagus[72], gastric distension [77], delayed gastric emptying [76, 78] – especially when dehydrated [79], increased intra-abdominal pressure in sports such as football, weightlifting and cycling [72], and increased mechanical stress by bouncing of organs [76].

Many symptoms are suggestive of GERD including retrosternal chest pain with radiation to the back, “heartburn,” eructation, water brash, and globus hystericus. The degree of discomfort may be substantial and often prevents the continuation of exercise. GERD may mimic anginal pain because impulses in afferent sensory nerves from the heart and esophagus are relayed by the same nerve roots (first through fifth thoracic roots) via the sympathetic nervous system [80]. GERD may also provoke or exacerbate EIB by either silent aspiration into the tracheobronchial tree or by stimulating an acid-mediated esophagobronchial reflex [81, 82]. In a study of asthmatics, 82% had reflux symptoms and 72% had GERD on esophageal pH testing [83]. In another study, 62% of asthmatics had evidence of asymptomatic GERD [84]. Acid reflux may also induce diffuse esophageal spasm that presents with symptoms similar to GERD.

Evaluation of potential GERD is accomplished via contrasted upper GI series, upper endoscopy (EGD), and consideration of distal pH-manometry to assess for mucosal evidence of reflux, inappropriately low distal esophageal pH, and evidence of esophageal dysmotility or poor relaxation.

Effective lifestyle modifications are a potent first line of treatment in athletes with GERD. These include separating dinner and bedtime by at least 4 h, avoiding post-prandial exercise, and limiting consumption of foods that worsen GERD – chocolate, peppermint, onions, high fat foods, alcohol, tobacco, coffee, and citrus products. Elevation of head of bed helps to enhance gravity-induced esophageal clearance.

Medications used to treat GERD primarily include H_2-receptor antagonists and proton pump inhibitors (PPI's). Although PPI's are effective in treating GERD and endoscopic negative reflux disease [85] and have been shown to be therapeutically superior to H_2-receptor antagonists [85–88], the literature on the efficacy of medications used to treat GERD in athletes is sparse. To address esophageal spasm and dysmotility, agents such as dicyclomine have been shown to decrease early postprandial reflux episodes [89].

Dysphagia

Esophageal dysphagia (ED) creates a chest pain typically localized to the sixth thoracic dermatome [90] several seconds after swallowing both solids and liquids. ED results from a variety of mechanical and inflammatory disorders affecting the esophageal body or its peristaltic function. Common causes for painful ED in athletes include esophagitis from acid reflux [75, 76] or from infectious causes including herpes simplex virus, cytomegalovirus, or *Candida* (more commonly seen in immunocompromised individuals). Caustic injury to the lower esophagus from bilious vomiting or "pill esophagitis" following treatment with tetracyclines, NSAID's, or alendronate may result in prominent ED as well. Persistent dysphagia necessitates further work-up and specialist evaluation.

Psychiatric Etiologies of Chest Pain

Chest pain in athletes may result from a variety of psychosocial stressors as well as psychiatric disorders such as anxiety, depression, panic disorder, and somatization.

Chest pain of psychogenic etiology occurs in 9–20% of adolescents [91], with adolescent girls far more likely than boys to suffer psychogenic chest pain. Pain may be vague, sometimes changing, and long-standing. Various associated symptoms may be reported, among them headaches and abdominal pain [91], dizziness and hyperventilation. A stressful event preceding the onset of chest pain can almost always be found [92].

Questions should be directed toward stressful life events which may correlate with the patient's chest pain. Issues such as loss, threat, or rejection are of particular importance [93]. Open questions are useful to elicit such factors, that is, "tell me about any changes or setbacks that occurred in the months before your symptoms began."

Two additional questions are highly sensitive for panic disorder [67]:

> In the past six months, did you ever have a spell or an attack when all of a sudden you felt frightened, anxious, or very uneasy?
>
> In the past six months, did you ever have a spell or an attack when for no reason your heart suddenly began to race, you felt faint, or you couldn't catch your breath?

A positive response to either question strongly suggests the presence of a panic disorder. The Diagnostic and Statistical Manual IV should be utilized for a definitive diagnosis of any psychiatric cause of chest pain.

Substance Abuse

Abuse of any of a number of legal and illicit substances may result in chest pain. The increasing use of psychostimulants for attention deficit disorder raises the likelihood of amphetamine-induced increases in heart rate and blood pressure with a resultant chest pain syndrome. Any athlete with unknown underlying cardiac disease may unexpectedly develop chest pain when stimulant therapy is used, particularly concomitantly with exercise. Supplemental stimulants and the use of energy drinks which contain large quantities of stimulants may similarly create such a risk. Illicit substances such as cocaine may dangerously elevate heart rate and blood pressure and induce myocardial ischemia. Excessive alcohol consumption superimposed on GI tract inflammation from high-level training or concomitant NSAID use may also create chest pain from dyspepsia or acid reflux.

Conclusion

Those who care for athletes will encounter a chief complaint of chest pain frequently in the course of their clinical work. Cardiac etiologies in this population are still uncommon and comprise less than 5% of total chest pain cases amongst athletes and active individuals. A thoughtful and efficient evaluation must be undertaken with each athlete to first determine the presence of cardiac or other potentially life-threatening conditions. In their absence, a wide array of alternative chest pain causes must be sought with an appreciation that pulmonary causes, most commonly exercise-induced bronchospasm, are most likely and that a large percentage of chest pain in this population is idiopathic. Comfort with the historical clues, unique physical exam features, and judicious use of directed ancillary testing are crucial for anyone caring for athletes. These basic components of the evaluation generally are sufficient to make the majority of chest pain diagnoses. Diligence in the evaluation and management of chest pain in sports medicine is an essential skill to help ensure the health and well-being of all who participate.

Clinical Cases

Case 1 (Fig. 7.4)

A 21-year-old collegiate football running back is pulled forward and downward by a tackler. As his shoulder contacts the ground, a second tackler dives on top of him and drives his chest and shoulder forcibly into the turf. As the players un-pile, the running back is in obvious distress on the field and begins clutching at his neck and upper chest. Initial assessment reveals an uncomfortable and anxious male. Once a basic assessment of airway, breathing, and circulation is completed, he is helped from the field for additional evaluation. After removal of his shoulder pads, physical examination reveals asymmetry of the sternoclavicular joints with prominence of the clavicular head anteriorly. The athlete is exquisitely tender to palpation in this area and a small degree of motion is discernible at the sternoclavicular joint. He demonstrates no stridor or apparent impairment in his cardiovascular status. After transport to an emergency facility, plain radiographs of the chest are interpreted as normal, but 40 degree cephalic angle radiographs reveal obvious sternoclavicular asymmetry consistent with *anterior* sternoclavicular dislocation. Cardiovascular compromise manifest by venous congestion and respiratory compromise manifest as stridor would suggest a *posterior* sternoclavicular dislocation which is a medical emergency requiring urgent relocation, often on-field.

Case 2 (Fig. 7.5)

A 19-year-old female cyclist is competing in a medium distance road race. While trying to navigate a sharp turn, she becomes entangled with another cyclist and falls from her bike, striking her chest on the back wheel of an adjacent bike. She has immediate sharp pain in the left side of her chest which causes her to splint her breathing. After resting for several minutes, she states that she feels better and tries to resume riding. As she picks up her pace, she becomes increasingly dyspneic and complains of worsening chest pain at the site of injury. Physical exam reveals a moderately uncomfortable woman who is gasping for breath as she supports her chest wall. Auscultation reveals diffusely diminished breath sounds on the left with hyperresonance to percussion. She is taken emergently to a medical facility where her chest X-ray reveals a large left-sided pneumothorax (Fig. 7.5).

References

1. Berger S, Kugler JD, Thomas JA, et al., *Chest pain in children and adolescents*. Pediatr Clin N Am, 2004. 51:1201–9.
2. Cava JR, Danduran MJ, Fedderly RT, et al., *Exercise recommendations and risk factors for sudden cardiac death*. Pediatr Clin N Am, 2004. 51: 1401–20.
3. Kachintorn U., *How do we define non-cardiac chest pain?* J Gastroenterol Hepatol, 2005. 20(Suppl): S2–S5.
4. Woodwell DA., *National ambulatory medical care survey: 1998 summary*. Adv Data, 1998. 19: 1–26.
5. Cherry DK, Woodwell DA, *National ambulatory medical care survey: 2000 summary*. Advance data from Vital and Health Statistics. Vol. 328. 2002, Hyattsville, MD: National Center for Health Statistics.
6. Selbst S., *Evaluation of chest pain in children*. Pediatr Rev, 1986. 8(2): 56–62.
7. Selbst SM, Ruddy RM, Clark BJ, *Pediatric chest pain: a prospective study*. Pediatrics, 1988. 82: 319–23.
8. Buntinx F, Knockaert D, Bruyninckx R, et al., *Chest pain in general practice or in the hospital emergency department: is it the same?* Fam Pract, 2001. 18: 586–9.
9. Klinkman MS, Stevens D, Gorenflo DW, *Episodes of care for chest pain: a preliminary report from MIRNET*. J Fam Pract, 1994. 38:345–52.
10. Pantell RH, Goodman BW, *Adolescent chest pain*. Pediatrics, 1983. 71:881–7.
11. Martin M., *Chest pain in adolescents: distinguishing cardiac from noncardiac causes*. Med Update Psych, 1997. 2(1):28–31.
12. Singh AM, McGregor RS, *Differential diagnosis of chest symptoms in the athlete*. Clin Rev Allergy Immunol, 2005. 29:87–96.
13. Cooke RA, Chambers JB, Anggiansah A, et al., *Chest pain and normal coronary arteries: a clinical evaluation with oesophageal function tests, exercise ECG, end tidal CO2 measurement and psychiatric scores*. Eur Heart J, 1991. 12(Suppl):103.
14. Fruergaard P, Launbjerg J, Hesse B, et al., *The diagnosis of patients admitted with acute chest pain but without myocardial infarction*. Eur Heart J, 1996. 17:1028–34.
15. Lawless CE, Best T, *Electrocardiograms in athletes: interpretation and diagnostic accuracy*. Med Sci Sports Exerc, 2008. 40(5):787–98.
16. Fikar CR, Koch S, *Etiologic factors of acute aortic dissection in children and young adults*. Clin Pediatr, 2000. 39:71–80.
17. Hatzaras I, Tranquilli M, Coady M, et al., *Weightlifting and aortic dissection: more evidence for a connection*. Cardiology, 2007. 107:103–6.
18. Wise CM, Semble EL, Dalton CB, *Musculoskeletal chest wall syndromes in patients with non-cardiac chest pain: a study of 100 patients*. Arch Phys Med Rehabil, 1992. 73:147–9.
19. Moore R., *Fracture of the first rib: an uncommon throwing injury*. Injury, 1991. 22:149–50.
20. Lorentzen JE, Movin M, *Fracture of the first rib*. Acta Orthop Scand, 1976. 47:623–43.
21. Aitken AP, Lincoln RE, *Fracture of the first rib due to muscle pull*. N Engl J Med, 1939. 220:1063–4.

22. Leung HY, Stirling A, *Stress fracture of the first rib without associated injuries*. Injury, 1991. 22(6):483–4.
23. Lin HC, Chou CS, Hsu TC, *Stress fractures of the ribs in amateur golf players*. Chung Hua I Hsueh Tsa Chih, 1994. 54(1):33–7.
24. Lord MJ, Ha KI, Song KS, *Stress fractures of the ribs in golfers*. Am J Sports Med, 1996. 24(1):118–22.
25. Goyal M, Kenney AJ, *Golfer's rib stress fracture (Duffer's fracture): scintigraphic appearance*. Clin Nucl Med, 1997. 22(7):503–4.
26. Read M., *Case report: stress fracture of the rib in a golfer*. Br J Sports Med, 1994. 28(3):206–7.
27. Gupta A, Jamshidi M, Robin TR, *Traumatic first rib fractures: is angiography necessary?* Cardiovasc Surg, 1997. 5:48–53.
28. Miles JW, Barrett GR, *Rib fractures in athletes*. Sports Med, 1991. 12(1):66–9.
29. Tullos HS, Erwin WD, Woods GW, et al., *Unusual lesions of the pitching arm*. Clin Orthop, 1972. 88:169–82.
30. Fererra PC, Williams CC, *Posterior sternoclavicular dislocation*. Phys Sportsmed, 1999. 27:105–13.
31. Lee FA, Gwinn JL, *Retrosternal dislocation of the clavicle*. Radiology, 1974. 110:631–4.
32. Cope R., *Dislocations of the sternoclavicular joint*. Skeletal Radiol, 1993. 22:233–8.
33. Fererra PC, Williams H, *Sternoclavicular joint injuries*. Am J Emerg Med, 2000. 18:58–61.
34. Destout JM, Gilula LA, Murphy WA, et al., *Computed tomography of the sternoclavicular joint and sternum*. Radiology, 1981. 138:123–8.
35. Fam AG, Smythe HA, *Musculoskeletal chest wall pain*. Can Med Assoc J, 1985. 133(5): 379–89.
36. Malghem J, Vande Berg B, Lecouvert F, et al., *Costal cartilage fractures as revealed on CT and sonography*. Am J Roentgenol, 2001. 176:429–32.
37. Gregory PL, Biswas AC, Batt ME, *Musculoskeletal problems of the chest wall in athletes*. Sports Med, 2002. 32(4):235–50.
38. Disla E, Rhim HR, Reddy A, et al., *Costochondritis: a prospective analysis in an emergency department setting*. Arch Int Med, 1994. 154(21):2466–9.
39. Arroyo JF, Vine R, Reynaud C, et al., *Slipping rib syndrome: don't be fooled*. Geriatrics, 1995. 50(3):46–9.
40. Mooney DP, Shorter NA, *Slipping rib syndrome in childhood*. J Pediatr Surg, 1997. 32(7): 1081–2.
41. Mitchell L, Schafermeyer RW, *Herniated cervical disc presenting as ischemic chest pain*. Am J Emerg Med, 1991. 9:457–9.
42. Billups D, Martin D, Swain RA, *Training room evaluation of chest pina in the adolescent athlete*. Southern Med J, 1995. 88(6):667–72.
43. Rowland TW, *Evaluating cardiac symptoms in the athlete*. Clin J Sport Med, 2005. 15(6): 417–20.
44. Cava JR, Sayger PL, *Chest pain in children and adolescents*. Pediatr Clin N Am, 2004. 51: 1553–68.
45. Wiens L, Sabath R, Ewing L, et al., *Chest pain in otherwise healthy children and adolescents is frequently caused by exercise-induced asthma*. Pediatrics, 1992. 90:350–3.
46. Bar-Or O, Rowland T, *Pediatric Exercise Medicine*. 2004, Champaign, IL: Human Kinetics Publishers. 139–161.
47. Orenstein D., *Asthma and sports*. The Child and Adolescent Athlete, ed. B.-O. O. 1996, Oxford: Blackwell Science. 433–454.
48. Abolnik IZ, Lossos IS, Gillis D, et al., *Primary spontaneous pneumothorax in men*. Am J Med Sci, 1993. 305:297–303.
49. Cvengros R, Lazor J, *Pneumothorax- a medical emergency*. J Ath Training, 1996. 31(2): 167–8.
50. Collins JC, Levine G, Waxman K, *Occult traumatic pneumothorax*. Am Surg, 1992. 58: 743–6.

51. Eckstein M., Henderson S, Markochick V, *Thoracic trauma*. Rosen's emergency medicine, ed. H.R. Marx JA, Walls RM. 2002, St. Louis, MO: Mosby. 381–414.
52. Brooks AP, Olson LK, *Computed tomography of the chest in the trauma patient*. Clin Radiol, 1989. 40:127–32.
53. Leiberman A., *Spontaneous pneumomediastinum in an adolescent patient*. J Adolesc Health Care, 1990. 11:170–2.
54. Moffatt K., Silberberg PJ, Gnarra DJ, *Pulmonary embolism in an adolescent soccer player: a case report*. Med Sci Sports Exerc, 2007. 39(6):899–902.
55. Freeman L., *Pulmonary embolism in a 13-year-old boy*. Pediatr Emerg Care, 1999. 15: 422–4.
56. Melanson SW, Silver B, Heller MB, *Deep vein thrombosis, pulmonary embolism, and white clot syndrome*. Am J Emerg Med, 1996. 14:558–60.
57. Rossdale M, Harvey JE, *Diagnosing pulmonary embolism in primary care*. BMJ, 2003. 327: 393.
58. Van Ommen CH, Heyboer H, Groothoff JW, et al., *Persistent tachypnea in children: keep pulmonary embolism in mind*. J Pediatr Hematol Oncol, 1998. 20:570–3.
59. Croyle PH, Place RA, Hilgenberg AD, *Massive pulmonary embolism in a high school wrestler*. JAMA, 1979. 241:827–8.
60. Wells PS, Anderson DR, Rodger M, et al., *Derivation of a simple clinical model to categorize patients probability of pulmonary embolism: increasing the models utility with the SimpliRED D-dimer*. Thromb Haemost, 2000. 83:416–20.
61. Stein PD, Hull RD, Patel KC, et al., *D-dimer for the exclusion of acute venous thrombosis and pulmonary embolism: a systematic review*. Ann Intern Med, 2004. 140:589–602.
62. Perrier A, Roy PM, Aujesky D, et al., *Diagnosing pulmonary embolism in outpatients with clinical assessment, D-dimer measurement, venous ultrasound, and helical computed tomography: a multicenter management study*. Am J Med, 2004. 116:291–9.
63. Metlay JP, Kapoor WN, Fine MJ, *Does this patient have community-acquired pneumonia? Diagnosing pneumonia by history and physical examination*. JAMA, 1997. 278:1440–5.
64. Diehr P, Wood RW, Bushyhead J, et al., *Prediction of pneumonia in outpatients with acute cough- a statistical approach*. J Chronic Dis, 1984. 37:215–25.
65. Bernhardt D, Landry G, *Chest pain in active young people*. Phys Sportsmed, 1994. 22(6): 70–82.
66. Karofsky P., *Hyperventilation syndrome in adolescent athletes*. Phys Sportsmed, 1987. 15(2):133–6.
67. Chambers J, Bass C, *Atypical chest pain: looking beyond the heart*. Q J Med, 1998. 91:239–44.
68. DeGuire S, Gevirtz R, Kawahara Y, et al., *Hyperventilation syndrome and the assessment of treatment for functional cardiac symptoms*. Am J Cardiol, 1992. 70:673–7.
69. Paterson WG, Abdollah H, Beck IT, et al., *Ambulatory esophageal manometry, pH-metry and Holter ECG monitoring in patients with atypical chest pain*. Dig Dis Sci, 1993. 38:795–802.
70. Casey E, Mistry DJ, MacKnight JM, *Training room management of medical conditions: sports gastroenterology*. Clin Sports Med, 2005. 24(3):525–40.
71. Shawdon A., *Gastro-oesophageal reflux and exercise. Important pathology to consider in the athletic population.* [*Review*] [*32 refs*]. Sports Med, 1995. 20(2):109–16.
72. Collings KL, et al., *Esophageal reflux in conditioned runners, cyclists, and weightlifters*. Med Sci Sports Exerc, 2003. 35(5):730–5.
73. Peters HPF, van Schelven FW, Verstappen PA, et al., *Gastrointestinal problems as a function of carbohydrate supplements and mode of exercise*. Med Sci Sports Exerc, 1993. 25:1211–24.
74. Parmelee-Peters K, Moeller JL, *Gastroesophageal reflux in athletes*. Curr Sports Med Reports, 2004. 3:107–11.
75. Soffer EE, et al., *Effect of graded exercise on esophageal motility and gastroesophageal reflux in trained athletes*. Dig Dis Sci, 1993. 38(2):220–4.
76. Van Nieuwenhoven MA, Brouns F, and Brummer RJ, *Gastrointestinal profile of symptomatic athletes at rest and during physical exercise*. Eur J Appl Physiol, 2004. 91(4):429–34.

77. Rehrer NJ, et al., *Gastrointestinal complaints in relation to dietary intake in triathletes*. Int J Sport Nutr, 1992. 2(1):48–59.
78. Van Nieuwenhoven MA, Vriens BEPJ, Brummer RJ, *Effect of dehydration on gastrointestinal function at rest and during exercise in humans*. Eur J Appl Physiol, 2000. 83:578–84.
79. Rehrer NJ., et al., *Effects of dehydration on gastric emptying and gastrointestinal distress while running*. Med Sci Sports Exerc, 1990. 22(6):790–5.
80. Waterfall WE, Craven MA, Allen CJ, *Gastroesophageal reflux: clinical presentations, diagnosis, and management*. CMAJ, 1986. 135:1101–9.
81. Boyle JT, *Pathogenic gastroesophageal reflux in infants and children*. Pract Gastroenetrol, 1990. 14:25–38.
82. Mathew JL, Singh M, Mittal SK, *Gastro-oesophageal reflux and bronchial asthma: current status and future directions.* [*Review*] [*60 refs*]. Postgrad Med J, 2004. 80(950):701–5.
83. Harding SM, Guzzo ME, Richter JE, *24-h esophageal pH testing in asthmatics: respiratory symptoms correlation with esophageal acid events*. Chest, 1999. 115:654–9.
84. Harding SM, Guzzo ME, Richter JE, *The prevalence of gastroesophageal reflux in asthma patients*. Am J Respir Care, 2000. 162:34–9.
85. van Pinxteren B, et al., *Short-term treatment with proton pump inhibitors, H2-receptor antagonists and prokinetics for gastro-oesophageal reflux disease-like symptoms and endoscopy negative reflux disease.* [*update of Cochrane Database Syst Rev. 2001;(4):CD002095; PMID: 11687139*]. [*Review*] [*63 refs*]. Cochrane Database Syst Rev, 2004. (4):CD002095.
86. Chiba N, et al., *Speed of healing and symptom relief in grade II to IV gastroesophageal reflux disease: a meta-analysis*. Gastroenterology, 1997. 112(6):1798–810.
87. Beck IT, et al., *The Second Canadian Consensus Conference on the Management of Patients with Gastroesophageal Reflux Disease.* [*Review*] [*65 refs*]. Can J Gastroenterol, 1997. 11(Suppl B):7B–20B.
88. Carlsson R., et al., *Prognostic factors influencing relapse of oesophagitis during maintenance therapy with antisecretory drugs: a meta-analysis of long-term omeprazole trials*. Aliment Pharmacol Therap, 1997. 11(3):473–82.
89. Koerselman J, et al., *Different effects of an oral anticholinergic drug on gastroesophageal reflux in upright and supine position in normal, ambulant subjects: a pilot study*. Am J Gastroenterol, 1999. 94(4):925–30.
90. DeGowin RL., *DeGowin & DeGowin's Bedside Diagnostic Examination*. 5th ed. 1987, New York: Macmillan Publishing Company. 139.
91. Anzai AK, Merkin TE, *Adolescent chest pain*. Am Fam Physician, 1996. 53(5):1682–8.
92. Asnes RS, Santulli R, Bemporad JR, *Psychogenic chest pain in children*. Clin Pediatr, 1981. 20(12):788–91.
93. Tennant K., *Life events and disorder*. Curr Opin Psychiat, 1994. 7:207–12.

Chapter 8
The Collapsed Athlete

Sanjeev Malik, George Chiampas, and William O. Roberts

As the field of sports medicine has evolved and expanded, emergency preparedness has become a critical skill in the repertoire of the sideline physician. While the large majority of medical encounters are nonemergent and self-limited, both quick recognition and appropriate response to life-threatening conditions are critical to a favorable outcome in a collapsed athlete. Although there are many reasons for an athlete to suddenly collapse to the ground, the basic differential diagnosis is relatively limited. Most cases will result from one of the following conditions to be discussed in this chapter: sudden cardiac arrest, exertional heat stroke (EHS), exercise-associated hyponatremia (EAH), hypoglycemia (insulin induced), anaphylaxis, and exercise-associated collapse (EAC).

Despite being sensationalized in the media, fatal athletic collapse is relatively rare. The incidence of nontraumatic fatal collapse is estimated to be 1/200,000 high school athletes/academic year; 78% are due to cardiac causes [1]. According to the National Center for Catastrophic Sports Injury Research, 59 nontraumatic fatalities occurred from 1983 to 2007 in high school spring sports [2]. In the marathon, the sudden cardiac death rate across the USA is approximately 1:75,000 finishers for years 2005 and 2006 (unpublished data – W. Roberts). This corresponds with the unpublished rates from Chicago, London, Marine Corps, and Twin Cities Marathons. Nonfatal collapse, however, occurs at a much more frequent rate. The true incidence is difficult to estimate due to variations amongst training conditions, weather, type of sport, and significant underreporting.

The approach to the collapsed athlete requires appropriate pre-event preparation. Recommendations from the Inter Association Task Force on Emergency Preparedness strongly urge that each athletic event and venue develop an emergency action plan (EAP), with quick access to an automated external defibrillator (AED) and application of the device within 3–5 min being an integral part of the plan [3]. A retrospective review of NCAA AED use demonstrated an average emergency medical response system (EMS) response time of 8.2 min when

S. Malik (✉)
Department of Emergency Medicine, Feinberg School of Medicine,
Northwestern University, 259 East Erie Street, Suite 100, IL 60611, Chicago
e-mail: sanjeev.malikmd@gmail.com

C.E. Lawless (ed.), *Sports Cardiology Essentials: Evaluation, Management and Case Studies*, DOI 10.1007/978-0-387-92775-6_8,

EMS was not onsite – exceeding the goal for early defibrillation. While collected data thus far has not shown a favorable outcome for the subgroup of intercollegiate athletes with sudden cardiac arrest, the presence of AEDs at NCAA athletic venues suggests in non-athletes successful resuscitation ([4], Chapter 1). Rapid defibrillation is also credited for saving several lives in marathons [5].

A mass participation event, such as a marathon, presents unique challenges to pre-event preparation due to the large number of athletes and length of the course (size of the "field of play"). Medical support services must be strategically placed, and preferably mobile, to maximize the accessibility to the collapsed athlete. For example, the Bank of America Chicago Marathon, which annually has 45,000 registered entrants and ≈35,000 actual starters, organizes over 700 medical volunteers excluding EMS personnel. In 2006, medical resources included 39 ambulances, 5 medical golf carts, 4 bike teams, and 2 medical vans strategically placed amongst the main medical tent and the 18 aid stations on the course to optimize response times.

In large scale events, communication between medical staff, race staff, and participants is essential to a successful and safe race. In the days preceding the race and as race conditions change through the day, a system to communicate new dangers (environmental, bioterrorism, or otherwise) to the athletes should be available. In 2008, the Bank of America Chicago Marathon piloted an expanded color coded event alert system (Table 8.1) with favorable initial feedback. Further validation of this system in other venues is in process.

In addition to event preparation and communication, medical volunteers should have resources available to stabilize and treat common event-specific conditions. Medical tents at key locations such as the finish area (high numbers of medical encounters) should be equipped with supplies needed to diagnose and treat these problems that might otherwise overload the area hospitals. These tents should be outfitted with defibrillators, rectal thermometers, IV fluids (including 0.9% NS and 3% NS), onsite point-of-care testing devices for blood glucose and sodium levels, and a method to warm or cool post-race casualties.

Table 8.1 Bank of America Chicago Marathon Event Alert System (reproduced with permission from the Bank of America)

Alert level	Event conditions	Recommended actions	Temperature
Extreme	Event cancelled/ extreme and dangerous conditions	Participation stopped/ follow event official instruction	WBGT > 82°f
High	Potentially dangerous conditions	Slow down/observe course changes/follow event official instruction/ consider stopping	WBGT 73–82°F
Moderate	Less than ideal conditions	Slow down/be prepared for worsening conditions	WBGT 65–73°F
Low	Good conditions	Enjoy the event/be alert	WBGT 40–65°F

WBGT = Wet bulbglobe temperature

Approach to the Down Athlete

Athletic collapse is defined as the loss of postural tone and altered level of consciousness. Various medical conditions can result in the collapse of an athlete from a life-threatening dysrhythmia to benign EAC. As with all emergent conditions, the approach to the down athlete begins with stabilization of the ABCs – airway, breathing, and circulation supplemented with early AED application. An algorithm for the approach to undifferentiated collapse used in the Chicago Marathon is shown in Fig. 8.1.

Compromise of the ABCs warrants emergent initiation of advanced cardiac life support (ACLS) protocols and activation of the EMS. An AED should be applied and defibrillation performed if warranted. The 2005 revised ACLS guidelines stress the importance of minimizing interruptions in CPR. In athletes with downtime greater than 4–5 min, the medical provider should consider CPR prior to defibrillation. Furthermore, CPR should be resumed immediately after a single defibrillation for 2 min prior to pulse check. This is a dramatic change from the 2000 AHA recommendations for three initial repeated shocks based on outcome studies showing improved efficacy of newer biphasic defibrillators [6, 7].

In athletes with relatively stable cardiopulmonary status and preserved mentation, a focused history and physical can direct appropriate management. Relevant historical information may include: fluid intake during the race, pre- and post-race weights, level of training, acclimatization, previous racing experience, prior history of athletic collapse, presence of neurologic or cardiac symptoms, history of trauma, or history of chronic diseases like coronary artery disease or diabetes. In severe cases, a complete set of vital signs including a rectal temperature as well as onsite assessment of oxygen saturation, glucose, and sodium/BUN/hematocrit may be necessary to establish the appropriate diagnosis and initiate the correct treatment. The most common conditions resulting in collapse will be explored further in the remainder of this chapter.

Cardiac Causes

Various cardiac conditions can lead to fatal and nonfatal sudden cardiac arrest during athletic competition. By far, the most common cause of cardiac arrest in mass participation events is due to coronary artery disease although hypertrophic cardiomyopathy, anomalous coronary arteries, and channelopathies like long QT syndrome may lead to sudden cardiac arrest in younger (<30 years old) athletes. Individual topics are discussed in more detail in previous chapters. CPR with early defibrillation, ACLS protocol, and rapid transport to an emergency facility that can provide immediate intervention are the mainstays of sideline treatment of cardiac conditions and have shown significant mortality reduction [5].

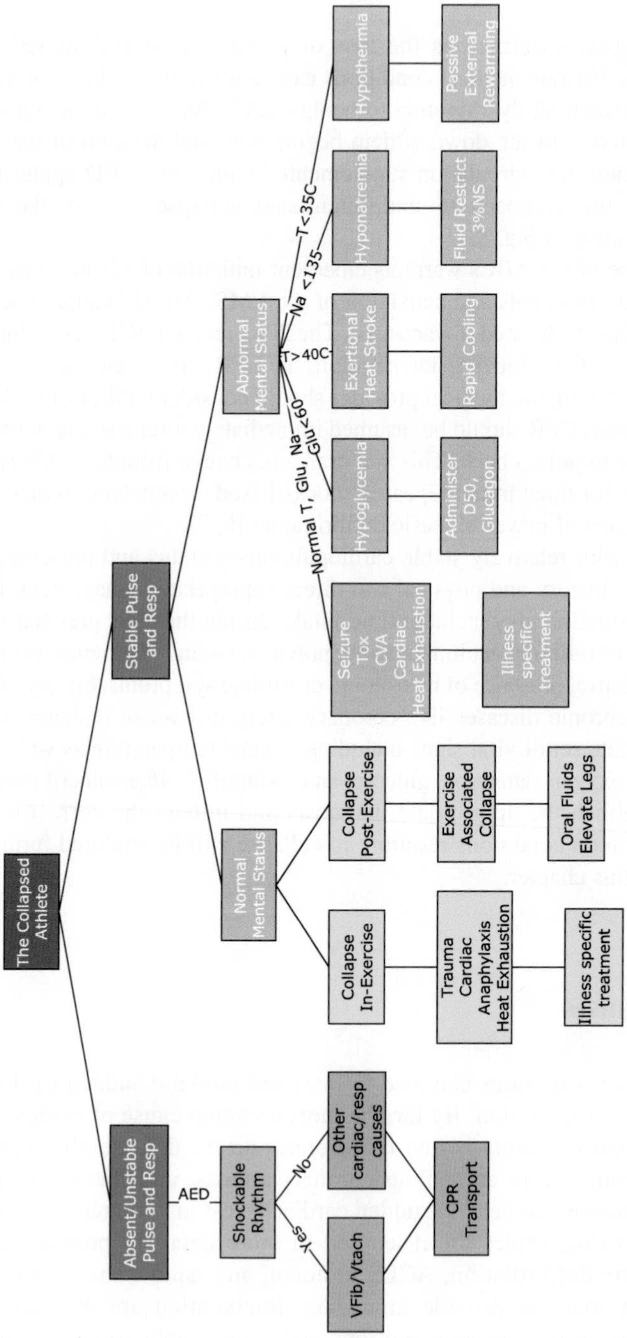

Fig. 8.1 Clinical decision algorithm. Approach to the collapsed athlete in endurance events

Hyperthermia/Exertional Heat Stroke

Exertional heat stroke (EHS) can be a frequent cause of collapse and accounts for the third highest number of deaths in athletes [8]. Exertional heat illness (EHI) refers to the spectrum of heat-induced illnesses, including exercise-associated muscle cramping, heat exhaustion, exertional hyperthermia, and EHS.

Elevations in core temperature >40°C meet the defined criteria for exertional hyperthermia [9, 10]. Prolonged exposure to elevated core temperatures place the athlete at risk for EHS. EHS is defined as an elevation of core temperature >40°C associated with signs of central nervous system (CNS) dysfunction or other organ system failure. The most common clinical presentation involves CNS signs and mental status changes in the presence of hyperthermia [9].

Background

While the true incidence of heat-related illness has been difficult to determine, few in the sports medicine community would doubt the associated morbidity for athletes participating in hot humid conditions. Heat exhaustion rates of 14/10,000 individuals/day have been reported in a 14 km race with ambient temperatures 11–20°C [11]. Similarly, the occurrence rates of exertional hyperthermia and heat stroke are unclear and likely underreported. A review of American football from the 7-year period of 1995–2002 reported 21 heat-related deaths – an incidence of fatal EHS in 1:350,000 participants [12].

Multiple factors affect the incidence of heat illness including ambient temperature, relative humidity, cloud cover, and both the intensity and duration of activity. The incidence of EHS in an annual 7.1 mile road race run in wet bulb globe temperatures (WBGT) 70–80°F has been approximately 1–2 per 1,000 finishers. The incidence of EHS at the Twin Cities Marathon is about 1:10,000 finishers with WBGT 40–55°F [13], but increases significantly to 12–15 per 10,000 finishers with WBGT in the 70°F range (unpublished data, W. Roberts).

An athlete's ability to protect from exertional hyperthermia and heat stroke depends on the ability to dissipate heat at a rate equivalent to metabolic heat generation. During intense exercise, heat production by exercising skeletal muscles can be 15–20 times greater than resting levels. Without heat dissipation, this metabolic heat will result in a rise in core temperature of 1°C/5 min of activity [9]. Heat dissipation occurs via sweat vaporization and a combination of conduction and convection heat exchange with the air. Radiant heat losses may occur as well, more commonly in cold conditions. The vascular system transports heat from exercising muscle and the core to the body shell; increased skin blood flow facilitates heat exchange with the environment. This heat exchange is dependent on the core to skin temperature gradient, the ability to vaporize sweat to transfer heat from the body, the amount of radiant heat added to the body, and the ability to transfer heat to the air via convection and conduction.

As ambient temperature increases, the core to skin gradient decreases and less heat can be transferred to the environment. The brain may compensate by allowing the core body temperature to drift upward to maintain a core to skin temperature gradient. Furthermore, as humidity increases, evaporative heat loss is impaired. Both factors contribute to a summative increase in core temperature. Elevated core temperatures may then progress to CNS hyperthermia, resulting in decreased cerebral blood flow and an increase in perceived exertion. If this perceived exertion increase is ignored and core temperature rises to critical levels, cardiovascular collapse ensues. This ultimately results in athletic collapse [14]. While some athletes have been reported to tolerate core temperatures up to 41.9°C without adverse effect, the large majority of athletes will terminate exercise due to fatigue at core temperatures below 40°C [9, 15, 16].

The most important predictive determinant of an athlete's risk of EHI remains high intensity or prolonged duration of exercise in high ambient temperatures and humidity, especially in unacclimatized participants. The gold standard for measurement of heat stress is the WBGT, which incorporates the sum of wet bulb (0.7), black globe (0.2), and ambient (0.1) temperature measurements. Data from the Boston Marathon and Twin Cities Marathon suggest a direct relationship between both the start and the peak WBGT and risk of medical encounters [13]. This marathon data suggests that optimal environmental conditions occur in the 4.4–15°C WBGT range. Elevations in WBGT above 15.5°C correlated with a higher incidence of collapse and EHIs. Guidelines from the American College of Sports Medicine (ACSM) recommend postponement of high risk events with WBGT >28°C [9, 13].

Recommendations for activity modification are shown in Table 8.2. Other factors that have been associated with increased risk of exertional heat-related illness are relative dehydration, lack of acclimatization, history of sickle cell trait, stimulant medicine, obesity, recent febrile illness, and insulating equipment or clothing [9, 16, 17].

Diagnosis

Recognition of EHS signs and symptoms is essential to prompt diagnosis of hyperthermia and EHS. A rectal (core) temperature >40°C with altered mental status is consistent with the diagnosis of EHS. Rectal temperature measurements should be used as oral, aural canal (TM), temporal artery, and skin temperature measurements consistently underestimate core temperature and have been proven unreliable [18, 19].

The presence of neurologic symptoms including headache, confusion, disorientation, or ataxia should raise the clinical suspicion for EHS. Athletes may also present with vomiting, diarrhea, hematochezia, seizures, and/or coma secondary to complications from EHS. EHS may occur in cooler climates and conditions that are generally considered low risk [20].

Table 8.2 Risk of heat-related illness with temperature (reproduced with permission from Roberts et al. [13])

Temperature [°C] (°F)	Flag	ACSM road race 1996 [1]	Military guide[a] [2]
<10 (50)	White	Increased hypothermia risk; EHS can occur	
10–18 (50–65)	Green	Low risk hyperthermia and hypothermia; EHS can occur	
18–23 (65–73)	Yellow	Caution (moderate hyperthermia risk); EHS risk rises	
23–28 (73–82)	Red	Extreme caution (high hyperthermia risk)	Caution for heat stroke
>28 (82)	Black	Extreme high hyperthermia risk; cancel or postpone	Discretion in unseasoned participants; no heavy exercise
>30 (85)			Suspend exercise <3 weeks training
>31 (88)			Curtail <12 weeks hot weather training
>32 (90)			Suspend all training and exercises

ACSM American College for Sports Medicine, *EHS* exertional heat stroke

[a]The current military doctrine (TBMED507) provides guidance based on weather and intensity of activity with the use of work rest ratios to minimize the likelihood that someone will fallout during activity due to heat stress, but does not allow for continuous activity in hot conditions

Athletes with heat exhaustion typically have rectal temperatures in the 37–40°C range with preserved mental status and relatively stable vitals, unless there is significant dehydration. Milder cases may present with muscle cramping, fatigue, and dehydration. Some athletes may even suffer collapse to the ground due to the extreme fatigue, relative dehydration, and postural hypotension. Heat exhaustion will typically respond to conservative measures of hydration and cooling.

Athletes should be assessed for concurrent hypoglycemia or hyponatremia as the etiology for the altered mental status, especially if the rectal temperature is not elevated into the heat stroke range.

Treatment

With prompt recognition and rapid cooling, morbidity and mortality from heat-related illnesses is preventable. Morbidity is directly related to the duration that core temperature is elevated above 40.5°C [21]. Most individuals with EHS will tolerate approximately 60°C per min above this threshold [9]. Guidelines adopted by the ACSM and National Athletic Trainers Association recommend cooling below 40°C within 30 min of collapse, preferably below 38°C [21].

Onsite cooling should be initiated as soon as possible and should not be delayed for transportation to the hospital. Multiple methods for onsite cooling exist and their cooling rates are shown in Fig. 8.2 below [22]. The gold standard for cooling is cold-water immersion (CWI), with typical rates of 0.16–0.20°C/min depending on water temperature. Opponents to CWI have raised concerns of drowning, sanitation, and inaccessibility for AED use as potential drawbacks to this methodology. However, the superior cooling rates compared to other modalities have led the ACSM to advocate the use of CWI as the preferred method of cooling unless unavailable [9].

Other methods of cooling have been proven to be effective as well. Rapidly alternating ice water-soaked towels or sheets applied to the head, trunk, and extremities have been successfully used in marathon medical tents with cooling rates of 0.12–0.16°C/min [23]. Other modalities including ice packs to the central arteries in the neck, axilla, and groin have been effective, but at approximately half the rate of ice water immersion [9, 24].

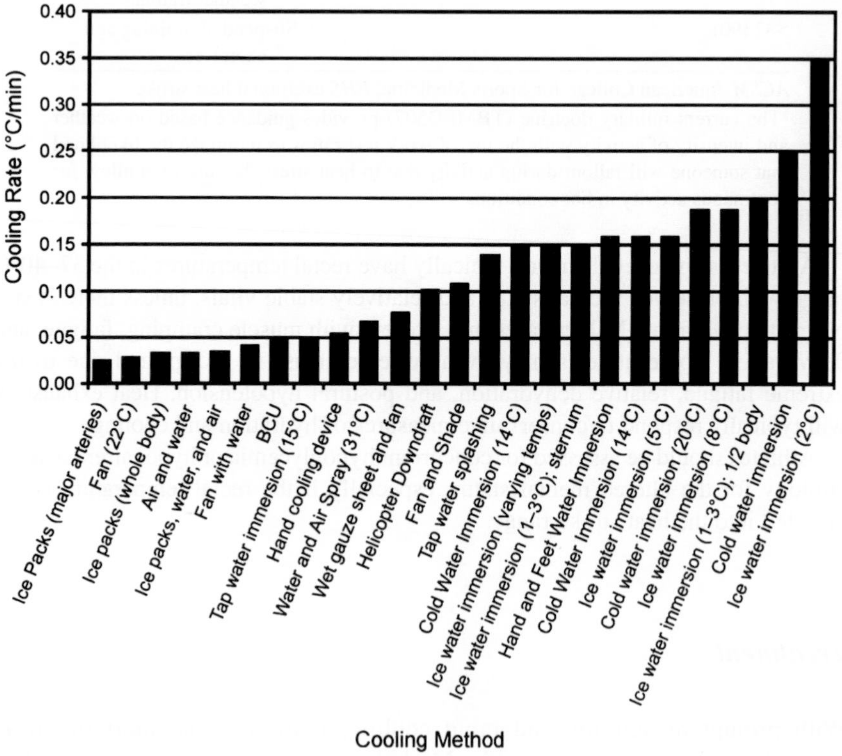

Fig. 8.2 Cooling rates by method (reprinted with permission from Casa et al. [22])

In refractory cases, more invasive hospital-based maneuvers for cooling may be implemented including cooling blankets, extracorporeal blood exchange, peritoneal lavage, cold saline intravenous infusions, nasogastric lavage with cold saline, or bladder irrigation with cold saline. Dantrolene may be indicated in cases where heat exchange modalities are not effective as carriers of the R1RY gene associated with malignant hyperthermia may be more prone to EHS and resistant to usual treatments. Although there is no known morbidity associated with cooling to or just below normal body temperatures, practitioners should be careful not to overcool [28]. However, future research may be done to explore the benefits of cooling to subnormal levels in severe cases to protect neurologic recovery as has been done with cardiac arrest and spinal cord injuries.

Hypothermia

Albeit a less common cause of athletic collapse, the spectrum of cold-related illness may have significant morbidity to the athlete as well. Exercise in cold weather conditions may result in a variety of injuries from mild self-limited cold-induced diuresis to life-threatening hypothermia. Hypothermia is defined as a core temperature of <35°C, classified into three categories by severity: mild, moderate, and severe(Table 8.3).

Mild hypothermia (33–35°C) may present with tachycardia, decreased manual dexterity, lethargy, apathy, and shivering. Moderate hypothermia (30–32°C) presents with more profound neurologic impairment including weakness, ataxia, and decreased level of consciousness, associated with bradycardia. Athletes with moderate hypothermia may present with decreased shivering. In cases of severe hypothermia (<30°C), the athlete will have profound impairment including impaired consciousness, hypotension, bradycardia, apnea, and complete impairment of both the thermoregulatory system and shivering mechanism. The risk of ventricular arrhythmia increases as the core temperature

Table 8.3 Field diagnosis and treatment of hypothermia

	Mild hypothermia	Moderate hypothermia	Severe hypothermia
Core temperature	33–35°C	30–33°C	<30°C
Shivering	Present	Decreased	Absent
Mental status	Fatigue, lethargy	Apathy	Impaired level of consciousness
Cardiac abnormalities	Tachycardic	Bradycardic	Myocardial irritability
Field interventions	PER, walking, warm PO fluids	PER, warm IV fluids	PER, warm IV fluids
Transport to ED	No, unless poor response to field treatment	Yes	Yes, immediate

PER passive external rewarming

drops below 28°C [25]. Mild to moderate hypothermia is relatively common in long distance events that are held in the 4–10°C temperature range with precipitation that "wets" the participants.

Background

Hypothermia occurs in athletes when heat loss exceeds basal heat production, and the thermoregulatory system cannot conserve body heat to ward off hypothermia. This happens most frequently in CWI, sweat soaked cotton clothing, or cold rainy conditions where heat transfer out of the body exceeds the metabolic heat production. In response to a cold stimulus, the body attempts to compensate by increasing relative heat production and heat conservation. Increases in heat production are promoted by shivering thermogenesis (regulated by the hypothalamus) which may result in a two- to fivefold increase in basal metabolic rate. Additionally, heat production may be maintained by the release of norepinephrine and thyroxine [26]. A cold stimulus of below 34–35°C triggers a thermoregulatory response resulting in peripheral vasoconstriction. This compensatory mechanism preserves core body temperature at the expense of peripheral skin and muscle temperature and improves insulation of the body shell [25]. Vasoconstriction induces a relative intravascular "overload" and generates a renal response with diuresis leaving the athlete with an increased fluid deficit during rewarming.

Heat loss occurs via four mechanisms – conduction, convection, radiation, and evaporation. In cold, dry conditions, radiation may account for 50% of heat loss, but is rarely a cause of hypothermia in athletes who are properly dressed. Heat loss that leads to hypothermia during athletic activity usually involves a combination of conductive, convective, and evaporative losses when the clothing is wet with sweat or precipitation. Body heat is conducted directly to the outer layer of clothing where exchange occurs rapidly in cold conditions. CWI causes very rapid heat loss due to conduction and convention, and immersion in water below 10°C will rapidly cool the body to near fatal levels [26, 27].

Intuitively, athletes in outdoor cold-weather sports are at risk for hypothermia, but this rarely occurs in athletes who are prepared for the conditions. Athletes at highest risk include those unexpectedly caught in cold, wet, rainy conditions and cold-water swimmers who have high convective heat losses as they move through the water. The convective heat losses in water are 28- to 32-fold greater than that of air [27]. Heat loss is directly proportional to the body surface area exposed for heat exchange, and athletes immersed in water have a more rapid decline in core body temperature than those exposed to cold air at the same temperature [29]. Similarly, wet cotton clothing in contact with skin can approach water immersion heat losses. Slow runners can lose more heat than they produce, even in relatively mild conditions if they are wet and not wearing adequate clothing. Athletes who choose cotton materials over the more technical clothing are at greater risk. Other risk factors include extremes of age (decreased thermoregulation in older athletes, increased body surface area to mass ratio in children), low body fat percentage (decreased insulation), and low intensity activity (decreased heat production).

Diagnosis

Appropriate diagnosis of hypothermia depends on early recognition of classic symptoms in conjunction with clinical suspicion in appropriate environmental conditions. As discussed in the previous section on heat-related illnesses, a rectal temperature is the gold standard for assessing core temperature. Oral, tympanic, and skin temperature measurements have been proven unreliable [19, 30]. Care should be taken to ensure low-temperature thermometers capable of measuring lower than 32°C are available for accurate assessment of core temperature [27].

Treatment

Mild hypothermia may be appropriately managed in the field setting. Passive external rewarming (PER) is the treatment of choice in these situations and often the most readily available option. PER may be accomplished by applying an insulating material such as dry clothing and blankets to the affected athlete. The athlete should be removed from wet, windy, and rainy conditions and wet clothes should be removed to prevent further heat loss. In the marathon road race setting, runners who are able to walk coming into the medical area often warm fast with continued walking, dry clothes, warmed blankets, and warm fluids. Clinicians should be careful to consider and treat concomitant hypovolemia and hypoglycemia [27].

Although moderate to severe hypothermia is rare in most athletic venues, these athletes are at increased risk for deadly ventricular dysrhythmias. The management needs exceed the capabilities of most field settings and casualties should be transferred to the nearest Emergency Department for more aggressive rewarming measures. Hospital-based interventions include active external rewarming (AER) and active core rewarming (ACR). Onsite care should consist of stabilization of the ABCs, initiation of PER (to central areas such as head, neck, axilla, and groin where vasodilation is minimized), warmed IV saline, and transport. As opposed to the EHS victim where "treat first, then transfer" is the most prudent course, the hypothermia casualty should be approached with a "transfer first, then treat" protocol.

Application of heat packs to the periphery may result in a paradoxical drop in core temperature by allowing circulating blood into cold peripheral tissue where the blood is cooled and returned to the core. In severe hypothermia casualties, care should be taken to avoid excessive patient movement as this has been theorized to trigger ventricular dysrhythmia in the cold irritable myocardium. However, a 2007 animal study by Grueskin suggested 5/7 cases of fatal dysrhythmias with severe induced hypothermia occurred in the absence of mechanical stimulation [31]. Rewarming should ideally occur at a rate of 0.5–2°C/h to reduce the risk of inducing ventricular fibrillation [27].

In the truly pulseless athlete, the airway should be secured while CPR and available rewarming methods are initiated. Caution is advised to ensure that the athlete is truly pulseless and not simply suffering from profound bradycardia. The unnecessary initiation of closed chest compressions may precipitate ventricular fibrillation. If available, an AED or electrocardiogram monitor should be applied to detect cardiac activity which may slow to exceedingly low rates in profound hypothermia. If the monitor pads will not stick to the cold skin, a needle can be passed through the pad into the skin and subcutaneous tissue to improve the electrical conduction. After rhythm identification, defibrillation may be performed if indicated. Successful defibrillation has been reported at body temperatures as low as 20°C, but defibrillation is routinely unsuccessful until core temperature has reached a minimum of 28°C [26, 32]. Resuscitation must be continued until the patient has become normothermic by all available rewarming methods as successful resuscitations have been reported up to 6.5 h from initiation of CPR and rewarming [33]. For this reason, the victim should not be pronounced dead, "until warm and dead" and the core temperature has been raised into the 32–35°C range. In the hospital setting, ACR for severe hypothermia may be performed by humidified air, mediastinal or peritoneal lavage, bladder irrigation, and extracorporeal cardiopulmonary bypass

Exercise-Associated Hyponatremia

Over the last 10–15 years, the sports medicine community has become acutely aware of exercise-associated hyponatremia (EAH) as a life-threatening cause of athletic collapse with at least ten reported fatalities in the last 20 years – four of which were civilians in marathons [34]. EAH seems to occur almost exclusively in long duration events such as marathons and triathlons and may affect up to 13% of participants [35]. Hyponatremia is defined by a serum sodium level <135 mmol/L and may be classified into asymptomatic and symptomatic categories. The actual sodium level may not be as predictive of symptoms as the change in sodium from pre- to post-activity. Runners with sodium levels of 131 mmol/L have developed encephalopathy (personal communication – J.C. Ayrus).

Background

Since the first reported case of EAH in a young South African woman in 1981, EAH has been reported in several venues and is most often secondary to overhydration with hypotonic fluids. An example of the correlation between aggressive hydration and hyponatremia occurred in 1990 when the US military adopted hydration guidelines aimed at reducing heat illness. Military personnel were instructed to ingest 1.8 L fluid/h when ambient temperature was >30°C. Unfortunately, an alarming 125 cases of EAH requiring hospitalization and six deaths occurred during a 7-year span. These rates dramatically fell when the US military guidelines for fluid ingestion were adjusted to more precisely match sweat losses [36, 37].

While overhydration with hypotonic fluids appears to be the most consistent risk factor published in the literature, a prospective study of 488 participants in the Boston Marathon in 2002 showed additional risk factors included female gender, BMI < 20, race duration >4 h, ingestion of >3 L fluid, and elevated post-race weights [35]. The authors also demonstrated that sports drinks did not protect from dilutional hyponatremia. Other studies have postulated that NSAID use may affect the development of EAH but studies to date have had conflicting results [38].

The true cause of EAH is likely multifactorial. Excessive oral rehydration with water or commercially available sports drinks associated with a decrease in renal water clearance due to loss vasopressin suppression is believed to be the main physiologic cause of EAH. While sports drinks do contain a minimal amount of electrolytes, they are still relatively hypotonic (10–20 mmol Na/L) compared to body fluid and contribute to a dilutional hyponatremia. In the presence of hyponatremia, one would expect maximally suppressed ADH levels. While ADH has not conclusively been elevated in EAH, case reports of elevated urinary osmolarity in athletes with EAH suggest a contributory role of inappropriate ADH suppression in the development of hyponatremia [39].

Diagnosis

Onsite diagnosis of EAH requires point-of-care electrolyte testing. Many athletes with sodium levels <135 mmol/L will be asymptomatic. Diagnosis in these individuals may be both difficult and unnecessary as these patients self-correct without intervention and simple fluid restriction. All athletes with symptoms suggestive of EAH should have onsite sodium testing if available [39]. While lower sodium levels are associated with increased risk of complications, classification of EAH should only be defined by the severity of the clinical symptoms. Clinical symptoms of hyponatremia may range from mild nonspecific neurologic symptoms such as headache, nausea, and fatigue to severe sequelae consistent with hyponatremic encephalopathy including confusion, seizures, and severe mental status changes. According to 2003 data collected by Hew in the Houston Marathon, vomiting was found to be the only statistically significant symptom that was more pronounced in hyponatremic athletes compared to normonatremic athletes [40]. Additionally, athletes with hyponatremia typically exhibit clinical signs of euvolemia or hypervolemia including extremity or facial puffiness, shortness of breath due to noncardiogenic pulmonary edema, lack of expected race weight loss, or increased post-race weight compared to pre-race weight.

Treatment

Treatment of EAH varies with the severity of clinical symptoms. The Second International Conference on EAH recommends onsite treatment for EAH be initiated as soon as the diagnosis is established. For mild symptomatic hyponatremia, oral fluid intake should be restricted until the athlete urinates [39]. Athletes with symptoms of exercise-associated hyponatremic encephalopathy (EAHE) secondary to cerebral edema should be given a 100 mL intravenous bolus of 3% NaCl solution. This may be repeated every 10 min until symptoms have improved. Hypertonic saline has been utilized onsite at multiple marathon events and has been effective in the prevention of mortality from EAHE. Most reported deaths from EAHE have occurred in patients treated initially with 0.9% NS [39].

Many practitioners have expressed reservations regarding the dangers of hypertonic saline outside of the hospital setting and the risk of central pontine myelinolysis (CPM) due to rapid correction of hyponatremia. However, these concerns do not apply to the acute hyponatremia in athletes and have not been supported in the literature. There have been no reported deaths due to EAHE or CPM with the onsite initiation of hypertonic saline [41]. Athletes with EAH should be transferred to the local emergency department for continuation of treatment and/or neuroimaging as indicated. A 2001 study by Davis in San Diego showed in-hospital continuation or initiation of hypertonic saline has also been effective at reducing morbidity from EAHE [38].

As the dangers of EAH have been publicized in the medical and running communities, it has become clear that prevention is the most effective treatment. As illustrated by the declining incidence of EAH in the US army after adoption of less aggressive fluid replacement guidelines, education of athletes and race directors regarding the dangers of overhydration is of paramount importance. The EAH consensus group recommends the placement of fluid stations in a typical marathon every 5 km and encourages athletes only to "drink to thirst." Athletes are also encouraged to measure pre- and post-race weights while training to document sweat losses and develop a rational fluid replacement plan to avoid excessive dehydration [39, 42].

Hypoglycemia

Another relatively rare, but commonly overlooked cause of athletic collapse is hypoglycemia. Hypoglycemia is defined as a serum glucose <60 mg/dL associated with characteristic symptoms that resolve with administration of glucose.

Background

Diabetic athletes, particularly insulin-dependent diabetics, are at the greatest risk for hypoglycemic events. However, hypoglycemia may occur in nondiabetics using performance-enhancing drugs such as human growth hormone (HGH), insulin growth factor I (IGF-I), and insulin [43]. A 2006 survey of known anabolic steroid users reported a 25% rate of insulin abuse, increased from 2% in 1997 [44]. Insulin has been proven to improve strength and endurance by promoting muscle glucose uptake and increasing muscle glycogen stores, thereby sparing muscle protein.

Furthermore, exercise alone has been postulated to improve insulin sensitivity perhaps leading to an increased relative risk of hypoglycemia. Evaluation of 19 well-trained Dutch cyclists showed transient hypoglycemia in 33% of participants at an average of 20 min of exercise with a gradual return to normoglycemic levels [45]. However, none of those athletes had hypoglycemic events resulting in collapse; this transient phenomenon is most likely clinically insignificant in the non-diabetic population.

Diagnosis

The major pitfall to the delayed diagnosis of hypoglycemia is the absence of clinical suspicion. Hypoglycemia has variable presenting signs and must be considered in the evaluation of the collapsed athlete. Hypoglycemic athletes may present with mental status changes, confusion, or coma. They may also exhibit adrenergic signs such as sweating, tremulousness, nausea, and palpitations. As evident in the diagnostic algorithm in Fig. 8.1, a point-of-care blood glucose analysis should be performed on all collapsed athletes with mental status changes. Alternatively, if onsite serum glucose testing is unavailable, empiric treatment with dextrose should be initiated as the adverse consequences of empiric therapy are exceedingly low. Resolution of symptoms with dextrose administration can confirm the diagnosis of hypoglycemia in the absence of serum glucose detection. Caution must be taken to consider concurrent etiologies of mental status changes and/or collapse in the hypoglycemic athlete that does not clinically respond to appropriate treatment.

Treatment

Prompt administration of glucose is essential to the rapid treatment of hypoglycemia. In mildly symptomatic patients, glucose may be safely replaced by oral route. Glucose tablets or gel, orange juice, and crackers are a few of the many effective treatment options. In the unconscious athlete, glucose must be administered parenterally. The intravenous administration of 50 mL of 50% dextrose in water solution (D50) is preferred in adults, while pediatric athletes should be given 2 mL/kg of 25% dextrose in water (D25) solution. Alternatively, glucagon 1 mg (0.03 mg/kg pediatric) may be administered intramuscularly if IV access is not obtainable.

Patients should be observed for rebound hypoglycemia. Patients on oral hypoglycemic medications or with unclear etiology of hypoglycemia should be transferred to the hospital for observation and monitoring. Race directors should encourage diabetic athletes to wear medical alert tags for prompt identification of hypoglycemic symptoms.

Exercise-Associated Collapse

While the onsite physician must be careful to consider life-threatening causes of athletic collapse, the large majority of athletes that present to a medical tent suffer from an entity known as exercise-associated collapse (EAC). EAC occurs in approximately 1.13% of race entrants in the Twin Cities Marathon and the rate significantly increases with race duration greater than 3.5 h, temperature, and humidity [46–48].

Initially, the EAC care matrix as defined by Roberts in 1989 was created as a broad-based classification and treatment matrix that includes postural hypotension, exhaustion, hypothermia, and hyperthermia to assist in the onsite management of collapse [49]. The classification speeds the care of hyperthermic, hypothermic, and normothermic casualties who present in large numbers in a narrow window of time at mass participation events. More recently, the term exercise-associated collapse has also been adopted in reference to benign athletic collapse resulting from inadequate peripheral vasoconstriction upon the cessation of exercise [50]. This corresponds to the normothermic and mildly hypo/hyperthermic categories in the EAC classification and treatment matrix.

Background

At rest, skeletal muscle blood flow accounts for approximately 20% of cardiac output. With exercise, skeletal muscle oxygen requirements increase and the body may compensate by a 20-fold increase in skeletal blood flow. In endurance events, skeletal blood flow may account for 60–80% of total cardiac output. Abrupt cessation of exercise results in a sudden decrease in venous return as the muscles, which have been acting as a secondary heart, cease to force blood back to the heart. The decrease in venous return combined with low post-exercise peripheral vascular resistance (PVR) and persistent skin and muscle vasodilatation result in a reduced pre-load. This phenomenon contributes to postural hypotension and collapse. While relative dehydration (decreased intravascular volume) and heat exhaustion (peripheral vasodilatation) may predispose to EAC, the causes of EAC are multifactorial [49, 51].

Diagnosis

Diagnosis of EAC is dependent on a classic history of collapse upon cessation of exercise in combination with stable vital signs and normal mental status. Clinical symptoms may include fatigue, generalized weakness, nausea, and lightheadedness. Clinical signs include rapid return to normal pulse and blood pressure, an intense "diamond" of vasoconstriction around the mouth (peri-oral pallor), and closed eyes. EAC is always a diagnosis of exclusion, and athletes should be evaluated for alternative etiologies of collapse if they do not respond to simple measures outlined below [49, 52].

Treatment

The athlete with the presumptive diagnosis of EAC should be placed in the supine position with the legs and pelvis elevated above the level of the heart. This may be started while other causes of collapse are eliminated. Oral rehydration fluids may be given as determined by athlete's thirst, unless the athlete exhibits signs of volume overload. The athlete may be reassessed in approximately 15–30 min [1]. Most collapse secondary to EAC will have marked improvement within this time frame.

Athletes with stable vitals, symptomatic resolution, and ability to walk unassisted may be safely discharged from the medical tent. Athletes who do not respond to conservative measures within 15–30 min should be further evaluated for heat illness, dehydration, or other concurrent problems. A complete set of vitals including a rectal temperature should be obtained and onsite testing of sodium and glucose are advised if available. Those athletes with tachycardia, hypotension, or inability to tolerate oral liquids should be considered for IV fluids with 5% dextrose (D5) in 0.9% saline solution (NS) [50]. Athletes who continue to show no improvement should be transferred to the local emergency department for further treatment.

Seizures

Another consideration in the differential of the collapsed athlete is seizure. While multiple types of seizures exist, generalized tonic–clonic seizures are the most common type resulting in collapse. Ictal activity is often self-limited and lasts less than 5 min. Affected individuals may have both tonic (rigid) and clonic (convulsive) motions. They may experience tongue biting and urinary or fecal incontinence during the episode. Afterwards, individuals usually experience a transient post-ictal period characterized by headache, slow mentation, fatigue, and a gradual return to baseline [53].

However, collapse from other etiologies may be misdiagnosed as a seizure and convulsive syncope should be considered in the differential of a suspected seizure. Classic historical features of convulsions and urinary incontinence are not specific to seizures. A 2007 Canadian review of 1,506 patients referred to an epilepsy center with the provisional diagnosis of seizure showed that 12.9% were ultimately diagnosed with neurocardiogenic syncope [54].

The managing physician should be well versed in the acute stabilization and management of seizures. Most seizures are self-limited and require only supportive care. During the event, athletes should be assisted to the ground and protected from dangerous objects. Cushioning near the head will minimize head trauma.

Occasionally, airway support with a chin lift or jaw thrust maneuver is required to maintain ventilation.

For persistent seizures greater than 2–5 min, administration of IV or rectal benzodiazepines such as diazepam may be considered. AED application for cardiac rhythm identification may also be appropriate to exclude dysrhythmia from the differential. Point-of-care testing for hypoglycemia and hyponatremia may also be appropriate, particularly in endurance events or in athletes with no prior seizure history. If present, hypoglycemia and hyponatremia must be treated concurrently with the seizure for optimal management. All athletes with new-onset seizure or secondary seizures should be transported to the emergency department for further evaluation [55].

Trauma

Acute traumatic injuries may also be the source of athletic collapse. In the event of an unwitnessed collapse of an athlete, the provider should quickly assess for secondary signs of head or neck trauma that may be a precipitant or resultant factor of the collapse. In the unconscious athlete, a cervical spine injury should be presumed until proven otherwise. The athlete should remain on the field with cervical spine precautions until appropriate backboard and cervical spine immobilization can be applied or until the athlete has regained consciousness to the level that cervical spine injury may be excluded clinically. On-field management of life-threatening traumatic injuries should consist of attention to the ABCs, initiation of Advanced Trauma Life Support (ATLS) protocols, and prompt activation of the EMS system. Further discussion of ATLS protocols and traumatic injuries are beyond the scope of this chapter.

Case #1

Time: 11:59 AM
Race time 3:59 h

Twenty-year-old male presents to the Main Medical Tent at the Chicago Marathon by field team after a witnessed collapse at the finish line. There was no evidence of trauma. Initially unconscious, the patient responds to pain and loud verbal stimuli upon arrival to medical tent. He is unable to give any further history due to impaired mentation.

PMH: Unknown

Initial Assessment by Field Team

- Airway: intact
- Breathing: intact
- Circulation: tachycardic, present pulses
- Neuro: lethargic, responds only to pain

Initial Assessment at Main Medical

- VS: T_R–108.3, P 150, RR 18, BP 110/75

Blood sugar 94, Istat Na-145

- Focused Physical Exam
  - Neuro: lethargic, responsive to painful stimuli, spontaneous movements of all extremities, +Gag reflex
  - HEENT: dry mucous membranes, atraumatic
  - CV: tachycardic, RR, no murmurs
  - RESP: Lungs clear
  - SKIN: cool, clammy, sweaty
  - CLOTHES: two t-shirts, basketball shorts over top of compression shorts.

Diagnosis: EHS
Algorithm

- Stable vitals (tachy) → altered mental status → elevated temperature = EHS Medical Tent Interventions
- 12:10 PM: Pt cooled with ice packs to axilla and groin and rapidly alternating ice water soaked towels to head, trunk, and extremities
- 12:17 PM: IV started, cool 0.9NS infusing
- 12:30 PM: Repeat Rectal Temp 100.8, pt with clearing mentation. Oral rehydration given.
- 1:30 PM: Pt tolerating PO, asymptomatic. Discharged with family.

Summary

The ability to manage sideline emergencies is critical to participant safety. Fatal athletic collapse, though rare, requires advance preparation for prompt evaluation and management for a favorable outcome in these highly publicized occurrences. An EAP with immediate access to an AED reduces the risk of a fatal SCA. The initial evaluation of a collapsed athlete must focus on the ABCs and early defibrillation when appropriate. In addition, utilization of a simple algorithmic approach similar to that presented in Fig. 8.1 will assist in the evaluation and treatment of the collapsed athletes. In endurance events, EAC is the most common cause of collapse. However, one must be familiar with diagnosis and field management of life-threatening events such as sudden cardiac arrest, EHS, and EAH.

References

1. Blue AG. The collapsed athlete. *Orthop Clin North Am* 2002;33(3):471–8.
2. Annual Report: National Center for Castrophic Sports Injury Research. http://www.unc.edu/depts/nccsi/AllSport.htm. Accessed August 23, 2008.

3. Drezner JA, Courson RW, Roberts WO, Mosesso VN Jr, Link MS, Maron BJ, Inter Association Task Force. Inter Association Task Force recommendations on emergency preparedness and management of sudden cardiac arrest in high school and college athletic programs: a consensus statement. *Prehosp Emerg Care* 2007;11(3):253–71.
4. Drezner JA et al. Use of automated external defibrillators at NCAA Division I universities. *Med Sci Sports Exerc* 2005;37(9):1487–92.
5. Roberts WO, Maron BJ. Evidence for decreasing occurrence of sudden cardiac death associated with the marathon. *J Am Coll Cardiol* 2005;46(7):1373–4.
6. Mary Fran Hazinski RN, Nadkarni VM, Hickey RW, O'Connor R, Becker LB, Zaritsky A. Major changes in the 2005 AHA Guidelines for CPR and ECC: reaching the tipping point for change. *Circulation* 2005;112(24 Suppl):IV206–11.
7. ECC Committee, Subcommittees and Task Forces of the American Heart Association. 2005 American Heart Association Guidelines for cardiopulmonary resuscitation and emergency cardiovascular care. *Circulation* 2005;112(24 Suppl):IV1–203.
8. Howe AS. Heat-related illness in athletes. *Am J Sports Med* 2007;35:1384.
9. Armstrong LE et al. American College of Sports Medicine Position Stand. Exertional heat illness during training and competition. *Med Sci Sports Exerc* 2007;39(3):556–72.
10. Hubbard RW et al. Rapid hypothermia subsequent to oral nicotinic acid ingestion and immersion in warm (30 degrees C) water. *Am J Emerg Med* 1988;6(3):316–7.
11. Richards R, Richards D. Exertion-induced heat exhaustion and other medical aspects of the city to surf fun runs 1978–1984. *Med J Australia* 1984;141:799–805.
12. Bergeron MF et al. Youth football: heat stress and injury risk. *Med Sci Sports Exerc* 2005;37(8):1421–30.
13. Roberts WO. Heat and cold, what does the environment do to marathon injury? *Sports Med* 2007;37(4–5):400–3.
14. Nielson B, Nybo L. Cerebral changes during exercise in the heat. *Sports Med* 2003;33:1–11.
15. Gonzalez-Alonso J,Teller C, Anderson S et al. Influence of body temperature on the development of fatigue during prolonged exercise in the heat. *J Appl Physiol* 1999;86(3):1032–9.
16. Sawka MN, Young AJ, Latzka WA et al. Human tolerance to heat strain during exercise: influence of hydration. *J Appl Physiol* 1992;73(1):368–75.
17. Luke AC et al. Heat injury prevention practices in high school football. *Clin J Sport Med* 2007;17(6):488–93.
18. Armstrong LE, Maresh CM, Crago AE, Adams R, Roberts WO. Interpretation of aural temperatures during exercise, hyperthermia, and cooling therapy. *Med Exerc Nutr Health* 1994;3(1):9–16.
19. Ronneberg K, Roberts WO, McBean AD, Center BA. Temporal artery and rectal temperature measurements in collapsed marathon runners. *Med Sci Sports Exerc* 2008;40(8):1373–5.
20. Roberts WO. Exertional heat stroke during a cool weather marathon: a case study. *Med Sci Sports Exerc* 2006;38(7):1197–202.
21. Casa DJ, Anderson JM, Armstrong LE, Maresh CM. Survival strategy: acute treatment of exertional heat stroke. *J Strength Cond Res* 2006;20:462.
22. Casa DJ et al. Exertional heat stroke in competitive athletes. *Current Sports Med Rep* 2005;4(6):309–17.
23. Roberts WO. Exertional heat stroke in the marathon. *Sports Med* 2007;37(4–5):440–3.
24. Armstrong LE, Crago AE, Adams R, Roberts WO, Maresh CM. Whole-body cooling of hyperthermic runners: comparison of two field therapies. *Am J Emerg Med* 1996;14(4):355–8.
25. Seto CK, Way D, O'Connor N. Environmental illness in athletes. *Clin Sports Med* 2005;24(3):695–718.
26. Danzl DF. Accidental hypothermia In: Marx J (ed.) Rosens Emergency Medicine Concepts and Clinical Practice, 5th Edition. Philadelphia: Mosby; 2002:1979–94.
27. Castellani JW, Young AJ, Ducharme MB, Giesbrecht GG, Glickman E, Sallis RE, American College of Sports Medicine. American College of Sports Medicine position stand: prevention of cold injuries during exercise. *Med Sci Sports Exerc* 2006;38(11):2012–29.
28. Proulx CI et al. Safe cooling limits from exercise induced hyperthermia. *Eur J Appl Physiol* 2006;96(4):434–45.

29. Lee DT, Toner MM, McArdle WD, Vrabas JS, Pandolf KB. Thermal and metabolic responses to cold-water immersion at knee, hip and shoulder levels. *J Appl Physiol* 1997;82:1523–30.
30. Casa DJ et al. Validity of devices that assess body temperature during outdoor exercise in the heat. *J Athl Train* 2007;42(3):333–42.
31. Grueskin J, Tanen DA, Harvey P, Dos Santos F, Richardson WH 3rd, Riffenburgh RH. A pilot study of mechanical stimulation and cardiac dysrhythmias in a porcine model of induced hypothermia. *Wilderness Environ Med* 2007;18(2):133–7.
32. Sakkas P et al. Pharmacotherapy of neuroleptic malignant syndrome. *Psychiatry Ann* 1991;21:157.
33. Lexow K. Severe accidental hypothermia: survival after 6 hours 30 minutes of cardiopulmonary resuscitation. *Arctic Med Res* 1991;50(Suppl 6):112–4.
34. Rosner KH, Kirven J. Exercise associated hyponatremia. *Clin J Am Soc Nephrol* 2007;2:151–61.
35. Almond CS et al. Hyponatremia among runners in the Boston Marathon. *N Engl J Med* 2005;352(15):1550–6.
36. Gardner JW. Death by water intoxication. *Mil Med* 2002;167:432–4.
37. Noakes TD et al. Case proven: exercise associated hyponatraemia is due to overdrinking. So why did it take 20 years before the original evidence was accepted? *Br J Sports Med* 2006;40(7):567–72.
38. Davis DP et al. Exercise-associated hyponatremia in marathon runners: a two year experience. *J Emerg Med* 2001;21(1):47–57.
39. Hew-Butler T et al. Statement of the second international exercise-associated hyponatremia consensus development conference, New Zealand 2007. *Clin J Sport Med* 2008;18:111–21.
40. Hew TD et al. The incidence, risk factors, and clinical manifestations of hyponatremia in marathon runners. *Clin J Sport Med* 2003;13(1):41–7.
41. Cheng JC, Zikos D, Skopicki HA et al. Long-term neurological outcome in psychogenic water drinkers with severe symptomatic hyponatremia: the effect of rapid correction. *Am J Med* 1990;88:561–6.
42. www.overhydration.org. Accessed September 7, 2008.
43. Holt RI. Growth hormone, IGF-1, and insulin and their abuse in sport. *Br J Pharmacol* 2008;154(3):542–56.
44. Parkinson AB, Evans NA. Anabolic angrogenic steroids: a survey of 500 users. *Med Sci Sports Exerc* 2006;38(4):644–51.
45. Kuipers H, Fransen EJ, Keizer HA. Pre-exercise ingestion of carbohydrate and transient hypoglycemia during exercise. *Int J Sports Med* 1999;20(4):227–31.
46. Roberts WO. A 12 year profile of medical injury and illness for the twin cities marathon. *Med Sci Sports Exerc* 2000;32:1549–55.
47. O'Conner FG, Pyne S, Brennan FH, Adirim T. Exercise associated collapse: an algorithmic approach to race day management. *Am J Med Sports* 2003;5:212–7, 229.
48. Sallis R. Dehydration and rehydration. SSE #95: collapse in the endurance athlete. Accessed September 1, 2008. http://www.gssiweb.com/Article_Detail.aspx?articleid=699.
49. Roberts WO. Exercise-associated collapse in endurance events: a classification system. *Phys Sportsmed* 1989;17(5):49–55.
50. Brennan FH, O'Connor FG. Emergency triage of collapsed endurance athletes: a stepwise approach to on-site treatment. *Phys Sportsmed* 2005;33:3.
51. Kenefick RW, Sawka MN. Heat exhaustion and dehydration as causes of marathon collapse. *Sports Med* 2007;37(4–5):378–81.
52. Holtzhausen LM, Noakes TD. Collapsed ultraendurance athlete: proposed mechanisms and an approach to management. *Clin J Sport Med* 1997;7(4):292–301.
53. Ko DY. Tonic–clonic seizures. http://www.emedicine.com/NEURO/topic376.htm. Updated April 5, 2007.
54. Josephson CB et al. Neurocardiogenic syncope: frequency and consequences of its misdiagnosis as epilepsy. *Can J Neurol Sci* 2007;34(2):221–4.
55. Dimberg EL, Burns TM. Management of common neurologic conditions in sports. *Clin Sports Med* 2005;24(3):637–62, ix.

Chapter 9
Syncope/Presyncope in the Competitive Athlete

Chad A. Asplund, Francis G. O'Connor, and Benjamin D. Levine

Introduction

Syncope is a relatively common event in the general population and is not infrequently encountered in athletes. The pathophysiology of all forms of syncope consists of a sudden decrease in cerebral blood flow, though there are many other mechanisms for transient loss of consciousness (TLOC). Syncope, albeit common and disabling, can be associated with an increased risk of sudden death depending on the setting and underlying mechanism. Although syncope is generally a benign event in young adults (less than 35 years of age), in many cases, exercise-related syncope (ERS) may be a prodromal sign of a more ominous condition.

In the young (<35 years of age), congenital cardiomyopathies are the most common cause of sudden death during physical exertion [1]. Hypertrophic cardiomyopathy is the most important cause that has been studied in particular in young American athletes [1]. In some Mediterranean countries, arrhythmogenic right ventricular dysplasia (ARVD) is important and is becoming more widely studied [2]. In the US military, autopsy studies have demonstrated that coronary anomalies are the leading cause of nontraumatic exertional sudden death in recruits, with cardiomyopathies and myocarditis being the next most common, respectively [3]. In children, aortic stenosis is a well-known cause of syncope and exercise-related sudden death [4].

The sports medicine physician is often the first clinician to evaluate and manage patients with ERS and must quickly assess the risk and expedite an appropriate workup. Syncope is a particularly challenging symptom in young athletes that requires careful investigation to resolve critical distinctions between physiologic events such as neurally mediated ("vasovagal") syncope and those related to underlying heart disease. This chapter reviews the differential diagnosis of ERS in young athletes (Fig. 9.1) and outlines a format for evaluation and management.

C.A. Asplund (✉)
Primary Care Sports Medicine, Department of Family Medicine,
Eisenhower Army Medical Center, Fort Gordon, GA 30905
e-mail: chad.asplund@gmail.com

C.E. Lawless (ed.), *Sports Cardiology Essentials: Evaluation, Management and Case Studies*, DOI 10.1007/978-0-387-92775-6_9,

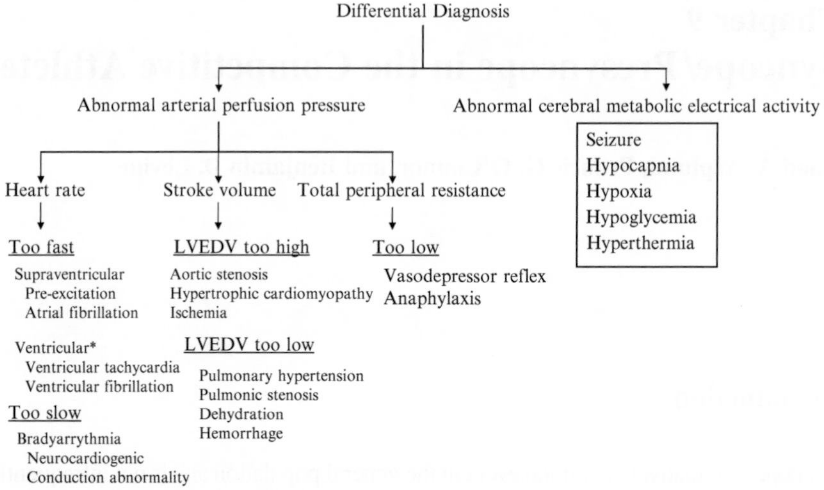

Fig. 9.1 Differential diagnosis of exercise related syncope in athletes. Etiologies of ventricular tachycardia or fibrillation include hypertrophic cardiomyopathy, arrythmogenic right ventricular dysplasia, long QT syndrome, drugs, and ischemia. Adapted from Levine et al. [18]

Definitions

Syncope/Presyncope

Syncope is best defined as a TLOC due to cerebral hypoperfusion, from which recovery is spontaneous [5, 6]. The pathophysiology of all forms of syncope consists of a sudden decrease in cerebral blood flow. Syncope is common, disabling when frequent, and possibly associated with a risk of sudden death, but its causes are difficult to diagnose [5].Presyncope is described as a feeling of lightheadedness that nearly causes collapse, while dizziness is a less well-defined symptom that can be characterized by any sort of abnormal sensation in the head or body. Recent American Heart Association (AHA) guidelines direct that any history of syncope or presyncope in the athlete, especially during exertion, warrants further cardiac preparticipation screening to include, at a minimum, an electrocardiogram [7].

Competitive Athlete

A competitive athlete is defined as one who participates in an organized team or individual sport that requires regular competition against others as a central component, places a high premium on excellence and achievement, and requires some form of systematic (and usually intense) training [8]. Therefore, organized competitive sports are regarded as a distinctive activity and lifestyle. An important component of defining a competitive sports activity concerns whether athletes are able to properly judge when it is prudent to terminate physical exertion or activity.

Exercise-Related Syncope

ERS is syncope that can occur either *during* or *immediately after* a period of exercise. The sports medicine literature also recognizes the term exercise-associated collapse (EAC) to describe athletes who are unable to stand or walk unaided as a result of light-headedness, faintness, dizziness, or syncope causing a collapse that occurs *after* completion of an exertional event [9]. EAC is generally the result of orthostatic hypotension or exhaustion and is usually benign, while ERS is more concerning and deserves further workup. While all exertional syncopal and presyncopal symptoms warrant a clinician's utmost attention, the sports medicine literature is clear in its message that collapse occurring during an exercise event tends to be more ominous than that occurring after event completion.

Epidemiology

In the general population, the most common cause of syncope is neurally mediated, i.e., associated with acute alterations in autonomic nervous system function, generally sympathetic withdrawal with or without increased vagal tone; arrhythmias of multiple etiologies are the next most common cause [5]. Other names for neurally mediated syncope include vasodepressor and vasovagal syncope.

The causes of syncope are highly age dependent [10]. Pediatric and young patients are most likely to have neurally mediated syncope, conversion reactions (psychiatric causes), and primary arrhythmic causes, such as the long QT syndrome (LQTS), and Wolff–Parkinson–White syndrome. In middle age, neurally mediated syncope remains the most frequent cause of syncope. Syncope related to other forms of neurally mediated syncope such as micturition, defecation, and cough, as well as orthostasis and panic disorders, are more common in the middle-aged or elderly patients than in younger patients. In contrast to younger and middle aged patients, elderly patients have a higher frequency of syncope caused by cardiovascular diseases, such as obstructions to cardiac output, e.g., aortic stenosis and pulmonary embolus, and arrhythmias resulting from underlying heart disease [10].

Very little is known about the prevalence of isolated ERS in the normal population, or within the subpopulation of athletes. To date, ERS has not been explicitly characterized in any major epidemiological studies on syncope [11]. However, Colivicchi et al. recently reported in a study of almost 7,500 athletes that

6.2% had reported a syncopal episode in the preceding 5 years. Of these cases of syncope, 87.7% were unrelated to exercise, 12.0% were postexertional, and 1.3% of these were exertional [12].

Syncope seldom occurs during effort. For example, in one recent study [13], syncope during effort was reported in only 17 (5%) of 341 patients referred to three Syncope Units for evaluation of unexplained syncope. In the patients with structural heart disease, syncope during effort was a significant predictor of a cardiac cause of syncope (with an odds ratio of 3.1) with a specificity of 96% [13].

Although there is limited evidence to support the etiology of ERS, several themes are consistent. First, only a minority of syncopal events are associated with physical activity, accounting for only 3–20% of cases [5, 14]. Second, although most cases of syncope in athletes are benign, those athletes who present with exertional syncope (during exertion) have a greater probability of cardiac causes [5, 7].

One study that evaluated collapse following the finish of an ultra marathon found that 85% of the syncope occurred after the runners crossed the finish line. The 15% of those who collapsed during the event were more likely to have an identifiable medical condition, such as heat stroke or hyponatremia. This study strengthens the assertion that collapse following the completion of an event is more likely to be benign and collapse during an event warrants further investigation [15].

Pathophysiology of Exercise-Related Syncope

During exercise, increases in heart rate (HR) and stroke volume (SV) with a decrease in total peripheral resistance (TPR) result in a rise in cardiac output that is proportional to the oxygen uptake and is especially large in endurance athletes [16]. Muscular activity is crucial to maintaining this cardiac output because muscle contractions act as a "second heart" facilitating venous return. After exercise, without this muscular activity to increase venous return, cardiac filling may decrease dramatically because of the reduction in left ventricular end-diastolic volume (LVEDP) and SV, thus temporarily decreasing cerebral blood flow.

Further, the chronic volume loading of and cardiac adaptation of endurance training result in increased effective ventricular compliance and alter the pressure–volume relationship and therefore Starling (SV/LVEDP) relation of the athlete's heart [17]. Such an increased chamber compliance and steep Starling curve are very beneficial to an athlete during participation, facilitating the delivery of large volumes of blood to exercising skeletal muscle. However, this adaptation may be a distinct disadvantage during periods of orthostasis, resulting in a larger effective decrease in SV when filling pressure is reduced.

This underscores the importance of SV in the "triple product" of blood pressure control (HR × SV × TPR). Several studies have suggested that SV might be an important independent factor not under the exclusive control of the autonomic nervous system and therefore an important pathophysiologic factor in ERS [18]. This theory does not exclude autonomic influences on ventricular filling and

Table 9.1 Cause of syncope

Cause of syncope	Mean prevalence (range)
Neurally mediated	
Vasovagal	18% (8–37)
Situational	5% (1–8)
Carotid sinus	1% (0–4)
Psychiatric disorders	2% (1–7)
Medications	3% (1–7)
Neurological disease	10% (3–32)
Cardiac syncope	
Organic heart disease	4% (1–8)
Arrythmias	14% (4–38)
Unknown	34% (13–41)

Adapted from Linzer et al. [22]

contractility but does show that adaptations affecting mechanical diastolic properties of the athlete's heart can explain a significant component of the orthostatic intolerance seen in this group.

Differential Diagnosis

While syncope has an extensive differential diagnosis with many classification systems, ERS in young athletes suggests a more limited set of possibilities (Table 9.1). The most important question to the provider who is evaluating an athlete with syncope or presyncope is "did the episode occur after finishing exercise or during the event?" Those episodes occurring after exercise are much less likely to be caused by structural heart disease.

The majority of syncope that occurs *after* exercise falls into two related categories: (1) neurally mediated syncope, and (2) exaggerated post exercise hypotension. It is possible that neurally mediated syncope is triggered by the hypotension. Both of these categories of syncope affect all ages, although younger athletes are more involved in competitive sports and therefore more represented.

Neurally Mediated Causes

Neurally mediated syncope is generally regarded as the most common cause of syncope in young adults. Neurally mediated syncope occurs when there is a loss of consciousness secondary to a sudden reflex vasodilation or bradycardia, or both. While most causes of neurally mediated syncope in young adults are triggered by situational stressors, neurally mediated mechanisms are also implicated in the majority of exercise-related syncopal events, particularly those that occur after exercise.

Athletes are believed to be particularly predisposed to neurally mediated syncope. High levels of resting vagal tone found in well-trained athletes may sensitize the efferent limb of the neurally mediated reflex. In addition, hemodynamic changes that are beneficial during training may put athletes at greater risk for orthostatic intolerance, making them more susceptible to syncope. Neurally mediated syncope in athletes is generally benign and has a favorable long-term prognosis.

The proper diagnosis of neurally mediated syncope requires the clinician to perform a thorough history and physical examination and incorporate selected testing to specifically exclude known cardiologic entities.

Cardiac Causes

Syncope or presyncope may indicate left ventricular outflow tract obstruction, or arrhythmia. Patients with organic heart diseases – such as coronary, valvular, or congenital heart diseases – or cardiomyopathy are easier to diagnose than patients with cardiac conduction system disease (arrhythmia). Since arrhythmia may be episodic, finding asymptomatic brief arrhythmias or the lack of finding such arrhythmia does not exclude a rhythmic disturbance as a cause of the syncope.

ARVD also termed right ventricular cardiomyopathy, may also be a possible cause of syncope. Although rare, this condition affects otherwise healthy young persons and can be fatal. Clinicians must have a high degree of suspicion in order to diagnose this condition, since the physical examination is often unremarkable. The classic electrocardiogram demonstrates inverted T waves in the right precordial leads, but it may be read as normal. Since this condition often only grossly affects the right ventricle, especially early in the disease process, the diagnosis may be missed on echocardiography. Subtle abnormalities of this chamber may be overlooked unless the reader of the echocardiogram is alerted to the suspicion of right ventricular dysplasia [19, 20].

We believe that in those cases where a cardiac cause for syncope during exertion is entertained, all patients deserve a thorough workup, including electrocardiography, echocardiography, with careful attention to the right ventricle, and a provocative test for arrhythmias such as an exercise stress test or an electrophysiologic study, before the condition is attributed to neurally mediated syncope.

Evaluation

In order to make the cardiac evaluation of ERS simpler and less expensive, several guidelines have been compiled. According to the guidelines on syncope of the European Society of Cardiology (ESC) [21] and a similar statement of the AHA [9], the initial evaluation of patients with syncope is based on a thorough history and physical examination, supine and upright blood pressure measurement, and standard electrocardiogram. Subsequently, three questions should be addressed:

(a) Is it a true syncope (loss of consciousness attributable to cerebral hypoperfusion)? (b) Does the initial evaluation lead to certain diagnosis, suspected diagnosis, or unexplained diagnosis? (c) Is heart disease present? [10, 21]

The approach to the patient with syncope begins with a thorough history (Table 9.2). In most patients, the cause of syncope can be determined with great accuracy from a careful history and physical examination, although the exact mechanism of syncope remains unexplained in approximately 35% of episodes [22].

Various aspects of the history help to establish the diagnosis (Table 9.3). The observations of onlookers are important. The occurrence of tonic-clonic, seizure-like activity may be associated with both cardiac and neurological causes of syncope. It is important to recognize that seizure-like activity that occurs prior to loss of consciousness or postural tone may be due to seizures, but tonic-clonic jerking that occurs after the patient has fallen to the ground and even incontinence may be the final common manifestation of cerebral hypoperfusion and should not necessitate a detailed neurological work-up in all such individuals. Episodes of neurally mediated syncope are typically associated with post episode fatigue or weakness, whereas the absence of a prodrome is consistent with cardiac arrhythmia. Auras, premonitions, postictal confusion, and focal neurological signs and symptoms suggest a neurological cause. A history of myocardial infarction with or without left ventricular dysfunction or repaired congenital heart disease raises the possibility of ventricular arrhythmias. A history of head trauma in a younger person without underlying heart disease may suggest a neurological origin, whereas syncope precipitated by neck turning raises the possibility of carotid sinus hypersensitivity.

Table 9.2 Historical clues for exercise related syncope

General
Prior syncope
Use of supplements/ergogenic aids
History of eating disorder
Cardiac
Age >35
Family history of sudden death
Syncope at rest
Prior cardiac disease
Chest Pain
Syncope during exercise
No prodromal symptoms
Neurological/metabolic
Headaches
Confusion
Dysarthria
Visual symptoms
History of seizure disorder
Anaphalaxis
Pruritis

Adapted from Linzer et al. [22]

Table 9.3 Differentiating cardiac from non-cardiac causes

	Neurally mediated	Possibly cardiac	Possibly neurological
Prodrome	Lightheaded, warmth, nausea	None	Aura, disturbance of vision or smell
Number of episodes	Multiple	Few	Few
Situation	Recent completion of prolonged endurance event, on feet for prolonged period	During exertional event	Anytime
Post syncopal symptoms	Fatigue	None	Fatigue, confusion, amnesia, tongue biting, loss of bowel or bladder function, focal neurological deficits
Structural heart disease	Rare	Common	Rare

Adapted from Link MS, Wang PJ, Estes NA III. Ventricular arrhythmias in the athlete. Curr Opin Cardiol 2001; 16: 33

The patient should be asked specifically if there is a positive family history for unexpected sudden cardiac death.

The history is also useful for identifying aggravating and alleviating factors. The practice of high-risk behaviors such as recreational drug use or eating disorders should be carefully investigated, although athletes may not always openly acknowledge such activity. A comprehensive medication list, including over-the-counter medications and ergogenic aids [23], is necessary for evaluation. Finally, a family history of sudden death is critical and, if present, may identify very-high-risk subgroups with hypertrophic cardiomyopathy, LQTS, or ARVD. It is especially important to have the family create a specific family tree in order to ensure the accurate recollection of all family members who may have died suddenly or unexpectedly at a young age.

Physical Examination

During the evaluation of syncope, a careful physical examination is second only to the history (Table 9.4). Orthostatic hypotension, autonomic dysfunction, and sometimes organic heart disease can be identified by measuring blood pressure and pulse rate in the upper and lower extremities and in the supine and upright positions after at least 3–5 min standing. Carotid bruits raise the question of impaired cerebral blood flow and underlying coronary artery disease. The physical examination can also suggest the presence of pulmonary hypertension, left ventricular dysfunction, valvular heart disease, or other forms of organic heart disease. Abnormalities of cognition and speech, visual fields, motor strength, sensation, tremor, and gait disturbance suggest an underlying neurological disorder.

Table 9.4 Physical examination findings suggestive of cause of ERS

Physical examination finding	Possible diagnosis
Difference in blood pressure between arms	Subclavian steal or aortic dissection
Syncope and murmur with change from sitting to lying	Atrial myxoma or thrombus
Associated with change in position from seated to standing	Orthostatic/postural orthostatic tachycardia
Abnormal dynamic cardiac examination	Structural cardiac disease
Abnormal peripheral vascular examination	
Pulsus paradoxus	Coarctation of the aorta
Slow rising pulse	Aortic stenosis
Bifid pulse	Hypertrophic cardiomyopathy
Wheezing	Anaphalaxis/Asthma
Pectus deformity	Marfan syndrome
High arched palate	
Extreme long wingspan	
Kyphoscoliosis	

In the field, immediately following an event, postsyncopal athletes are best evaluated in a head-down, legs-up position as this may be therapeutic for EAC [24]. The assessment of the collapsed athlete should, of course, begin with assessment of mentation and circulatory status. If the patient is unresponsive and no pulse is confirmed, chest compressions should be started until an automatic or manual defibrillator can be applied and a stable rhythm is confirmed as suggested by the new cardiopulmonary resuscitation guidelines. Once cardiorespiratory status has been established, a thorough history should be obtained, with a particular focus on any presyncopal symptoms and prior episodes.

Physical examination should include a comprehensive neurologic assessment, especially with regard to cognitive function. Vital statistics should be obtained, with the caveat that a rectal temperature is the most reliable means of assessing core temperature after exertion if heat stroke is suspected as a cause for the syncopal episode. Blood pressure in both arms, pulse, and hydration status will provide additional immediate clues. Cardiac and pulmonary examinations should attempt to identify any structural cardiac abnormalities. Careful evaluation of the carotid or radial pulse may demonstrate the bifid pulse (two systolic peaks) of hypertrophic cardiomyopathy or the slow rising pulse (pulsus parvus et tardus) of aortic stenosis.

The cardiac examination begins with chest palpation in an attempt to identify the point of maximal impulse, as well as any thrills or heaves that may identify pathologic conditions. Auscultation should be performed with the patient in the supine, seated, and standing positions. Murmurs, gallops and pathologic splitting should all be noted. Listening to the patient during squatting, while standing, and during a Valsalva maneuver may help to rule out dynamic outflow obstruction. A systolic murmur that gets louder with standing or during a Valsalva maneuver suggests the obstruction of hypertrophic cardiomyopathy. A patient with an identified systolic murmur and a systolic pressure gradient between the upper and lower extremities of greater than 10 mmHg should suggest a diagnosis of aortic stenosis [25].

Electrocardiography (ECG) offers additional information for the physician evaluating syncope, and it is especially helpful if it is entirely normal as this finding is a strong evidence against life-threatening cardiovascular disease (Table 9.5). It has been recognized, however, that abnormal ECGs are common in athletes [26]. The spectrum of abnormalities includes sinus bradycardia, first-and-second degree heart block, early repolarization, left ventricular hypertrophy, and T-wave inversion [27]. However, certain ECG abnormalities are associated with heart disease, and in increased risk of life-threatening arrhythmias, therefore, careful evaluation and a high level of suspicion for abnormalities are needed. Table 9.5 lists some common ECG changes and the conditions that they may represent.

A history, a physical examination, and an electrocardiogram are often sufficient to identify the presence of heart disease. In the setting of an abnormal ECG or with a high suspicion for structural heart disease, echocardiography should be considered. Echocardiography should be performed for the evaluation of murmurs that are diastolic, continuous, holosystolic, or of intensity grade 3 or greater.

If ECG monitoring is unrevealing, either through the inability to record an event or if there is no arrhythmia with symptoms, referral for echocardiogram and/or stress testing may be considered.

Table 9.5 Common ECG changes found in various conditions associated with syncope

ECG abnormalities	Likely condition
Normal	Neurocardiogenic syncope
	Anomalous coronary arteries
Left ventricular hypertrophy	Hypertrophic cardiomyopathy
Q-waves anteriorly	
Rarely normal	
Pre-excitation	Supraventricular tachycardia
Left bundle branch block	Idiopathic dilated cardiomyopathy
Prolonged QT	
Can be normal	
Prolonged QT	Prolonged QT syndrome
Abnormal appearance ST segment	
Right bundle branch block (complete or incomplete)	Brugada syndrome
Anterior ST elevation	
Changes vary with time	
Short PR interval	Wolf–Parkinson–White syndrome
Delta waves	
Pseudoinfarct pattern	
Left ventricular hypertrophy	Aortic stenosis
T wave inversion V1-V3	Right ventricular dysplasia
Epsilon wave	
Pre-ventricular contractions	
Left bundle branch block	

Echocardiography

In other patients with recurrent syncope and a normal baseline assessment, the initial investigations should be aimed at identifying occult structural heart disease. Because structural heart disease is a strong predictor of mortality among patients with syncope, an echocardiogram, a stress test, or both are needed when the presence or absence of underlying cardiac disease cannot be determined clinically. Echocardiography should precede exercise-stress testing, and it allows the clinician to assess ventricular size and function, estimate pulmonary pressures, and rule out valvular dysfunction.

Echocardiogram should only be used in the patient suspected of a structural abnormality, and it is not recommended as a screening tool for sudden cardiac death [28].Echocardiograms rarely reveal unsuspected abnormalities of cardiac function (in 5–10% of patients), and the discovery of such abnormalities does not necessarily lead to the diagnosis of a cause [29].

In the young athlete, echocardiography can specifically assist in making the diagnosis of hypertrophic cardiomyopathy, aortic stenosis, and pulmonary hypertension. The echocardiogram should be specifically examined for the presence of the left coronary ostium, which should arise from the left sinus of Valsalva. If present, it excludes an important congenital coronary anomaly often reported to cause sudden cardiac death. If not clearly identified further testing could be required.

The exercise stress test should be performed after the echocardiogram. Rather than a standard Bruce protocol, a test should be designed to reproduce the conditions that provoked the specific syncopal event and challenge the individual athlete, for example, a stuttering start–stop test for a basketball or soccer player or a prolonged high-intensity tests for a runner. The exercise electrocardiogram should also be examined for appropriate shortening of the QT interval. Further testing should be ordered only as indicated and in consultation with the appropriate specialist.

Further Diagnostic Testing

A serious problem in the evaluation of syncope is the lack of a gold standard against which the results of diagnostic tests can be assessed. Thus, measurements of the sensitivity and specificity of these tests are often not possible [30]. Since syncope is a symptom and not a disease, the diagnostic evaluation has focused on physiologic states that could plausibly cause a sudden loss of consciousness. This type of reasoning leads to uncertainty in the diagnosis unless pathophysiologic abnormalities are found during the occurrence of the episode, which happens rarely.

Long-term ECG monitoring with Holter monitors can be useful in those patients with frequent reproducible symptoms. Athletes with intermittent symptoms are best evaluated with a continuous loop monitor.

Ambulatory Monitoring

In studies of ambulatory (Holter) monitoring, symptoms are found to occur in conjunction with arrhythmias in only 4% of patients (leading to a diagnosis of arrhythmic syncope), and symptoms occur without arrhythmias in 17% (potentially ruling out arrhythmic syncope). In 79% of patients, either brief arrhythmias or no arrhythmias are found [31]. Arrhythmic syncope cannot be excluded in these patients, because arrhythmias may be episodic. A recent study found, however, that increasing the duration of monitoring to periods as long as 72 h did not increase the yield for symptomatic arrhythmias [22]. Thus in patients with exertional syncope occurring rarely (or only once), the key to establishing that an arrhythmia is not the cause of syncope is to make a recording during an event, either directly observed during exercise testing, or with much more prolonged periods of recording.

Continuous-Loop Event Monitoring

Continuous-loop recorders are used for long-term monitoring (lasting weeks or months). The patient or an observer can activate the monitor after symptoms occur, thereby freezing in its memory the readings from the previous 2–5 min and the subsequent 60 s. In patients with frequently recurring syncope (a median of 15–30 episodes per patient), arrhythmias were found during syncope in 8–20%, and normal rhythm was found during symptoms in 12–27% [22]. The limitations of this test are the need for compliance on the part of the patient and the potential for errors in using the device and problems with transmission.

Recently, an implantable continuous-loop recorder that is inserted subcutaneously and has the capability of performing cardiac monitoring for up to 18 months was used in patients with recurrent syncope of undiagnosed cause [32]. Among the 85 patients studied, 18 with bradycardia and 3 with tachycardia were identified when symptoms recurred at a mean of 2.3 months after implantation [32]. This method of monitoring is likely to be applicable in a small percentage of cases, but further studies are needed to define its role.

Tilt Table

For neurally mediated syncope associated with exercise, tilt table testing and exercise testing have been suggested. However, the diagnostic value of tilt table testing may be low since symptoms are not often reproducible [33]. In addition, since athletes have a unique susceptibility to orthostatic hypotension and tilt-induced syncope [34], positive tilt results should not be used to rule out other potential diagnoses, in particular hypertrophic cardiomyopathy [35]. As above, ECG, echocardiography, and exercise testing should be performed in all cases of exertional syncope.

Upright tilt-table testing, which is frequently used in the evaluation of nonathletes with syncope of undetermined etiology, is not useful in well-trained athletes because orthostatic stress may cause a positive result in many athletes with no clinical history of syncope [33]. In fact, reliance on tilt-table testing to make a diagnosis of neurally mediated syncope in an athlete may provide a false sense of security with potentially catastrophic consequences [36]. Given the high likelihood of false positives in athletes, it is our recommendation that tilt table testing should be used with great caution in the evaluation of ERS in the athlete.

In conclusion, in the absence of structural heart disease, syncope occurring during or immediately after exercise is generally a benign condition, either in athletes or in the sedentary population; its etiology is likely to be neutrally mediated irrespective of the result of tilt testing. There is no reason to consider athletes different from sedentary subjects. The absence of structural heart disease is the strongest predictor of good outcome. No other test seems useful for risk stratification as no test adds more to the prognostic significance given by the absence of heart disease; thus, several investigations could be safely avoided.

Electrophysiologic Studies

The yield of electrophysiologic tests depends on whether there is an abnormal ECG or presence of structural heart disease. Among patients with heart disease, approximately 21% have inducible ventricular tachycardia and 34% have bradycardia (14% have multiple diagnoses). In patients with abnormal electrocardiograms (revealing conduction abnormalities), 3% have inducible ventricular tachycardia and 19% have bradycardia [37]. In patients with a normal heart and a normal electrocardiogram, only 1% have ventricular tachycardia and 10% have bradycardia [37]. It has been found that while electrophysiologic tests are good at detecting tachyarrhythmia, they have poor sensitivity and specificity for bradyarrhythmias [38]. See Chapter 10 for discussion of the role of electrophysiology in the approach to the athlete with syncope.

Management of Syncope

The clinical approach to a patient with syncope is determined by the mode of presentation (Fig. 9.2) The most likely cause in the athletic population is vasovagal syncope, and in a patient with a characteristic history, and a normal physical examination and ECG, no further investigation is necessary. Patients should not participate in athletics during this evaluation [39].

The treatment should be aimed initially at increasing salt and fluid intake. The patient should be encouraged to maintain hydration. If the prodrome of an episode is recognized, the patient should lie flat until the episode passes. These measures, along with patient education, will frequently be all that is required.

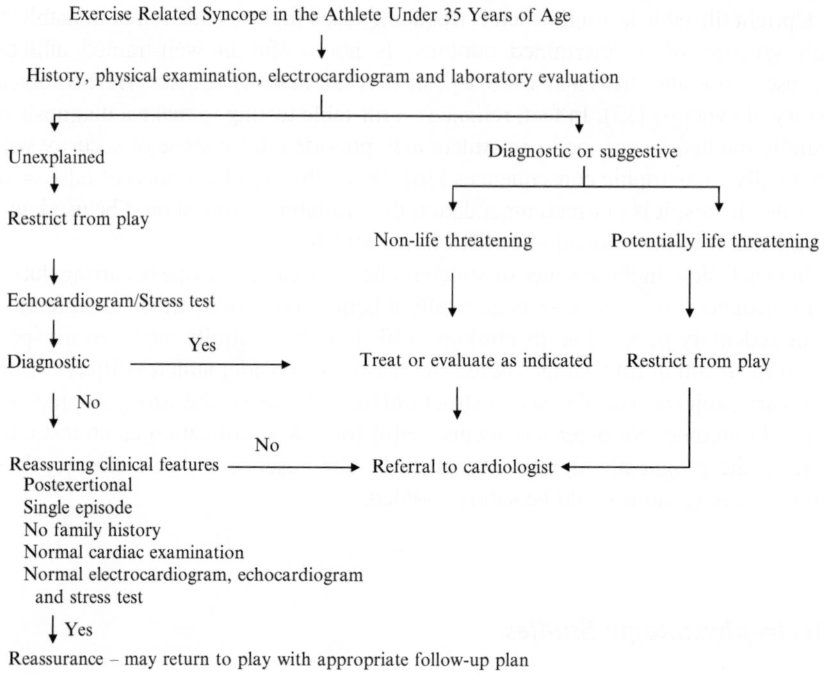

Fig. 9.2 Evaluation of exercise related syncope. Adapted from O'Connor et al. [39]

Management of neurally mediated syncope in competitive athletes is controversial. The condition is optimally managed by a consultant who is familiar with this population. While pharmacologic therapy may be warranted in carefully selected cases, the use of any medication in the management of neurally mediated syncope is controversial, and physicians should be reluctant to prescribe any drugs in these conditions [20].

In a few select patients in whom episodes are frequent, pharmacological therapy may be required. Beta blockers are usually recommended as first-line therapy, but the effect on athletic performance may be unacceptable and recent clinical trials suggest that they do not prevent syncope. Moreover, beta blockers are considered banned substances in certain sports. Alternative approaches include plasma volume expanders such as fludrocortisone, vasoconstrictors such as midodrine, and serotonin reuptake inhibitors such as sertraline or fluoxetine. These latter compounds act by modulating the brainstem reflexes that underlie fainting. Because pharmacologic therapy is controversial, specialist referral should probably be advised.

The baseline assessment of the patient may rarely be diagnostic in other circumstances. For example, the surface ECG may reveal complete heart block, or an account from a witness may strongly suggest a seizure disorder. More commonly in patients with diagnoses other than obvious vasovagal syncope, the initial assessment will be normal and further investigation will be required. These patients merit referral for specialist evaluation. Patients with obvious structural heart disease, for example, a history of ischemic heart disease or cardiomyopathy, should be referred to a specialist immediately. If syncope or presyncope remains unexplained, the patient should be referred to a cardiologist. Symptomatic patients should be evaluated thoroughly before returning to athletic participation [40, 41].

Return to Play

A critical decision for the sports medicine provider who encounters a case of ERS is, "Can the athlete safely return to play?" Generally, for athletes without structural cardiac defects, in whom syncope occurred after exercise, return to play is likely. In a recent study of 17 athletes with the correct diagnosis of exercise-induced vasodepressor syncope, who were followed for a mean of 35 months, it was found that with appropriate management, neither recreational nor competitive athletes needed to eliminate or modify their athletic activities [42].

Those athletes with structural or electrical defects noted on exam or those with syncope during exertion should be restricted until definitive diagnosis is made, and return-to-play decision should be made with appropriate specialty consultation [8].

When making eligibility-and-disqualification decisions, it is important to follow current clinical guidelines, such as the ESC or AHA guidelines. Often there are pressures from athletes, parents, or coaches to maintain athletes' eligibility. However, the law supports limiting high school and college athletes with cardiovascular abnormalities from participation in competitive sports if there are unacceptable medical risks [43]. This type of decision making however is quite complex and may not always be clear, especially for professional athletes for whom exclusion represents the loss of livliehood [44].

Conclusion

Athletes with syncope warrant a full evaluation. Athletes will commonly have benign neurally mediated syncope, which is the most frequent cause of syncope in the young. However, it is possible that exertion may unmask underlying heart disease, either electrical or structural, and that these athletes may be at increased risk of sudden death. The key for the clinician is to determine correctly benign versus serious causes of ERS. Those with benign conditions may return to play and those with more serious conditions should be restricted according to current guidelines. Athletes for whom syncope could be situationally life threatening for themselves or others (i.e., bicyclists or mountaineers) should be made aware of these dangers and possibly advised to take additional safety measures or, if not possible, cease athletics. The diagnosis, treatment, and management of ERS and presyncope offer a challenge to the sports medicine provider, but with a thorough, well-guided approach, safe return to sports may be possible.

References

1. Maron BJ. Cardiovascular risks to the young person on the athletic field. Ann Int Med 1998; 129(5): 379–386.
2. Ananthasubramaniam K, Khaja F. Arrhythmogenic right ventricular dysplasia/cardiomyopathy: review for the clinician. Prog Cardiovasc Dis 1998; 41: 237–246.
3. Eckart RE, Scoville SL, Campbell CL, et al. Sudden death in young adults: a 25-year review of autopsies in military recruits. Ann Intern Med 2004; 141: 829–834.
4. Maron, BJ. Sudden death in young athletes. N Engl J Med 2003; 349: 1064–1075.
5. Kapoor W. Syncope. N Engl J Med 2000; 343(25): 1856–1862.
6. Thijs RD, Wieling W, Kaufmann H, et al. Defining and classifying syncope. Clin Auton Res 2004; 14(S1): 4–8.
7. Maron BJ, Thompson PD, Ackerman MJ, et al. Recommendations and considerations related to preparticipation screening for cardiovascular abnormalities in competitive athletes: 2007 update. Circulation 2007; 115: 1643–1655.
8. Mitchell JH, Haskell W, Snell P, et al. Task Force 8: classification of sports. 36th Bethesda Conference: eligibility recommendations for competitive athletes with cardiovascular abnormalities. J Am Coll Cardiol 2005; 45: 1364–1367.
9. Roberts WO. Exercise-associated collapse in endurance events. A classification system. Phys Sportsmed 1989; 17: 49–57.
10. Strickberger SA, Benson DW, Biaggioni I, et al. AHA/ACCF Scientific Statement on the evaluation of syncope: from the American Heart Association Councils on Clinical Cardiology, Cardiovascular Nursing, Cardiovascular Disease in the Young, and Stroke, and the Quality of Care and Outcomes Research Interdisciplinary Working Group; and the American College of Cardiology Foundation: in collaboration with the Heart Rhythm Society: endorsed by the American Autonomic Society. Circulation 2006; 113: 316–327.
11. Sarasin FP, Louis-Simonet M, Carballo D, et al. Prospective evaluation of patients with syncope. Am J Med 2001; 111: 177–184.
12. Colivicchi F, Ammirati F, Santini M, et al. Epidemiology and prognostic implications of syncope in young competing athletes. Eur Heart J 2004; 25: 1749–1753.
13. Alboni P, Brignole M, Menozzi C et al. The diagnostic value of history in patients with syncope with or without heart disease. J Am Coll Cardiol 2001; 37: 1921–1928.
14. Driscoll DJ, Jacobsen SJ, Porter CJ, et al. Syncope in children and adolescents. J Am Coll Cardiol 1997; 29(5): 1039–1045.
15. Holtzhausen L, Noakes TD, Kroning B, et al. Clinical and biochemical characteristics of collapsed ultramarathon runners. Med Sci Sports Exerc 1994; 26: 1095–1101.
16. Levine BD. VO2max: What do we know, and what do we still need to know? J Physiol 2008; 586.1: 25–34.
17. Levine BD, Lane LD, Buckey JC Jr, et al. Left ventricular pressure-volume and Frank-Starling relations in endurance athletes: implication for orthostatic tolerance and exercise performance. Circulation 1991; 84: 1016–1023.
18. Levine BD, Buckey JC, Fritsch JM, et al. Physical fitness and cardiovascular regulation: mechanisms of orthostatic intolerance. J Appl Physiol 1991; 70: 112–122.
19. Corrado D, Basso C, Schiavon M et al. Screening for hypertrophic cardiomyopathy in young athletes. N Engl J Med 1998; 339: 364–369.
20. Marcus FI, Fontaine GH, Guiraudon G, et al. Right ventricular dysplasia: a report of 24 adult cases. Circulation 1982; 65: 384–398.
21. Brignole M, Alboni P, Benditt DG, et al. Guidelines on management (diagnosis and treatment) of syncope – update 2004. Europace 2004; 6: 467–537.
22. Linzer M, Pritchett ELC, Pontinen M, et al. Incremental diagnostic yield of loop electrocardiographic recorders in unexplained syncope. Am J Cardiol 1990; 66: 214–219.
23. Nasir JM, Durning SJ, Ferguson M, et al. Exercise-induced syncope associated with qt prolongation and ephedra-free xenadrine. Mayo Clin Proc 2004; 79(8): 1059–1062.

24. McAward KJ, Moriarty JM. Exertional syncope and presyncope. Phys Sportsmed 2005; 33: 7–20, 41.
25. Ing FF, Stare TJ, Griffiths SP, et al. Early diagnosis of coarctation of the aorta in children: a continuing dilemma. Pediatrics 1996; 98(3): 378–382.
26. Pellicia A, Maron BJ, Cuasso F, et al. Clinical significance of abnormal electrocardiographic patterns in trained athletes. Circulation 2000; 102: 278–284.
27. Zehender M, Meinertz T, Keul J, et al. ECG variants and cardiac arrythmias in athletes: clinical relevance and prognostic importance. Am Heart J 1990; 119: 1378–1391.
28. Ritter S, Tani LY, Etheridge SP, et al. What is the yield of screening echocardiography in pediatric syncope? Pediatrics 2000; 105(5): e58.
29. Recchia D, Barzilai B. Echocardiography in the evaluation of patients with syncope. J Gen Intern Med 1995; 10: 649–655.
30. Linzer M, Yang EH, Estes NA, et al. Diagnosing syncope. Part 1: value of history, physical examination, and electrocardiography. Clinical efficacy assessment project of the American College of Physicians. Ann Intern Med 1997; 126(12): 989–996.
31. Bass EB, Curtiss EI, Arena VC, et al. The duration of Holter monitoring in patients with syncope: is 24 hours enough? Arch Intern Med 1990; 150: 1073–1078.
32. Krahn AD, Klein GJ, Yee R, et al. Use of an extended monitoring strategy in patients with problematic syncope. Circulation 1999; 99: 406–410.
33. Kosinski D, Brubb BP, Karas BJ, et al. Clinical data, pathophysiological aspects, and potential role of tilt table testing. Europace 2000; 2: 77–82.
34. Grubb BP, Temesy-Armos PN, Samoil D, et al. Tilt table testing in the evaluation and management of athletes with recurrent exercise induced syncope. Med Sci Sports Exerc 1993; 25(1): 24–28.
35. Raven PB, Pawelczyk JA. Chronic endurance exercise training: a condition of inadequate blood pressure regulation and reduced tolerance to LBNP: Symposium. Med Sci Sports Exerc 1993; 25(6): 713–721.
36. Johnson WO. Heart of the matter. Sports Illus 1993; 24: 36–41.
37. Linzer M, Yang EH, Estes NA, et al. Diagnosing syncope. Part 2: unexplained syncope. Clinical efficacy assessment project of the American College of Physicians. Ann Intern Med 1997; 127(1): 76–86.
38. Fujimura O, Yee R, Klein GJ, et al. The diagnostic sensitivity of electrophysiologic testing in patients with syncope caused by transient bradycardia. N Engl J Med 1989; 321: 1703–1707.
39. O'Connor FG, Oriscello RG, Levine BD. Exercise-related syncope in the young athlete: reassurance, restriction or referral? Am Fam Physician 1999; 60(7): 2001–2008.
40. Maron BJ, Zipes DP. Introduction: eligibility recommendations for competitive athletes with cardiovascular abnormalities-general considerations. J Am Coll Cardiol 2005; 45: 1318–1321.
41. American Academy of Pediatrics Committee on Sports Medicine and Fitness. Cardiac dysrhythmias and sports. Pediatrics 1995; 95: 786–788.
42. Calkins H, Seifert M, Morady F. Clinical presentation and long-term follow-up of athletes with exercise-induced vasodepressor syncope. Am Heart J 1995; 129: 1159–1164.
43. Paterick TE, Paterick TJ, Fletcher GF, et al. Medical and legal issues in the cardiovascular evaluation of competitive athletes. JAMA 2005; 294: 3011–308.
44. Levine BD, Stray-Gundersen J. The medical care of competitive athletes: the role of the physician and individual assumption of risk. Med Sci Sports Exerc 1994; 26: 1190–1192.

Chapter 10
Electrophysiological Approach to Syncope and Near-Syncope in the Athlete

Rakesh Gopinathannair and Brian Olshansky

Case

A 20-year-old male college basketball player passes out 2 minutes after finishing a training session. He recovers consciousness in a few seconds without confusion, nausea, or vomiting but does not remember anything that happened. Vital signs on recovery are normal. No seizure activity was noted by teammates and a coach who was present. He denies any previous episodes as well as a family history of sudden death. However, he does mention being dizzy recently while practicing but this was very transient. He reminds his physician that he has a national level tournament coming up next week and insists on playing.

This scenario highlights the often dramatic, potentially dangerous, symptom of syncope in the athlete and the challenges faced by the evaluating physician. This chapter discusses the significance, etiology, evaluation, and management of syncope in the athlete. Several illustrative cases are presented towards the end of the chapter to highlight the myriad causes as well as complexities involved in diagnosing and managing athletes with arrhythmic causes of syncope.

Introduction

Syncope, by definition, is a transient loss of consciousness associated with a loss of postural tone followed usually by rapid and complete recovery. This usually results from sudden cerebral hypoperfusion, specifically to the reticular activating system. Syncope should be differentiated from *aborted sudden cardiac death* where there is no rapid and complete recovery and usually requires advanced cardiac life support. This is very essential as *aborted sudden cardiac death* carries a worse prognosis and has significant implications on treatment and quality of life.

R. Gopinathannair (✉)
Assistant Professor of Medicine, Division of Cardiology,
Section of Electrophysiology, University of Louisville Hospitals, Louisviller, KY 40202
e-mail: DRRAKESHG@YAHOO.com

C.E. Lawless (ed.), *Sports Cardiology Essentials: Evaluation, Management and Case Studies*, DOI 10.1007/978-0-387-92775-6_10,

Syncope is a nonspecific symptom with multiple causes ranging from benign causes such as vasovagal (i.e., neurocardiogenic) syncope to life-threatening ventricular arrhythmias. Syncope in the athlete is a dramatic event and often leads to tremendous concern. A policy conference [1] concerning arrhythmias and the athlete concluded that despite considerable advances in the knowledge regarding the mechanism, diagnosis, and therapy of arrhythmias in the athlete, much remains unknown. This is particularly true with the problem of syncope. Despite guidelines and recommendations [1–3], most of our knowledge comes from anecdotal case reports and our fear of what might occur in an athlete with syncope.

Significance of Syncope and Near-Syncope in the Athlete

The problem with syncope in the athlete is that there can be recurrent symptoms, i.e., they can pass out and hurt themselves during continued athletic events; there can be risk of injury from syncope but, most importantly, syncope may be a premonitory sign for arrhythmic or other types of cardiovascular or noncardiovascular deaths.

There are specific reasons to consider that athletes are different than other individuals who pass out. This is because the athlete is highly visible and syncope is a frightening event. The problem is further compounded by the fact that athletes have a drive to push themselves beyond standard amounts of exertion and they can deny that they have a problem. Therefore, it is possible, and even likely, that an athlete may have had near-syncope or even frank syncope and continue high levels of physical activity despite the fact that they may be at increased risk. In addition, athletes have specific physiological adaptations and stresses that may accentuate the risk of adverse cardiovascular consequences.

Syncope in the athlete can be associated with harmful and potentially life-threatening cardiovascular consequences. It must be taken seriously in every athlete who passes out during an athletic event. In fact, syncope precedes sudden death in up to 17–23% of athletes who ultimately die [4, 5]. In a study of 44 soldiers who had syncope, 16% had syncope during exercise and sudden death during exertion occurred in 86% of these cases [5], illustrating the importance of syncope during exertion.

The prognostic significance of syncope has been related primarily to its specific cause and to the presence of structural heart disease [6, 7]. The presence of structural heart disease has been associated with increased mortality in patients with syncope [8, 9]. The Framingham study [6] indicated that there is a relationship between the presumed cause for syncope and its prognosis. Presumed cardiac syncope was an independent predictor of the risk of death (HR 2.01, $p < 0.001$). Vasovagal (neurocardiogenic) syncope was associated with a benign prognosis, while syncope of unknown cause carried an intermediate risk for all-cause mortality (HR 1.32, $p < 0.01$). From these data, it remained unclear whether syncope was causally related to the risk of death or an unrelated marker of poor prognosis.

Syncope, as a prognostic indicator, may be disease-dependent. Syncope indicates a particularly high risk of death in patients with specific genetic cardiac disorders such as arrhythmogenic cardiomyopathies, short and long QT syndromes, and Brugada syndrome [10–13]. When present along with other noninvasive risk factors, recurrent syncope has been generally accepted as an indicator of increased sudden death in patients with hypertrophic cardiomyopathy [14]. Recent prospective data indicate that in patients with structural heart disease, syncope is an independent predictor of all cause and cardiovascular mortality and that this excess risk may not be ameliorated by therapeutic modalities like Implantable defibrillators (ICDs) and antiarrhythmic drugs like amiodarone [15]. Whether this is true in the athlete with structural heart disease and syncope is not clear.

However, all syncope does not necessarily portend a poor prognosis. It can also depend on the age of the athlete, the type of athletic event, and the time relationship between syncope and the athletic event. For example, a proportion of young patients, including athletes, who die suddenly have long QT syndrome. However, they most often die when they are not involved in an athletic event or when they are not even involved with any physical exertion at all [16].

In addition, there is some evidence that syncope per se is not a real concern in the athlete. In a study by Colivicchi et al. of 7,568 athletes, only 6.2% ($n = 474$) had syncope. Of the athletes with syncope, 12% had post-exertional syncope, 1.3% had exertional syncope, and the rest had non-exertional syncope. Of those athletes with syncope unrelated to exercise, the great majority had neurally mediated or situational types of syncope by history. Post-exertional syncope was generally due to post-exertional postural hypotension. In the six athletes with exertional syncope (1.3%), the diagnosis was made of a significant structural heart disease in two (33%) and the remaining four had exercise-induced neurally mediated syncope [17].

Overall, only 2 out of 474 athletes with syncope had underlying heart disease and both had exercise-induced syncope. Of the athletes with non-exertional and post-exertional syncope ($n = 468$) and those without history of syncope, none had underlying heart disease. However, it should be mentioned that this assessment was based on history, physical, 12-lead electrocardiogram, and limited exercise testing. Only those athletes with exercise-induced syncope ($n = 6$) underwent extensive cardiac testing involving echocardiogram, electrophysiology study, and tilt-table testing. Whether extensive cardiac evaluation in athletes with non-exertional and post-exertional syncope would have unearthed underlying structural cardiac disease with potential prognostic implications remain unclear but their long term prognosis was good.

Syncope-free survival was similar with non-exertional syncope and post-exertional syncope but there was not enough data to substantiate that exertional syncope had a similar outcome. No major adverse cardiovascular outcomes were noted in the entire study population at 6.4 ± 3.1 years of follow up [17]. These results need to be confirmed in other populations.

In a similar study, 33 athletes with recurrent exercise-related syncope (mean number of spells before evaluation: 4.66 ± 1.97) underwent extensive evaluation and were followed up over a period of 34 ± 17 months. Out of 33, the only structural heart disease noted was mitral valve prolapse in two. The majority of them had a positive response (syncope occurring in association with hypotension and/or bradycardia) to head-up tilt testing, which the authors considered as diagnostic for neurally mediated syncope. Over the follow-up period, 33% had recurrence of syncope, but no major adverse cardiovascular events were recorded in any subject. The authors concluded that recurrent exercise-related syncope is not associated with an adverse outcome in an athlete without significant heart disease [18].

Despite conflicting data, syncope should still be considered a "red flag" when it happens in an athlete, and especially during athletics or any exertion, in particular. It warrants a thorough evaluation to rule out underlying cardiac conditions that could be potentially life-threatening if the athlete were to continue his activities.

Epidemiology

In the United States general population, syncope is a common clinical problem that is responsible for approximately 1–6% of hospital admissions and 3% of emergency room visits [19]. The actual epidemiology and real risk of syncope in the athlete is not clearly known. The only epidemiological data available at present is from a study by Colivicchi et al. [17]. In this study of 7,568 competitive athletes, 6.2% (474) had a history of syncope. Of these, 87% (411) had syncope but not during exercise, 12% (57) had post-exertional syncope, and 1.3% (6) had exertional syncope [17]. These data are shown in Fig. 10.1.

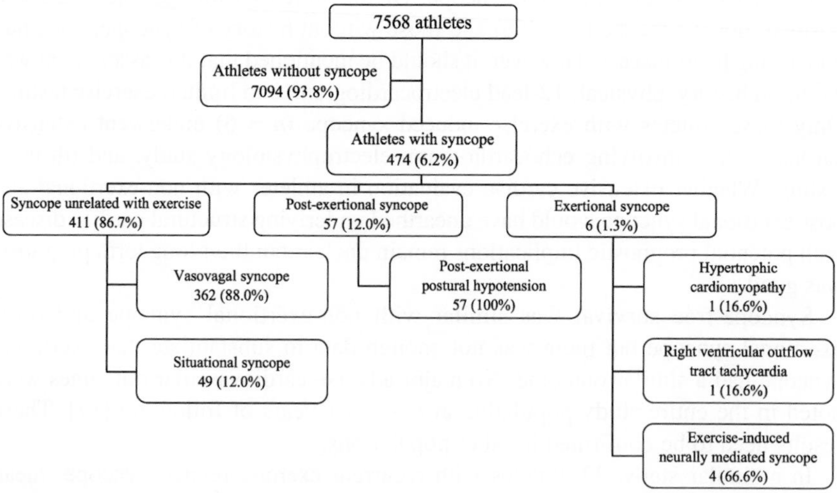

Fig. 10.1 Incidence and causes of syncope in 7,568 young athletes. Reproduced with permission from [17]

Mechanisms and Causes of Syncope and Near-Syncope in the Athlete

Like in the general population, the causes of syncope in the athlete can be divided into noncardiovascular, cardiovascular, and unexplained or unknown causes (Table 10.1). Since syncope precedes sudden death in up to 23% of the athletic population [4, 5], the causes of syncope are intertwined with causes of sudden cardiac death. In athletes <35 years of age, hypertrophic cardiomyopathy was the single largest cause of sudden cardiac death, followed by commotio cordis and anomalous coronary arteries [20]. In athletes >35 years of age, coronary artery disease stands out as the single most common cause of sudden cardiac death [20, 21].

Noncardiovascular causes for syncope predominate in the athlete. A common cause is dehydration, which is sometimes intentional as for example in the wrestler. Hyperventilation, leading to decreased pCO_2, can cause decreased cerebral blood flow by causing cerebral vasoconstriction leading to syncope. Valsalva maneuver, as can occur with sudden heavy lifting, results in reduced venous return to the left heart and can result in syncope. Loss of peripheral muscle pumps while stopping after a marathon can lead to syncope due to hypotension. Circulating mediators such as histamine or serotonin can cause vasodilatation and syncope. Various drugs and over-the-counter supplements such as Ma-huang [22], androgenic steroids, creatine, erythropoietin [23], ephedra and other sympathomimetic substances [24], and cocaine can trigger arrhythmias as well as fluid shifts that can lead to hypotension and loss of consciousness.

Neurocardiogenic (or, perhaps, better stated, neurally mediated exercise related) syncope is another potential cause for syncope but only rarely occurs during running or during aerobic activity in which the legs are moving. On the other hand, "autonomic failure," which is perhaps a form of neurocardiogenic syncope, may be more likely in the athlete during or after heavy physical exertion.

Cardiovascular causes for syncope can be due to hemodynamic collapse from conditions such as aortic stenosis which can lead to decreased blood flow as a result of mechanical obstruction from the stenotic valve or due to a neurocardiogenic reflex from machanoreceptor activation due to increased left ventricular wall stress from the valve obstruction [25]. Similarly, hypertrophic cardiomyopathy can lead to syncope from mechanical left ventricular outflow tract obstruction, ventricular arrhythmia, a neurocardiogenic reflex, or even from diastolic dysfunction [26]. Other cardiomyopathies, myocarditis, aortic dissection, acute pulmonary embolism, and other vascular abnormalities can lead to cardiovascular and hemodynamic collapse, resulting in syncope.

Various ischemic causes for syncope are known. These can be due to anomalous coronary artery and is more likely to occur in athletes <35 years of age [20, 27, 28]. The anomalies include a single or aberrant ostium, a tunneled or bridged left anterior descending artery, hypoplasia of the coronary arteries, or coronary spasm. In younger individuals, Kawasaki disease is another potential cause for ischemia-mediated

Table 10.1 Causes of syncope in the athlete

- Noncardiovascular
  - Reflex mechanisms
    - Vasovagal and vasodepressor syncope (neurocardiogenic syncope)
    - Carotid sinus hypersensitivity
    - Situational (micturition, defecation, deglutition, cough)
    - Valsalva maneuver (heavy lifting)
    - Trigeminal neuralgia
  - Orthostatic hypotension
    - Dysautonomias
      - Pure autonomic failure (Bradbury-Eggleston syndrome)
      - Multiple system atrophy (Shy-Drager syndrome)
    - Fluid depletion (possibly intentional)
    - Loss of peripheral muscle pump (e.g., stopping after a marathon)
    - Drugs (antidepressants, sympathetic blockers)
    - Postural orthostatic tachycardia syndrome
  - Psychogenic
    - Hysterical
    - Panic disorder
    - Anxiety disorder
  - Metabolic
    - Hypoglycemia
    - Hyperventilation (hypocapnea)
    - Hypoxemia
  - Primary neurogenic
    - Seizures
    - Major stroke
    - Migraine
    - Arnold-Chiari malformation
  - Drug-induced
    - Ma Huang
    - Steroids
    - Cocaine
    - Ephedra and other sympathomimetic agents
    - Creatine
    - Erythropoeitin
- Cardiovascular
  - Arrhythmic causes
    - Bradyarrhythmias
      - AV block with bradycardia
      - Sinus pauses with bradycardia
      - Pacemaker malfunction
    - Tachyarrhythmias
      - Supraventricular tachycardia
      - Atrial fibrillation/atrial flutter with rapid rates
      - Monomorphic ventricular tachycardia
      - Polymorphic ventricular tachycardia (Torsade de pointes)

(continued)

Table 10.1 (continued)

Nonarrhythmic causes
Hypertrophic cardiomyopathy
Aortic stenosis
Left atrial myxoma
Cardiac tamponade
Myocarditis
Mitral stenosis
Myocardial ischemia/infarction
Anomalous coronary artery (<35 years old)
Kawasaki disease
Coronary artery disease (>35 years old)
Aortic dissection
Acute pulmonary embolism
Pulmonary hypertension
Subclavian steal
Syncope of unknown origin

syncope during exertion [28]. For those over the age of 35, the most common cause for ischemic cardiovascular syncope with exertion are arrhythmias secondary to atherosclerotic coronary artery disease [20, 21, 29]. To date, the best method to assess a patient for one of these problems remains uncertain. Cardiac CT and MRI are being actively investigated and should be considered when there are suspicions for a coronary anomaly.

The other important group of cardiovascular causes for syncope includes arrhythmias. Ventricular tachycardia (VT), supraventricular tachycardia, atrial fibrillation with rapid rates, and bradycardia due to AV block or sinus arrest are all potential causes for syncope. These can be idiopathic or related to a variety of underlying structural heart diseases including long QT syndrome, hypertrophic cardiomyopathy, right ventricular cardiomyopathy, Brugada syndrome, Wolff-Parkinson-White syndrome, and various corrected and uncorrected congenital heart diseases [30].

Evaluation of the Athlete with Syncope and Near-Syncope

The 36th Bethesda Conference Task Force on "Arrhythmias in the Athlete" identified syncope as an important symptom that mandates a thorough evaluation [3]. No universally applicable "cookbook" approach exists to evaluate syncope in the athlete. Arrhythmic and nonarrhythmic cardiovascular causes should be carefully excluded by appropriate work up in all cases of syncope. A benign cause should be a diagnosis of exclusion. However, even after a careful and extensive evaluation, the cause for syncope can be difficult or even impossible to diagnose. An approach to evaluation is suggested in Fig. 10.2. The history and the physical exam are key towards reaching a diagnosis.

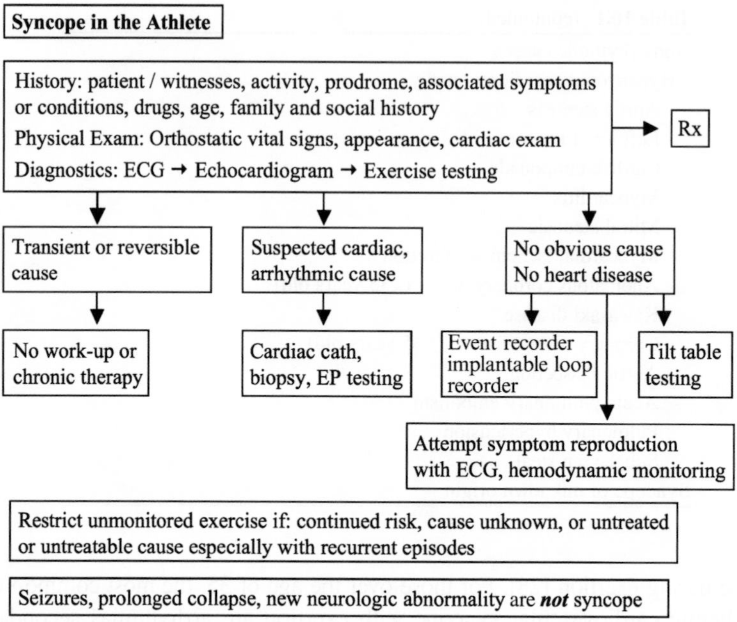

Fig. 10.2 Approach to evaluating syncope in the athlete

History

Taking a thorough history is vital to reaching a diagnosis in the athlete with syncope. The history should focus on establishing whether the event was truly a syncopal episode and to exclude conditions like seizures, pseudoseizures, and prolonged collapse. Once syncope is established, the next part of the history should focus on identifying clues that might point towards a specific etiology. It is important to identify how often and the circumstances under which the symptoms occurred. It is also important to obtain as much information as possible regarding witnessed accounts of what happened as well as any monitoring during the event. Old records (and outside records) should be reviewed for clues. A thorough family history should focus on syncope, unexplained or sudden death at a young age, and any congenital or structural heart disease as well as primary electrical disorders in immediate family members. Social history should note information on alcohol and drug abuse, dietary supplements, and performance-enhancing agents.

The following clinical features may indicate a higher risk for a cardiac cause for syncope: presence of structural heart disease, male gender, family history of syncope or sudden death, syncope during exertion or in supine position, blurred vision, and history of antecedent palpitations or chest pain [31]. On the other hand, syncope only after stopping exercise, during upright posture, associated with a clear situation or trigger, prodromal symptoms (light-headedness, warmth, abdominal discomfort, and nausea), postsyncopal nausea and fatigue, and multiple episodes, all point towards a neurally mediated or non-cardiac etiology [32].

Physical Examination

Physical examination can help determine if there is a vascular or cardiac cause for syncope by revealing a murmur suggestive of aortic stenosis, mitral stenosis, or hypertrophic cardiomyopathy, tumor "plop" suggestive of left atrial myxoma, palpable Pulmonary condition of second heart sound suggesting pulmonary hypertension, systemic or orthostatic hypotension, tachycardia or rhythm disturbances. Hypertrophic cardiomyopathy and aortic stenotic murmurs can be differentiated by physical maneuvers, with standing and Valsalva accentuating the former. Assessment should be made of any focal or global neurologic deficits. In the general population, it has been shown that a carefully performed history and physical examination can lead to a diagnosis in 45–50% of cases [33, 34]. Whether this is applicable in the athletic population is not known.

Diagnostic Testing

Further evaluation should be guided by clinical findings derived from the history and physical examination. Ruling out potentially life-threatening structural heart disease and electrical abnormalities should be the priority. Although the presence of structural heart disease does not always indicate that syncope has a cardiac cause, exertional syncope as well as sudden unexpected loss of consciousness without prodrome in an athlete is worrisome and could indicate an arrhythmic cause or sudden hemodynamic collapse. No symptom, however, appears to be able to predict mortality or syncope recurrence [33].

Noninvasive Testing

Following history and physical exam, a 12-lead electrocardiogram (ECG) as well as an echocardiogram should be the initial diagnostic tests in the further evaluation of syncope.

Electrocardiography

The ECG can help differentiate changes of athletic conditioning, which may be present in up to 40% of athletes [35], from abnormalities which may be the underlying cause of syncope. Resting sinus bradycardia, marked sinus arrhythmia, sinus pauses up to 3 s, first and second degree AV block are all secondary to increased vagal tone, usually resolves with activity, and so are considered benign in a conditioned athlete [1]. Other, much less common, benign abnormalities include high precordial lead voltages, Q-waves, and ST-T deviation indicating abnormal repolarization [35]. On the other hand, the ECG may show pathologic abnormalities like preexcitation indicating Wolff-Parkinson-White syndrome, complete heart block, Brugada pattern, ischemic changes, abnormal QT intervals, or right ventricular cardiomyopathy [32]. An abnormal ECG, by itself, is a nonspecific finding.

Electrocardiographic Monitoring (Holter Monitor, Event Monitor, Implantable Loop Recorder)

In patients with intermittent symptoms and no ECG abnormalities at baseline, correlating the event with a cardiac rhythm disturbance should be sought by means of monitoring. Ambulatory ECG monitoring, either continuous (24–48 h Holter) or patient-triggered event monitoring are of low value if the episodes are rare. A limitation of external loop monitoring is inability of many syncope patients to activate the device in a timely fashion. The diagnostic yield of external recording devices for arrhythmia detection has been recently improved by auto-triggering as well as by continuous ECG transmission to a central monitoring station (so-called mobile cardiac outpatient telemetry) [36, 37]. Implantable loop recorders, subcutaneous monitoring devices for arrhythmia detection, are effective for patients with infrequent symptoms and who have a suspected arrhythmia where other diagnostic testing is inconclusive [38, 39].

Echocardiogram

Echocardiography can help identify and characterize structural heart disease that may be responsible for syncope and differentiate pathological heart disease from cardiac structural changes that can be seen in a conditioned athlete. Significant abnormalities include dilated cardiomyopathy, hypertrophic cardiomyopathy, myocarditis, cardiac tamponade, arrhythmogenic right ventricular dysplasia, and congenital and valvular heart disease. Intracardiac shunts can be assessed by color doppler and by using saline contrast.

A careful transthoracic echo examination can help in identifying abnormal position of coronary ostia. If this diagnosis is suspected, further evaluation using transesophageal echo, cardiac catheterization, cardiac MRI, and/or CT coronary angiography should be performed for confirmation of anomalous coronary artery and to define its course. Similarly, patients suspected of having myocarditis or right ventricular dysplasia should undergo a cardiac MRI for further evaluation of scar or fatty infiltrates.

Different nonpathologic structural cardiac abnormalities can be seen in the athlete depending on the kind of physiological stresses the athlete is exposed to and myocardial adaptation to these stresses (so-called "athlete's heart"). This creates a tendency to overdiagnose these changes, which usually involve hypertrophy and chamber dilatation, as pathological [40].

Regarding cardiac hypertrophy, wall thickness ≥13 mm in an athlete is rare [41] except in rowers. Wall thickness ≥16 mm has not been described in the athlete and is considered pathological, raising suspicion of hypertrophic cardiomyopathy [41]. Between 12 and 15 mm is a "gray zone" where diastolic function assessment can be used to differentiate the rare athlete with physiological hypertrophy (intact diastolic function) from hypertrophic cardiomyopathy (abnormal diastolic function) [41, 42].

If the diagnosis is still uncertain, a period of deconditioning can be tried where physiological hypertrophy is expected to resolve [43]. On the other hand, not all the changes related to conditioning may be benign. Residual chamber dilatation was noted on echocardiography in about 20% of competitive athletes long after their retirement from competitive sports [44]. The significance of these residual structural abnormalities and their relation to syncope is not known.

Tilt-Table Testing

Upright tilt-table testing may be of value in young athletes in whom the diagnosis of neurocardiogenic syncope is suspected. Tilt testing should be considered in cases of unexplained single syncopal episodes in high-risk settings (occurrence of, or potential risk for physical injury), or recurrent episodes in the absence of organic heart disease, or, in the presence of structural heart disease, after cardiac causes of syncope have been excluded [45].

Tilt-table testing is not of value in the assessment of treatment for syncope, when only a single episode happens without injury and not in a high risk setting, and when clear cut vasovagal features are present by initial evaluation [45]. In athletes without structural heart disease in whom neurocardiogenic syncope is suspected, tilt-table testing can be diagnostic when spontaneous syncope is reproduced.

However, considerable debate exists over the sensitivity of tilt-table testing, especially in the athlete, with estimates ranging from 30 to 80%. The exact specificity is difficult to assess and depends on how closely the test represents the physiological response that results in neurocardiogenic syncope [46]. High vagal tone may facilitate the triggering of a neurocardiogenic response even if it is not responsible for syncope. In addition, it appears that high vagal tone actually prevents neurocardiogenic responses by some unknown mechanism. It is also possible to produce an abnormal response even in normal individuals when longer duration, steeper incline, and provocative drugs like nitroglycerin and isoproterenol are used [47]. As might have happened in the case of Boston Celtics basketball player Reggie Lewis, it is possible that a false-positive test may prevent the physician from exploring other life-threatening causes of syncope and expose the athlete to further risk by clearing him/her for competition.

In summary, optimal protocol, diagnostic value of a positive test other than reproduction of syncope and long-term prognostic significance of positive results, as well as optimal therapeutic strategy for patients with a positive test, remain to be determined. If employed, results of the tilt-table testing alone should not be relied upon to make the diagnosis.

Exercise Testing

Exercise testing is recommended [45] in patients who experience syncope during or shortly after exercise. Exercise testing should also be considered in the athlete >35 years of age if there is suspicion of coronary artery disease. The test is considered diagnostic when ECG and hemodynamic abnormalities are present and syncope is reproduced during or immediately after exercise. Similarly, development of Mobitz II second degree or third degree AV block during exercise is considered diagnostic even without syncope [45].

Chronotropic incompetence, even though uncommon in the young trained athlete, may suggest a rare genetic predisposition to sinus node dysfunction. Clues toward diagnosis can be found in athletes with history of syncope who demonstrate lack of shortening of QT interval with exercise, especially when a long QT interval is not apparent in the surface ECG. However, even if begun at a high level of exercise like Bruce stage 4, the treadmill exercise test may not necessarily reproduce the exact physiological circumstances and exertional demands of actual competition. For example, a weightlifter pushing several hundred pounds may have blood pressure peak up to 500 mmHg, potentially causing a neurocardiogenic response whereas this would not be expected to occur while dribbling down the basketball court.

Other Noninvasive Testing

ECG in patients with Brugada syndrome can change over time from being totally normal to one with typical Brugada characteristics. In athletes with syncope and a normal ECG but suspected Brugada syndrome, monitored intravenous infusion of a sodium channel blocker (Class I antiarrhythmic drugs such as flecainide or procainamide) can unmask the characteristic Brugada ECG changes and help establish a diagnosis [48].

Mutations in potassium channel genes KCNQ1 (LQT1 locus) and KCNH2 (LQT2 locus) and the sodium channel gene SCN5A (LQT3 locus) are the most common causes of the long QT syndrome. Identifying the locus by genetic testing has been shown to independently predict the risk of a first cardiac event (defined as the occurrence of syncope, cardiac arrest, or sudden death before age of 40) in patients with long QT syndrome [49].

The role of risk stratification methods such as signal-averaged ECG and microvolt T-wave alternans in evaluating syncope in the athlete is uncertain.

Invasive Testing

Electrophysiology Testing

An electrophysiologic (EP) study is an invasive procedure aimed at diagnosis and treatment of arrhythmias. The study is performed using a combination of local anesthesia and conscious sedation or, occasionally, under general anesthesia. The procedure involves inserting flexible electrode catheters into the femoral and/or internal jugular venous system and advancing them to various cardiac chambers under fluoroscopic guidance. Strategically placed electrode catheters provide valuable electrical information, which when combined with various pacing and pharmacological maneuvers, will help locate as well as assess mechanisms of arrhythmias. Once a definite diagnosis is achieved, various treatment modalities, including catheter ablation, drug therapy, and device therapy (pacemakers or defibrillators) can be instituted.

EP testing is indicated in selected athletes with unexplained syncope, especially when structural heart disease is present and there is concern of ventricular arrhythmias. However, the diagnostic and predictive value of the test is limited and disease-dependent, and normal findings on EP testing does not exclude an arrhythmic cause for syncope.

The test is most valuable in patients with coronary artery disease where inducible ventricular arrhythmias can predict prognosis and guide treatment [50]. In patients with coronary artery disease, EP testing has been shown to have high sensitivity (90–95%) and specificity (95% for inducible monomorphic VT) [51]. With respect to the type of induced ventricular tachyarrhythmia, inducible monomorphic VT is the most specific when compared to induction of nonsustained VT, polymorphic VT, and ventricular fibrillation [52].

EP testing is of some value in patients with arrhythmogenic right ventricular dysplasia, with sensitivities approaching 70–80% [32, 53], but specificity of EP testing in this disorder is not clearly known. Sensitivity and specificity of EP testing is low in patients who have hypertrophic cardiomyopathy, dilated cardiomyopathy, long QT syndrome, and congenital heart disease [32], which unfortunately are common causes in athletes with syncope and sudden death. Similarly EP testing is of limited value in evaluation of bradycardia [54, 55], except in athletes with high-degree AV block in whom a level of block cannot be determined.

In case of athletes with syncope and documented abnormalities by ECG monitoring, EP testing may be of benefit, even in the absence of structural heart disease, in confirming the diagnosis and providing treatment by catheter ablation. This can be the case with supraventricular arrhythmias like AV nodal reentrant tachycardia, AV reentrant tachycardia, atrial tachycardia, atrial fibrillation, and atrial flutter. Athletes with Wolff-Parkinson-White syndrome with syncope should also undergo EP testing to localize and ablate the accessory pathway [56].

Asymptomatic athletes with preexcitation are rarely restricted and whether they need EP testing is still a matter of debate, since the lifetime risk of a malignant arrhythmia is extremely low [57]. If performed, diagnosis of a bypass tract able to sustain a rapid arrhythmia with hemodynamic compromise should prompt ablation [58]. Similarly, EP testing showing refractory period of bypass tract <250 ms (as compared to antegrade refractory periods and location of bypass tract) in a young athlete with asymptomatic Wolff-Parkinson-White syndrome constitutes a high-risk group in whom prophylactic catheter ablation can provide long-term freedom from arrhythmia [59].

In athletes with documented spontaneous sustained VT, the sensitivity and specificity of invasive EP testing vary with the underlying etiology, with high utility in coronary artery disease, right ventricular cardiomyopathy, and idiopathic left and right VT [60].

In summary, EP testing is of limited diagnostic value in the athlete with syncope unless there is evidence of specific structural heart disease with suspected arrhythmic etiology where noninvasive evaluation has failed to demonstrate a cause. Positive findings should not be taken in isolation and should be evaluated in conjunction with the rest of the clinical picture.

Cardiac Catheterization

Cardiac catheterization is indicated in young athletes with syncope suspected to be due to anomalous coronary artery or in older athletes in whom atherosclerotic coronary artery disease and myocardial ischemia is suspected. CT coronary angiography can be used as a viable alternative to evaluate coronary arteries in these settings.

Coronary angiography alone is not diagnostic of the cause of syncope [45] and should be reserved for confirmation of the diagnosis suspected by prior noninvasive evaluation and for planning treatment.

Endomyocardial Biopsy

In athletes with cardiomyopathy suspected to be secondary to an infiltrative disease (arrhythmogenic right ventricular cardiomyopathy, sarcoidosis, amyloidosis, and giant cell myocarditis), endomyocardial biopsy can help establish the diagnosis and determine prognosis.

Management of Syncope in the Athlete

After a thorough initial evaluation involving a complete history, physical exam, and baseline testing including an ECG and an echocardiogram, no further workup or chronic therapy is needed if the episode appears to be transient and reversible. A suspected cardiac structural or arrhythmic cause needs further evaluation using ECG monitoring, cardiac catheterization, or EP testing. EP study may not be of value in the younger athlete without structural heart disease, and monitoring becomes more helpful. If there is no obvious cause for syncope from the initial evaluation, event-monitoring and/or implantable loop recorder, tilt-table testing, or exercise treadmill testing should be considered. However, each test has its own sensitivity and specificity, and any test by itself may not be diagnostic. The most useful test would be hemodynamic and ECG monitoring during an episode, but this is hard to achieve in the real world.

Treatment for syncope is directed by the specific cause. A detailed discussion of therapy for diseases that can lead to syncope in the athlete is beyond the scope of this chapter. Instead, a summary of treatment strategies for the important causes of syncope will be made (see Table 10.2). Definitive therapy for arrhythmic causes of syncope or arrhythmic substrate with potential for syncope should be accompanied by recommendation regarding eligibility for continued athletic activity based on the Bethesda guidelines [3].

Treatment of Neurocardiogenic Syncope

Therapeutic approach to the athlete with vasovagal or neurocardiogenic syncope should be individualized. The most important initial step is to educate the athlete and family on the need to avoid any known triggers (extreme exertion, heat, dehydration, and alcohol). The athlete should be advised to lie down at the onset of any prodromal symptoms and to allow at least 10 min after regaining consciousness before he/she gets up. Leg crossing and muscle tensing during the prodromal phase of syncope may be of value [61].

Management strategies consist of increasing salt and water consumption [62, 63]. Tilt training, where the patient stands with their back against the wall and their feet about a foot from the wall, has been suggested as an effective therapy by desensitizing the system to orthostatic stress [64]. Medical management consists of various agents including mineralocorticoids (fludrocortisone), beta-blockers, midodrine, and selective serotonin-reuptake inhibitors. In athletes with a significant bradycardic/asystolic component to their syncope episode who do not respond to the above measures, cardiac pacing may be helpful by prolonging the time from onset of symptoms to loss of consciousness [46]. None of these maneuvers have been proven to be effective, however, in the athlete to treat neurally mediated syncope due to exertion, and they must be used with caution due to adverse effects and lack of benefit. Conservative measures are generally the first-line approach.

Treatment of Arrhythmic Syncope

Sinus bradycardia, first-degree AV block, and Mobitz I second degree AV block at rest are usually physiologic in a trained athlete and do not require treatment if they

Table 10.2 NASPE policy conference guidelines on treatment and restriction for arrhythmias in the athlete [1]

Arrhythmia	Treatment options	Guidelines for athletic participation
Supraventricular arrhythmias		
APCs	Reassurance	No restriction
Atrial fibrillation, atrial flutter	Rate, rhythm control, warfarin, RFA	No bodily contact if on warfarin
Ventricular preexcitation (WPW) on ECG	No therapy. RFA if high risk	Consider EP testing to risk stratify
WPW with SVT	RFA, antiarrhythmics	No restrictions after 3–6 months without symptoms
AVNRT	RFA, antiarrhythmics	No restrictions after 3–6 months without symptoms
Ventricular arrhythmias		
PVCs	Reassurance, beta-blocker	No restrictions if no SHD
NSVT	If no SHD, reassurance	No restrictions if no SHD
Sustained VT	If no SHD, RFA If SHD, evaluate further for ICD vs. antiarrhythmics	No restrictions if successful ablation and no SHD; Low intensity sports otherwise
Cardiac arrest/VF	ICD, antiarrhythmics	Low intensity sports
Conditions associated with ventricular arrhythmias		
Condition	Treatment	Guidelines for athletic participation
HCM	AAD, ICD, myomectomy	Low intensity exercise only
ARVD	AAD, ICD	Low intensity exercise only
CAD	AAD, ICD	Low intensity exercise only
IDCM	AAD, ICD	Low intensity exercise only
LQTS	Beta-blocker, ICD	Low intensity exercise only
Anomalous CAD	CABG	No restrictions after CABG
Idiopathic LVT	RFA	No restrictions 3 months after RFA
Idiopathic RVT	RFA	No restrictions 3 months after RFA

AAD antiarrhythmic drugs, *APCs* atrial premature contractions, *ARVD* arrhythmogenic right ventricular dysplasia, *AVNRT* AV nodal reentrant tachycardia, *CABG* coronary artery bypass grafting, *CAD* coronary artery disease, *HCM* hypertrophic cardiomyopathy, *ICD* implantable cardioverter defibrillator, *IDCM* idiopathic dilated cardiomyopathy, *LV* left ventricular, *LQTS* long QT syndrome, *NSVT* nonsustained ventricular tachycardia, *PVCs* premature ventricular contractions, *RFA* radiofrequency ablation, *RV* right ventricular, *SHD* structural heart disease, *SVT* supraventricular tachycardia, *VF* ventricular fibrillation, *VT* ventricular tachycardia, *WPW* Wolff-Parkinson-White syndrome

are chronotropically competent with activity. Mobitz II or complete heart block usually requires permanent pacing. In athletes with syncope related to bradycardia, athletic participation should be restricted unless there is a period of 3–6 months of definitive therapy for the bradyarrhythmia [1].

Antiarrhythmics, beta-blockers, and other rate-controlling drugs, in addition to affecting exercise tolerance, are often banned in many competitive sports, making treatment of supraventricular arrhythmias difficult in the athlete. However, the advent of catheter ablation has made a tremendous impact in treatment of supraventricular arrhythmias in the young athlete, as the two most common forms of supraventricular arrhythmias (AV reentrant tachycardia and AV nodal reentrant tachycardia) are easily treated and can be cured by this modality. Catheter ablation also offers potential for cure and should be considered as first-line therapy for atrial flutter, atrial tachycardia, and select forms of focal atrial fibrillation in the absence of structural heart disease [65, 66].

Catheter ablation can achieve cure rates of up to 95% in idiopathic left and right VT [67, 68]. In general, nonsustained VT in the absence of structural heart disease does not carry an increased risk of sudden death and need not be treated [3]. However, athletes with nonsustained polymorphic VT may be at higher risk of sudden cardiac death and treatment in the form of beta-blockers, athletic restriction [60, 69], and ICDs in select instances may be needed [1]. Syncope secondary to ventricular arrhythmias in the setting of structural heart disease carries a high risk of sudden cardiac death, and the athlete should be considered for an ICD per current guidelines [70]. Structural heart disease treatment should be disease-specific as outlined in Table 10.2.

Implanted Devices in the Athlete

The safety of sports participation for athletes with ICDs and other implanted devices is unknown but is being actively investigated. See Chap. 18 for a detailed discussion of this issue.

Athletic Restrictions

It is important to consider restrictions if, after the initial evaluation, there is suspicion of a potentially dangerous structural heart or arrhythmic problem that could get worse with further athletic participation. Even though there is considerable debate, the 36th Bethesda Conference [2] provides eligibility recommendations for competitive athletes with cardiovascular abnormalities.

The Bethesda guidelines recommend that athletes with syncope or near-syncope should not participate in sports until the cause is determined and treated. If the athlete is asymptomatic for 2–3 months during treatment, he/she can then resume participation [3]. However, this depends on the underlying condition. For example, the 36th Bethesda guidelines indicate that if there is syncope in an athlete with diagnosed long QT interval syndrome, then restriction is appropriate. Diagnosis of long QT interval (QTc >470 ms in males and >480 ms in females) is also reason for athletic restriction, even in asymptomatic individuals. Even though risk stratification is suggested based on genotyping, sex, and QTc [49], considerable risk is still present even for the low-risk group to warrant restriction.

Similarly, established cardiac conditions like right ventricular cardiomyopathy, hypertrophic cardiomyopathy, coronary artery disease, and idiopathic dilated cardiomyopathy require some degree of permanent athletic restriction irrespective of presence of syncope and treatment of the condition.

In the consensus statement from the NASPE policy conference [1] on "Arrhythmias and the Athlete," restrictions have been made based on underlying diagnoses. For example, if there is a supraventricular tachycardia present, ablation may cure that problem and then the individual can participate in sports 4 weeks later. However, one has to be clear that this arrhythmia, which was treated, was the most likely cause of the athlete's syncopal episode. Guidelines are also made for ventricular arrhythmias and for underlying cardiovascular conditions as well (Table 10.2).

Illustrative Cases

The following cases exemplify some of the complexities of managing athletes with arrhythmic causes for syncope. Evaluation is as described earlier in the chapter, and management is often dictated by data derived from other populations and after careful discussion with patients.

Eighteen-Year-Old Female with Syncope

An 18-year-old female who has a full scholarship to the rowing team has recurrent episodes of transient loss of consciousness while rowing. She also had syncope when she was fluid depleted in a hot environment while kneeling. Her father had syncope especially when running marathons. His ECG suggests long QT interval syndrome. ECGs on our patient are also shown demonstrating lack of shortening of the QT interval with exercise (Fig. 10.3). Tilt-table test was positive for neurocardiogenic syncope. The patient was restricted from rowing, and an implantable loop recorder was placed. There were no further syncopal episodes over the next 1½ years while she was taking nadolol.

This case illustrates that it can be difficult to determine in an athlete with syncope during exertion and without exertion what the potential mechanisms and causes for syncope may be. Furthermore, the proper therapy can remain uncertain when long QT syndrome is apparent but not clearly the cause for syncope. Patients with long QT syndrome and syncope have potentially higher risk for sudden cardiac death and recurrent syncope so they should be restricted from activity and placed at least on a beta-blocker and perhaps have an ICD. This may also depend on the type of long QT syndrome [16]. Our patient underwent genetic screening, which was negative, but this does not necessarily provide solace as to the mechanism regarding syncope and the long-term prognosis.

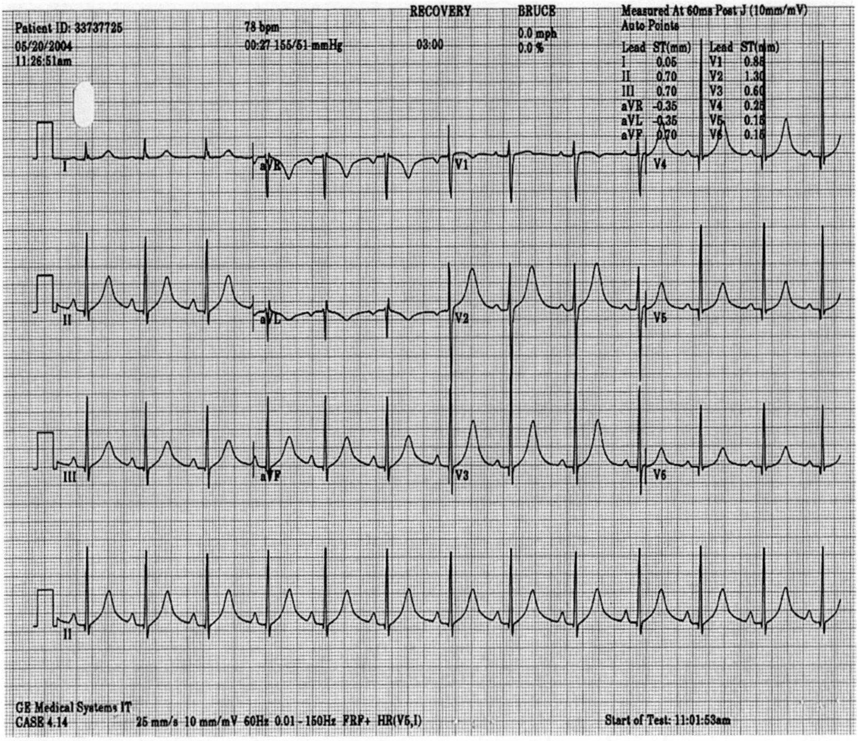

Fig. 10.3 Eighteen-year-old female with syncope

Nineteen-Year-Old Male Swimmer with Frequent Palpitations and Near Syncope

A competitive swimmer has recurrent episodes of frequent rapid palpitations associated with near syncope, and happens after he gets out of the pool from swimming. ECG is shown demonstrating a regular, narrow QRS tachycardia (Fig. 10.4). This patient had AV nodal reentry supraventricular tachycardia, but it may have also been orthodromic AV reciprocating tachycardia due to a concealed retrograde accessory pathway activation. In either case, ablation of the accessory pathway or the slow pathway responsible for the reentrant tachycardia will eliminate the problem and then our patient could return to swimming within a relatively short period of time.

The recent Bethesda guidelines have changed now indicating that a patient with structural heart disease who is status post catheter ablation for highly symptomatic supraventricular tachycardia can return to full competitive activity in 2–4 weeks. If no structural heart disease is present, an athlete with supraventricular tachycardia is allowed to return to full competition several days following ablation provided a follow-up EP study shows noninducibility [3].

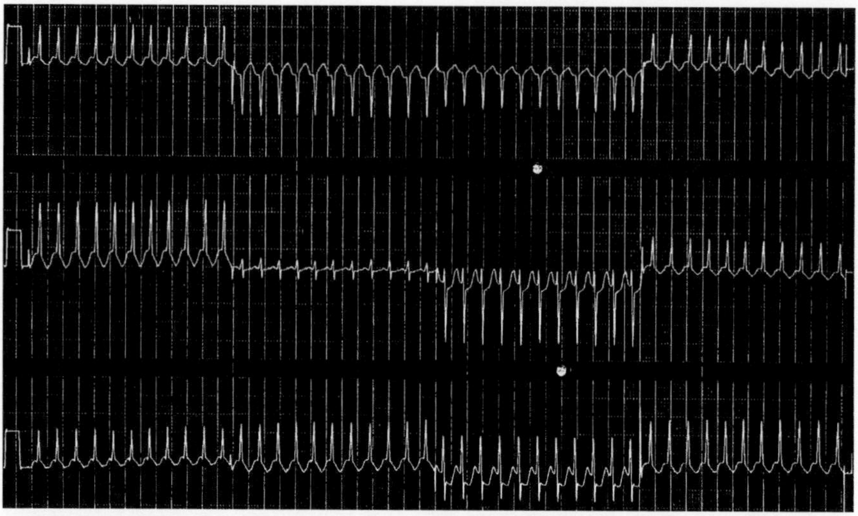

Fig. 10.4 Nineteen-year-old male swimmer with frequent palpitations and near syncope

Twenty-Year-Old Male with Syncope While Playing Basketball

A 20-year-old male is brought to the emergency room from a basketball game. After dribbling down the court, he suddenly lost consciousness. ECG obtained in the emergency room is shown in Fig. 10.5. This demonstrates atrial fibrillation with an irregular, but very rapid, ventricular response rate. The QRS complex is wide and at times narrow. This is consistent with Wolff–Parkinson–White syndrome. In this case, the accessory pathway appears to be a left posterior accessory pathway. This patient underwent ablation of the accessory pathway and then was able to return back to full competitive activity within 2–4 weeks [3].

Eighteen-Year-Old Male with Near Syncope and Palpitations During Basketball

During a basketball game, an 18-year-old male develops light-headedness and feels as though he is going to pass out. ECG in the emergency room is shown in Fig. 10.6. This demonstrates a wide QRS tachycardia that is regular with a right bundle branch block, inferior axis morphology. The patient required cardioversion for this arrhythmia. In follow-up, the patient had a normal echocardiogram and a normal ECG at baseline. A treadmill test was negative. Other attempts at reproducing the tachycardia failed. During EP testing, there was no evidence for inducible supraventricular or VT, as well as for aberrant conduction. On the

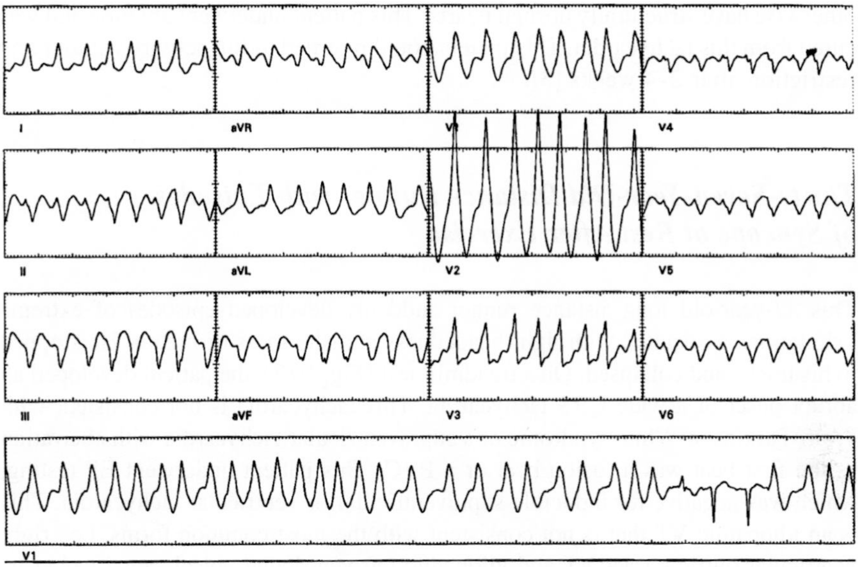

Fig. 10.5 Twenty-year-old male with syncope while playing basketball

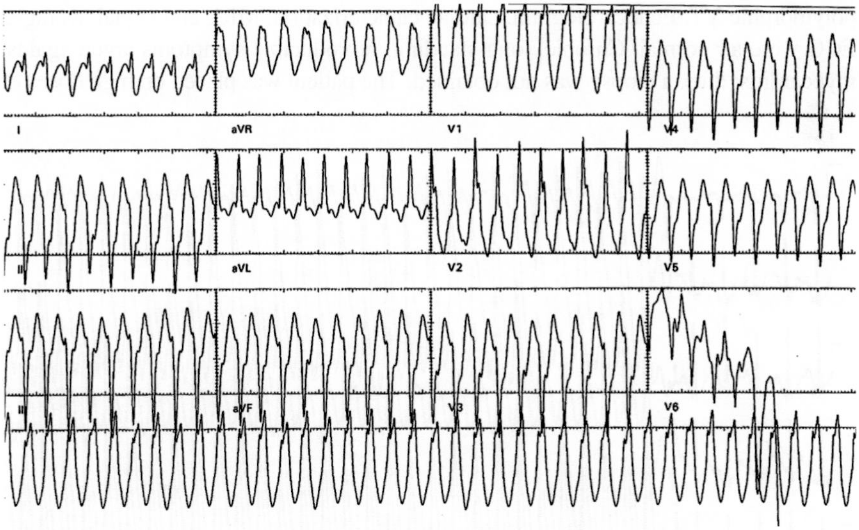

Fig. 10.6 Eighteen-year-old male with near syncope and palpitations during basketball

other hand, rapid pacing in the presence of isoproterenol induced this wide complex tachycardia showing AV dissociation consistent with an idiopathic left ventricular apical septal Purkinje VT. Idiopathic VT's tend to occur from the left ventricular apical septum or the right ventricular outflow tract. These patients otherwise have structurally normal hearts. This patient underwent ablation and was cured from this tachycardia. This patient could returned to full activity without any restriction after 2–4 weeks [3].

Thirty-Seven-Year-Old Distance Runner with Episodes of Syncope at Rest After Exercise

This 37-year-old long-distance runner suddenly developed episodes of extreme palpitations associated with light-headedness and shortness of breath. He stopped in his tracks and collapsed. On a treadmill test (Fig. 10.7), the patient developed an abrupt onset of a wide QRS tachycardia. This tachycardia is not consistent with Wolff-Parkinson-White syndrome or a supraventricular tachycardia with aberration as the first beat was a fusion beat or a PVC. This patient underwent EP testing, which was negative for inducible supraventricular or ventricular tachycardia. This is an idiopathic VT that is not consistent with the most common forms, i.e., right ventricular outflow tract VT and idiopathic left ventricular apical septal tachycardia. This tachycardia could not be induced, and there were no PVCs with or without isoproterenol infusion.

The monomorphic nature of the tachycardia is inconsistent with catecholaminergic polymorphic VT. Echocardiogram, cardiac catheterization, MRI, and signal averaged ECG were all normal. Chronic, long-standing, reproducible symptoms argue against myocarditis; thus, a biopsy was not obtained. The patient was placed on high doses of

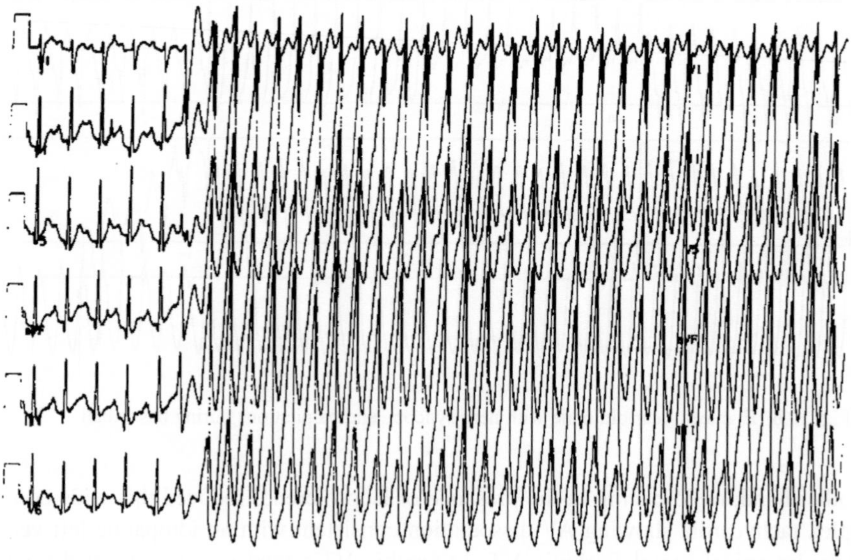

Fig. 10.7 Thirty-seven-year-old distance runner with episodes of syncope at rest after exercise

a beta-blocker. This patient had repeat treadmill testing off and on beta blockade, demonstrating reproducible VT off beta blockade and no VT on beta blockade. The patient refused to restrict his exercise activity and, over the years, remained asymptomatic with no recurrent tachycardia clinically and on treadmill testing. Over time, the patient attempted to stop beta blockade and was successful weaning it down over many years without recurrent tachycardia. The patient is presently not taking a beta-blocker and is asymptomatic.

Nine-Year-Old Female Who has Recurrent Collapse During Activity

A 9-year-old female has recurrent syncope at recess while running. The ECG is normal, and echocardiogram and an MRI confirm left ventricular hypertrophy. Monitoring during recess demonstrates the initiation of a wide complex tachycardia (Fig. 10.8). This patient has a rapid VT. This is consistent with VT in a patient with hypertrophic cardiomyopathy. This patient requires an ICD and should be restricted from physical activity. Over many years of follow-up, the patient never used the ICD and remained under activity restriction.

Nineteen-Year-Old with Syncope During Football

While running for a pass, our patient became light-headed and ultimately collapsed. It was a very hot day, and the patient had not been eating well and had nothing to drink. ECG was performed and is shown in Fig. 10.9. It demonstrates marked T-wave changes that are consistent with hypertrophic cardiomyopathy. Echocardiogram demonstrated hypertrophic cardiomyopathy with the septal thickness of 20 mm. There is no family history of sudden death. Holter monitor demonstrated rare premature ventricular contractions, but there were no episodes of syncope during monitoring. This patient most likely had syncope due to hypertrophic cardiomyopathy, but the exact mechanism of syncope in this patient remains uncertain. It may well be due to ventricular arrhythmia, but on the

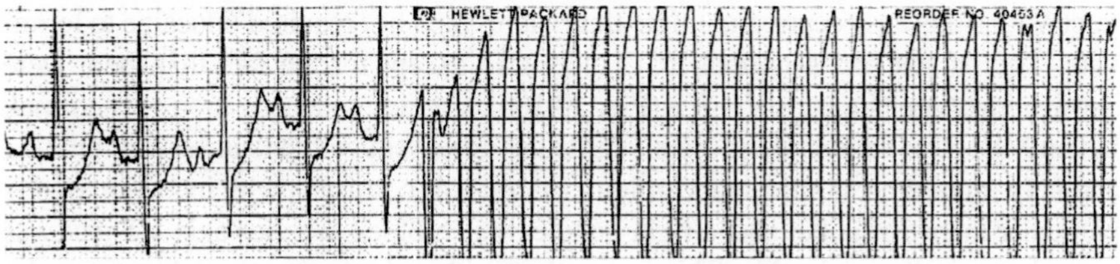

Fig. 10.8 Nine-year-old female who has recurrent collapse during activity

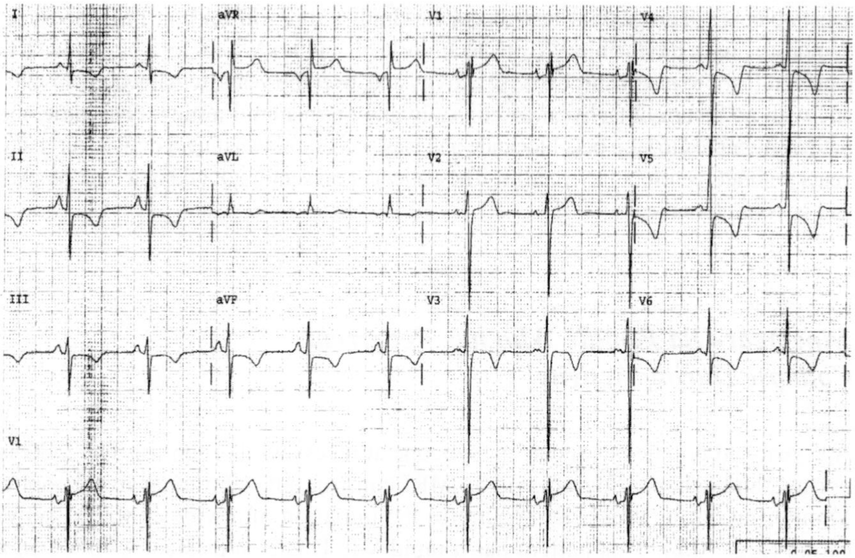

Fig. 10.9 Nineteen-year-old with syncope while playing football

other hand it also may be due to atrial fibrillation, diastolic dysfunction, or outflow tract obstruction [26]. While this patient has risk for recurrent syncope with physical activity, it is debatable whether this patient would necessarily need to undergo ICD implantation based on present guidelines [70]. This patient should, however, be restricted from heavy physical activity as this may put the patient at greater risk for not only recurrent syncope but sudden death while playing competitive sports. Beta blockade would also be appropriate for this patient.

Twenty-Year-Old Female with Syncope with Exertion

A 20-year-old female develops syncope with moderate jogging. She comes into the emergency room with the following tachycardia (Fig. 10.10a). This demonstrates a wide complex tachycardia with a left bundle branch block, marked rightward axis morphology consistent with idiopathic right ventricular outflow tract VT. However, this patient did not have the typical presentation of idiopathic right ventricular outflow tract VT, as this has occurred multiple times at rest and has required lidocaine to terminate. The patient had a normal ECG otherwise except for the fact that there were T-wave inversions in leads V1–V3 (Fig. 10.10b). Cardiac catheterization was normal, but an MRI scan demonstrated right ventricular aneurysm with dilatation and thinning and fatty replacement of the myocardium. EP test was consistent with induction of this particular tachycardia but also a right bundle branch block superior axis VT that was hemodynamically intolerable. This is a patient with arrhythmogenic right ventricular cardiomyopathy who has VT that mimics idiopathic VT. This patient underwent ICD

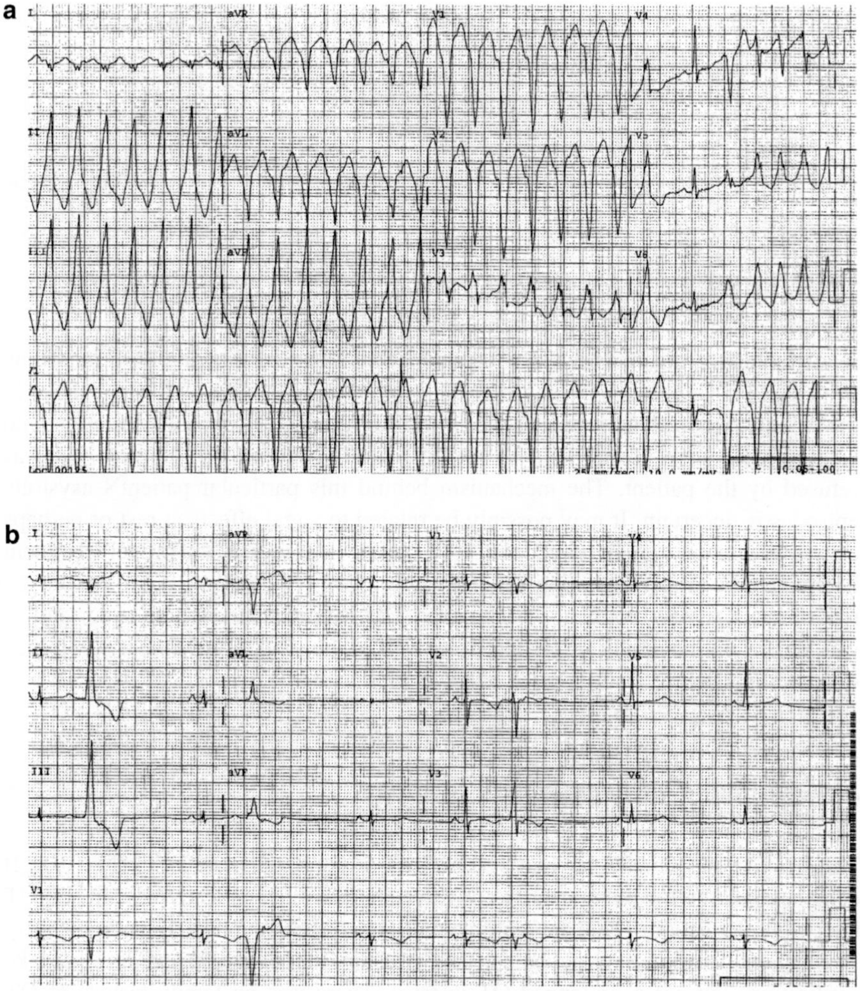

Fig. 10.10 (a) Twenty-year-old female with exertional syncope. (b) Baseline ECG of patient in (a)

implantation, had recurrent ICD shocks, and therefore was placed on sotalol therapy in addition. She has done well in the long term, and heavy physical activity is restricted.

Forty-Year-Old Male Physician Who Has Syncope at Rest While Examining Patients

This 40-year-old gastroenterologist bikes up to 500 miles per weekend and never passes out with exercise but only passes out at rest. His history, physical examination, and ECG are otherwise normal. A tilt-table test demonstrated hypotension and

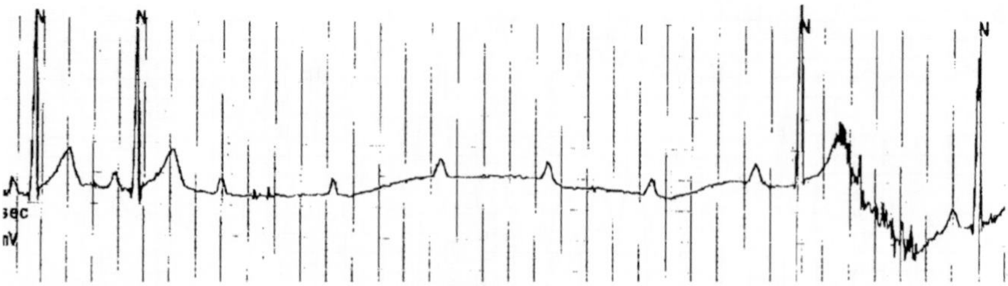

Fig. 10.11 Forty-year-old male physician who has syncope at rest while examining patients

relative bradycardia, and on a monitor the patient had the following ECG recording (Fig. 10.11). This shows paroxysmal AV block (many P waves with no change in the PP interval) with asystole at rest. Echocardiogram, cardiac catheterization, and cardiac MRI were all normal. An endomyocardial biopsy was advised but was refused by the patient. The mechanism behind this particular patient's asystolic episodes is uncertain. It may possibly be related to vagal effects at rest or perhaps excess adenosine causing paroxysmal AV block. In any case, the proper treatment here would be to restrict biking which may improve AV conduction and reduce the risk of syncope or to implant a pacemaker. The patient refused to do either and so was started on theophylline. He has done well in the long term without recurrence of symptoms and probably no AV block as well.

Sixteen-Year-Old Female with Syncope

This 16-year-old female has had sudden loss of consciousness. ECG (Fig. 10.12) demonstrated the following changes: T-wave abnormalities in leads V1–V3 and QT interval prolongation. There are multiple types of congenital long QT syndrome [16]. This patient does not have any underlying structural heart disease and does not take medications but has a prolonged QT interval. There was no family history of QT interval prolongation or sudden cardiac death. This patient should be placed on a beta-blocker, but the response to exercise and restriction from exercise will depend on the type of QT prolongation syndrome that she has. Patients with the LQT1 genotype have a high incidence of exercise-induced cardiac events, with swimming being a specific trigger. Patients with the LQT2 genotype are at high risk of having arrhythmic events triggered by a sudden loud noise. Patients with the LQT3 genotype experience events without emotional arousal during sleep or at rest [16, 72, 73].

Thirty-Five-Year-Old Male with Near Syncope Playing Hockey

This patient has only had syncope while playing hockey. He has had three to four episodes during intense physical activity. Echocardiogram, ECG, and treadmill test

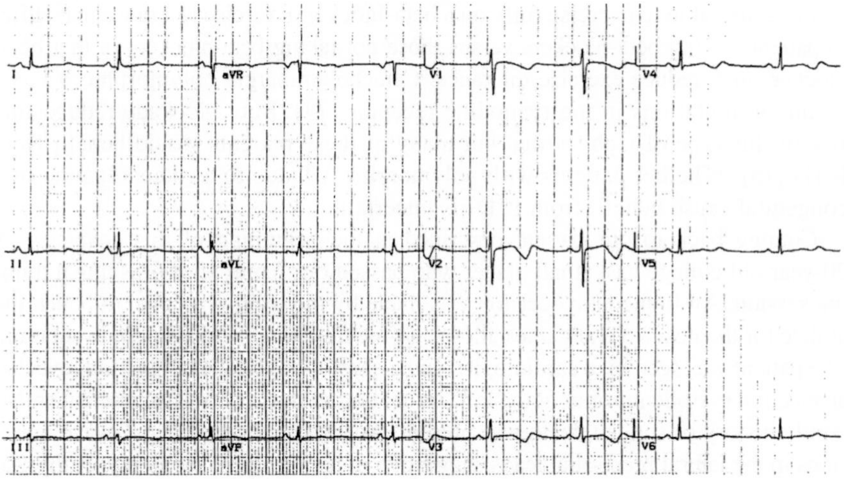

Fig. 10.12 Sixteen-year-old female with syncope

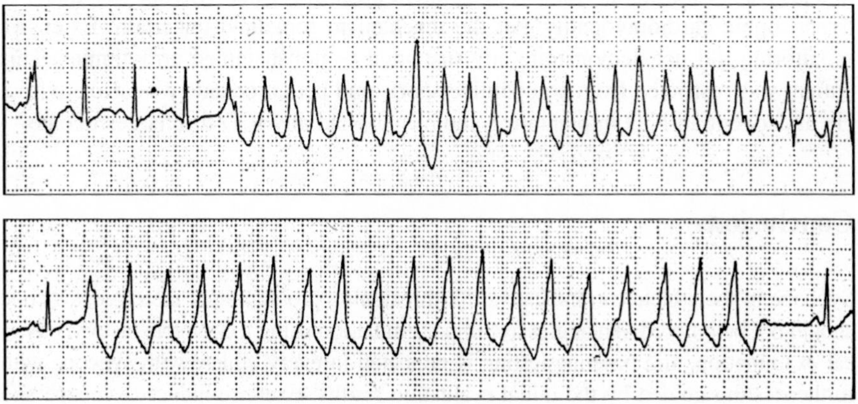

Fig. 10.13 Thirty five-year-old male with near syncope playing hockey

are all normal. MRI scan and cardiac catheterization were also normal. However, prior to these tests, Holter monitor was performed during hockey which demonstrates the following arrhythmia (Fig. 10.13). This patient has a polymorphic VT that is nonsustained and is associated with symptoms. Electrophysiology test was negative with or without isoproterenol infusion. This patient most likely has catecholaminergic polymorphic VT.

He would benefit from a beta-blocker, and if there are recurrent long episodes of this type of VT, he may also require an ICD. Ultimately, it would be in the best interest of this patient not to participate in competitive sports such as hockey. Restriction from hockey would be appropriate, but the patient refused to be restricted from hockey. The patient, however, was willing to take a beta-blocker and did not have recurrent episodes of syncope on a beta-blocker and was also able to exercise fully on a beta-blocker. Exercise tolerance may differ in patients taking beta-blockers versus those not taking beta-blockers in that beta-blockers may reduce exercise tolerance. Catecholaminergic polymorphic VT can be due to mutations in the ryanodine receptor [74]. Beta blockade reduces the risk of this type of tachycardia, but many of these patients would benefit from ICDs [75]. Whether patients with polymorphic VT due to a catecholamine or a congenital cause benefit from ICDs is uncertain.

Coming back to our patient described at the beginning of this chapter – A 20-year-old college basketball player who passed out 2 min after finishing a training session. An immediate decision was made by the team physician to bench the athlete for the next several games allowing time for a complete syncope evaluation. The patient was seen by a cardiologist, and a careful physical examination revealed an ejection systolic murmur at the left sternal border during Valsalva maneuver. No family history of sudden death was present. An ECG revealed deep T-wave inversions in the lateral precordial leads suggestive of hypertrophic cardiomyopathy. An echocardiogram revealed a septal wall thickness of 25 mm and an outflow tract gradient of 65 mmHg which increased to 110 mmHg with amyl nitrite. As described in a previous case in this chapter, this patient most likely had syncope secondary to hypertrophic cardiomyopathy, but the mechanism remained uncertain. Extensive monitoring did not demonstrate any sustained or nonsustained arrhythmias. This patient was restricted from competitive sports and beta blockade was also advised. He underwent an ICD implantation and has not had any ICD discharges to date.

Conclusions

Syncope in the athlete can indicate a life-threatening problem and, therefore, syncope should not be ignored. An aggressive initial evaluation using a complete history, physical examination, and baseline testing is indicated in every athlete with syncope with further testing guided by the initial evaluation results. Exercise-induced syncope and sudden collapse without a prodrome should be extensively evaluated. The goal in terms of diagnostic evaluation is to identify structural heart disease or an arrhythmia that can be potentially life-threatening. A benign cause should always be a diagnosis of exclusion, even though it is the predominant cause. However, diagnosis can be a challenge even after an extensive evaluation. The goal in management of syncope in the athlete is to prevent sudden cardiac death and recurrent episodes. In managing athletes with syncope, proper risk stratification is key in identifying the athlete who will need restriction. However, it may be possible that in some cases, restriction may be necessary despite treatment. A balance between athlete's desires and restriction is essential.

References

1. Estes NA III, Link MS, Cannom D, et al. Report of the NASPE policy conference on arrhythmias and the athlete. *J Cardiovasc Electrophysiol.* 2001;12(10):1208–1219.

2. Maron BJ, Zipes DP. Introduction: Eligibility recommendations for competitive athletes with cardiovascular abnormalities-general considerations. *J Am Coll Cardiol*. 2005;45(8): 1318–1321. 10.1016/j.jacc.2005.02.006.
3. Zipes DP, Ackerman MJ, Estes NA III, Grant AO, Myerburg RJ, Van Hare G. Task force 7: Arrhythmias. *J Am Coll Cardiol*. 2005;45(8):1354–1363. 10.1016/j.jacc.2005.02.014.
4. Maron BJ, Roberts WC, McAllister HA, Rosing DR, Epstein SE. Sudden death in young athletes. *Circulation*. 1980;62(2):218–229.
5. Kramer MR, Drori Y, Lev B. Sudden death in young soldiers. high incidence of syncope prior to death. *Chest*. 1988;93(2):345–347.
6. Soteriades ES, Evans JC, Larson MG, et al. Incidence and prognosis of syncope. *N Engl J Med*. 2002;347(12):878–885. 10.1056/NEJMoa012407.
7. Kapoor WN, Hanusa BH. Is syncope a risk factor for poor outcomes? comparison of patients with and without syncope. *Am J Med*. 1996;100(6):646–655.
8. Martin TP, Hanusa BH, Kapoor WN. Risk stratification of patients with syncope. *Ann Emerg Med*. 1997;29(4):459–466.
9. Olshansky B, Hahn EA, Hartz VL, Prater SP, Mason JW. Clinical significance of syncope in the electrophysiologic study versus electrocardiographic monitoring (ESVEM) trial. The ESVEM investigators. *Am Heart J*. 1999;137(5):878–886.
10. Turrini P, Corrado D, Basso C, Nava A, Thiene G. Noninvasive risk stratification in arrhythmogenic right ventricular cardiomyopathy. *Ann Noninvasive Electrocardiol*. 2003;8(2):161–169.
11. Brugada R, Hong K, Cordeiro JM, Dumaine R. Short QT syndrome. *CMAJ*. 2005;173(11): 1349–1354. 10.1503/cmaj.050596.
12. Vohra J. The long QT syndrome. *Heart Lung Circ*. 2007;16(Suppl 3):S5–S12. 10.1016/j.hlc.2007.05.008.
13. Antzelevitch C. Brugada syndrome. *Pacing Clin Electrophysiol*. 2006;29(10):1130–1159. 10.1111/j.1540–8159.2006.00507.x.
14. Behr ER, Elliott P, McKenna WJ. Role of invasive EP testing in the evaluation and management of hypertrophic cardiomyopathy. *Card Electrophysiol Rev*. 2002;6(4):482–486.
15. Olshansky B, Poole JE, Johnson G, et al. Syncope predicts the outcome of cardiomyopathy patients: Analysis of the SCD-HeFT study. *J Am Coll Cardiol*. 2008;51(13):1277–1282. 10.1016/j.jacc.2007.11.065.
16. Goldenberg I, Moss AJ. Long QT syndrome. *J Am Coll Cardiol*. 2008;51(24):2291–2300. 10.1016/j.jacc.2008.02.068.
17. Colivicchi F, Ammirati F, Santini M. Epidemiology and prognostic implications of syncope in young competing athletes. *Eur Heart J*. 2004;25(19):1749–1753. 10.1016/j.ehj.2004.07.011.
18. Colivicchi F, Ammirati F, Biffi A, Verdile L, Pelliccia A, Santini M. Exercise-related syncope in young competitive athletes without evidence of structural heart disease. Clinical presentation and long-term outcome. *Eur Heart J*. 2002;23(14):1125–1130.
19. Kapoor WN. Workup and management of patients with syncope. *Med Clin North Am*. 1995;79(5):1153–1170.
20. Maron BJ. Sudden death in young athletes. *N Engl J Med*. 2003;349(11):1064–1075. 10.1056/NEJMra022783.
21. Burke AP, Farb A, Virmani R. Causes of sudden death in athletes. *Cardiol Clin*. 1992;10(2): 303–317.
22. Samenuk D, Link MS, Homoud MK, et al. Adverse cardiovascular events temporally associated with ma huang, an herbal source of ephedrine. *Mayo Clin Proc*. 2002;77(1):12–16.
23. Ramotar J. Cyclists' deaths linked to erythropoietin? *Phys Sportsmed*. 1990;18:48.
24. Nasir JM, Durning SJ, Ferguson M, Barold HS, Haigney MC. Exercise-induced syncope associated with QT prolongation and ephedra-free xenadrine. *Mayo Clin Proc*. 2004;79(8): 1059–1062.
25. Somers VK, Abboud FM. Neurocardiogenic syncope. *Adv Intern Med*. 1996;41:399–435.
26. Manganelli F, Betocchi S, Ciampi Q, et al. Comparison of hemodynamic adaptation to orthostatic stress in patients with hypertrophic cardiomyopathy with or without syncope and in vasovagal syncope. *Am J Cardiol*. 2002;89(12):1405–1410.

27. Kumpf M, Sieverding L, Gass M, Kaulitz R, Ziemer G, Hofbeck M. Anomalous origin of left coronary artery in young athletes with syncope. *BMJ*. 2006;332(7550):1139–1141. 10.1136/bmj.332.7550.1139.
28. Corrado D, Thiene G, Cocco P, Frescura C. Non-atherosclerotic coronary artery disease and sudden death in the young. *Br Heart J*. 1992;68(6):601–607.
29. Futterman LG, Myerburg R. Sudden death in athletes: An update. *Sports Med*. 1998;26(5): 335–350.
30. Michaud GF, Wang PJ, Estes NAM. Syncope in the athlete. In: Estes NAM, Salem DN, Wang PJ, eds. *Sudden Cardiac Death in the Athlete*. Armonk, NY: Futura, 1998:419–440.
31. Alboni P, Brignole M, Menozzi C, et al. Diagnostic value of history in patients with syncope with or without heart disease. *J Am Coll Cardiol*. 2001;37(7):1921–1928.
32. Link MS, Wang PJ, Estes NA, III. Ventricular arrhythmias in the athlete. *Curr Opin Cardiol*. 2001;16(1):30–39.
33. Oh JH, Hanusa BH, Kapoor WN. Do symptoms predict cardiac arrhythmias and mortality in patients with syncope? *Arch Intern Med*. 1999;159(4):375–380.
34. Linzer M, Yang EH, Estes NA III, Wang P, Vorperian VR, Kapoor WN. Diagnosing syncope. part 1: Value of history, physical examination, and electrocardiography. clinical efficacy assessment project of the american college of physicians. *Ann Intern Med*. 1997;126(12):989–996.
35. Pelliccia A, Maron BJ, Culasso F, et al. Clinical significance of abnormal electrocardiographic patterns in trained athletes. *Circulation*. 2000;102(3):278–284.
36. Reiffel JA, Schwarzberg R, Murry M. Comparison of autotriggered memory loop recorders versus standard loop recorders versus 24-hour holter monitors for arrhythmia detection. *Am J Cardiol*. 2005;95(9):1055–1059. 10.1016/j.amjcard.2005.01.025.
37. Rothman SA, Laughlin JC, Seltzer J, et al. The diagnosis of cardiac arrhythmias: A prospective multi-center randomized study comparing mobile cardiac outpatient telemetry versus standard loop event monitoring. *J Cardiovasc Electrophysiol*. 2007;18(3):241–247.
38. Brignole M, Sutton R, Menozzi C, et al. Early application of an implantable loop recorder allows effective specific therapy in patients with recurrent suspected neurally mediated syncope. *Eur Heart J*. 2006;27(9):1085–1092. 10.1093/eurheartj/ehi842.
39. Krahn AD, Klein GJ, Yee R, Manda V. The high cost of syncope: Cost implications of a new insertable loop recorder in the investigation of recurrent syncope. *Am Heart J*. 1999;137(5):870–877.
40. Maron BJ, Pelliccia A, Spirito P. Cardiac disease in young trained athletes. Insights into methods for distinguishing athlete's heart from structural heart disease, with particular emphasis on hypertrophic cardiomyopathy. *Circulation*. 1995;91(5):1596–1601.
41. Pelliccia A, Maron BJ, Spataro A, Proschan MA, Spirito P. The upper limit of physiologic cardiac hypertrophy in highly trained elite athletes. *N Engl J Med*. 1991;324(5):295–301.
42. Maron BJ. Structural features of the athlete heart as defined by echocardiography. *J Am Coll Cardiol*. 1986;7(1):190–203.
43. Goldschlager N, Epstein AE, Grubb BP, et al. Etiologic considerations in the patient with syncope and an apparently normal heart. *Arch Intern Med*. 2003;163(2):151–162.
44. Pelliccia A, Maron BJ, De Luca R, Di Paolo FM, Spataro A, Culasso F. Remodeling of left ventricular hypertrophy in elite athletes after long-term deconditioning. *Circulation*. 2002;105(8):944–949.
45. Brignole M, Alboni P, Benditt D, et al. Guidelines on management (diagnosis and treatment) of syncope. *Eur Heart J*. 2001;22(15):1256–1306. 10.1053/euhj.2001.2739.
46. Grubb BP. Neurocardiogenic syncope. In: Grubb BP, Olshansky B, eds. *Syncope: Mechanisms and Management*. Armonk, NY: Futura, 1998:73–106.
47. Grubb BP, Temesy-Armos PN, Samoil D, Wolfe DA, Hahn H, Elliott L. Tilt table testing in the evaluation and management of athletes with recurrent exercise-induced syncope. *Med Sci Sports Exerc*. 1993;25(1):24–28.
48. Antzelevitch C. The brugada syndrome. *J Cardiovasc Electrophysiol*. 1998;9(5):513–516.
49. Priori SG, Schwartz PJ, Napolitano C, et al. Risk stratification in the long-QT syndrome. *N Engl J Med*. 2003;348(19):1866–1874. 10.1056/NEJMoa022147.

50. Brilakis ES, Shen WK, Hammill SC, et al. Role of programmed ventricular stimulation and implantable cardioverter defibrillators in patients with idiopathic dilated cardiomyopathy and syncope. *Pacing Clin Electrophysiol*. 2001;24(11):1623–1630.
51. Bigger JT Jr, Reiffel JA, Livelli FD Jr, Wang PJ. Sensitivity, specificity, and reproducibility of programmed ventricular stimulation. *Circulation*. 1986;73(2 Pt 2):II73–II78.
52. Brugada P, Green M, Abdollah H, Wellens HJ. Significance of ventricular arrhythmias initiated by programmed ventricular stimulation: The importance of the type of ventricular arrhythmia induced and the number of premature stimuli required. *Circulation*. 1984;69(1):87–92.
53. Peters S, Reil GH. Risk factors of cardiac arrest in arrhythmogenic right ventricular dysplasia. *Eur Heart J*. 1995;16(1):77–80.
54. Brignole M, Menozzi C, Moya A, et al. Mechanism of syncope in patients with bundle branch block and negative electrophysiological test. *Circulation*. 2001;104(17):2045–2050.
55. Menozzi C, Brignole M, Garcia-Civera R, et al. Mechanism of syncope in patients with heart disease and negative electrophysiologic test. *Circulation*. 2002;105(23):2741–2745.
56. Jackman WM, Wang XZ, Friday KJ, et al. Catheter ablation of accessory atrioventricular pathways (wolff-parkinson-white syndrome) by radiofrequency current. *N Engl J Med*. 1991; 324(23):1605–1611.
57. Zardini M, Yee R, Thakur RK, Klein GJ. Risk of sudden arrhythmic death in the wolff-parkinson-white syndrome: Current perspectives. *Pacing Clin Electrophysiol*. 1994;17(5 Pt 1):966–975.
58. Link MS, Homoud MK, Wang PJ, Estes NA III. Cardiac arrhythmias in the athlete. *Cardiol Rev*. 2001;9(1):21–30.
59. Pappone C, Santinelli V, Manguso F, et al. A randomized study of prophylactic catheter ablation in asymptomatic patients with the wolff-parkinson-white syndrome. *N Engl J Med*. 2003;349(19):1803–1811. 10.1056/NEJMoa035345.
60. Link MS, Estes NAM. Ventricular arrhythmias. In: Estes NAM, Salem DN, Wang PJ, eds. *Sudden Cardiac Death in the Athlete*. Armonk. NY: Futura, 1998:253–275.
61. Krediet CT, van Dijk N, Linzer M, van Lieshout JJ, Wieling W. Management of vasovagal syncope: Controlling or aborting faints by leg crossing and muscle tensing. *Circulation*. 2002;106(13):1684–1689.
62. Jordan J, Shannon JR, Black BK, et al. The pressor response to water drinking in humans: A sympathetic reflex? *Circulation*. 2000;101(5):504–509.
63. El-Sayed H, Hainsworth R. Salt supplement increases plasma volume and orthostatic tolerance in patients with unexplained syncope. *Heart*. 1996;75(2):134–140.
64. Reybrouck T, Heidbuchel H, Van De Werf F, Ector H. Long-term follow-up results of tilt training therapy in patients with recurrent neurocardiogenic syncope. *Pacing Clin Electrophysiol*. 2002;25(10):1441–1446.
65. Link MS, Homoud MK, Wang PJ, Estes NA III. Cardiac arrhythmias in the athlete: The evolving role of electrophysiology. *Curr Sports Med Rep*. 2002;1(2):75–85.
66. Haissaguerre M, Jais P, Shah DC, et al. Spontaneous initiation of atrial fibrillation by ectopic beats originating in the pulmonary veins. *N Engl J Med*. 1998;339(10):659–666.
67. Calkins H, Kalbfleisch SJ, el-Atassi R, Langberg JJ, Morady F. Relation between efficacy of radiofrequency catheter ablation and site of origin of idiopathic ventricular tachycardia. *Am J Cardiol*. 1993;71(10):827–833.
68. Klein LS, Miles WM. Ablative therapy for ventricular arrhythmias. *Prog Cardiovasc Dis*. 1995;37(4):225–242.
69. Eisenberg SJ, Scheinman MM, Dullet NK, et al. Sudden cardiac death and polymorphous ventricular tachycardia in patients with normal QT intervals and normal systolic cardiac function. *Am J Cardiol*. 1995;75(10):687–692.
70. European Heart Rhythm Association, Heart Rhythm Society, Zipes DP, et al. ACC/AHA/ESC 2006 guidelines for management of patients with ventricular arrhythmias and the prevention of sudden cardiac death: A report of the american college of Cardiology/American heart association task force and the european society of cardiology committee for practice guidelines (writing committee to develop guidelines for management of patients with ventricular

arrhythmias and the prevention of sudden cardiac death). *J Am Coll Cardiol*. 2006;48(5):e247–e346. 10.1016/j.jacc.2006.07.010.

71. Lampert R, Cannom D, Olshansky B. Safety of sports participation in patients with implantable cardioverter defibrillators: A survey of heart rhythm society members. *J Cardiovasc Electrophysiol*. 2006;17(1):11–15.
72. Schwartz PJ, Priori SG, Spazzolini C, et al. Genotype-phenotype correlation in the long-QT syndrome: Gene-specific triggers for life-threatening arrhythmias. *Circulation*. 2001; 103(1):89–95.
73. Moss AJ, Robinson JL, Gessman L, et al. Comparison of clinical and genetic variables of cardiac events associated with loud noise versus swimming among subjects with the long QT syndrome. *Am J Cardiol*. 1999;84(8):876–879.
74. Priori SG, Napolitano C, Tiso N, et al. Mutations in the cardiac ryanodine receptor gene (hRyR2) underlie catecholaminergic polymorphic ventricular tachycardia. *Circulation*. 2001;103(2):196–200.
75. Wilde AA, Bhuiyan ZA, Crotti L, et al. Left cardiac sympathetic denervation for catecholaminergic polymorphic ventricular tachycardia. *N Engl J Med*. 2008;358(19):2024–2029. 10.1056/NEJMoa0708006.

Chapter 11
Heart Murmurs

Robert E. Poley and Bryan M. White

Introduction

Family physicians, pediatricians, and internists all have regular contact with athletes in settings where a heart murmur may be discovered. This chapter discusses the diagnosis and management of a newly detected heart murmur in the athletic population and reviews current guidelines that allow for safe participation in sports [1].

Table 11.1 provides the basic classification of all murmur types. Murmurs are first described as systolic, diastolic, or continuous. Further classification into each of these categories provides additional information as to their etiology and is included in the table. Determining where in the cardiac cycle the murmur is audible is of paramount importance in determining workup, as is reflected in the algorithm provided in Fig. 11.1 [2].

Patient History

A thorough history is the essential first step when encountering an athlete with a cardiac murmur. Symptoms that could be attributable to a murmur include shortness of breath, chest pain, palpitations (the sensation of skipped or forceful heartbeats), syncope or near-syncope, dizziness, early fatigue, and peripheral edema. Any symptom uncovered should then be discussed in detail with attention to *duration, onset, provoking factors, palliating factors, quality, severity, location, radiation, and associated symptoms* [3, 4].

Once a detailed symptom history has been obtained, it is important to gather the remainder of the historical information. Has the patient ever experienced these symptoms before? The past medical history should review symptoms of exercise-associated syncope or near syncope. Any chronic or previous medical conditions or hospitalizations are important. Sometimes, an adolescent or young adult mentions

R.E. Poley (✉)
Division of Sports Medicine, William Beaumont Hospital, Troy, MI, USA
e-mail: dr_poley@yahoo.com

C.E. Lawless (ed.), *Sports Cardiology Essentials: Evaluation, Management and Case Studies*, DOI 10.1007/978-0-387-92775-6_11,

Table 11.1 Classification of cardiac murmurs

Systolic murmurs	(a) Holosystolic (pan-systolic) murmurs
	(b) Mid-systolic (systolic ejection) murmurs
	(c) Early systolic murmurs
	(d) Mid- to late-systolic murmurs
Diastolic murmurs	(a) Early high-pitched diastolic murmurs
	(b) Mid-diastolic murmurs
	(c) Presystolic murmurs
Continuous murmurs	

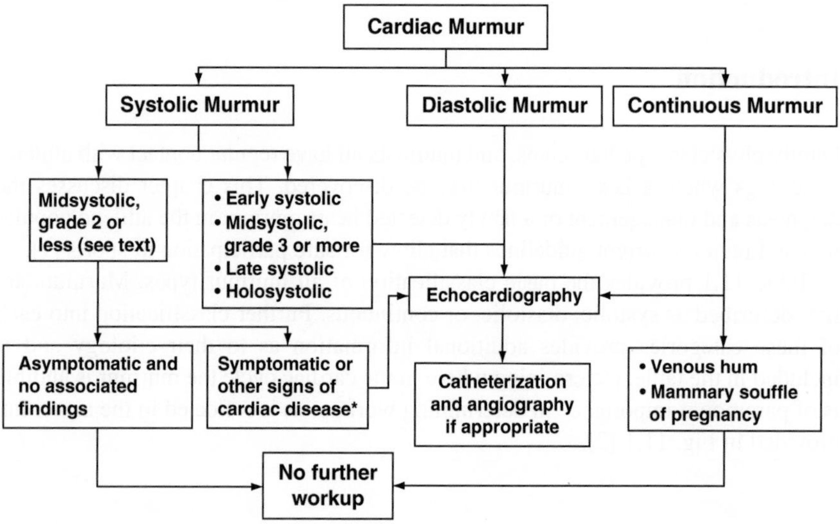

Fig. 11.1 Algorithim for workup of newly detected cardiac murmurs [2]. From: ACC/AHA 2006 Guidelines for the Management of Patients with Valvular Heart Disease. Reprinted with Permission. Circulation 2006 114: e84–e231. ©2006 American Heart Association, Inc

a history of a murmur as a young child which resolved or seemed to go away. In this instance, obtaining more information including physician progress notes or test results may be necessary.

A directed but detailed family history should be obtained. Specific questions should inquire as to the presence of congenital heart disease, history of arrhythmias in relatives, early sudden cardiac death (under the age of 50 years), Marfan's syndrome, and any instance of valvular disease or history of deep vein thrombosis or pulmonary embolism.

In the adolescent athlete and college athlete especially, the social history is of importance to identify substance use that may contribute to the athlete's complaints. Recreational drugs, over-the-counter medications, herbal and alternative supplements, energy drinks, as well as tobacco and alcohol use can have a direct or indirect effect on the heart.

Finally, a comprehensive review of systems is necessary to identify any underlying or contributing medical conditions that may be at work. For example, recent upper respiratory infections preceding chest pain or shortness of breath could indicate myocarditis. Unexplained fevers could suggest an underlying infection such as bacterial endocarditis.

Physical Examination

The physical examination is often curtailed to the setting in which the athlete first presents. In the training room, a brief cardiopulmonary examination is performed with further follow-up planned in a more formal setting. In the office, time, assistance, and resources are more available and allow for a more comprehensive examination. This would include measurement of blood pressure, respirations, pulse rate and pulse oximetry, height, weight, electrocardiogram, and sometimes X-ray if readily available.

The patient's history can be used to direct some aspects of the examination to areas of highest concern. The initial exam along with the presenting history is often all that the practitioner has to make a determination on clearance for participation. Pulling an athlete from any sports activity until additional workup is performed is often prudent. If a specific cause can be identified that does not jeopardize the athlete's health, step-by-step return to sport can be allowed with appropriate treatment and with close monitoring of the athlete's symptoms.

The approach to the physical examination, especially the cardiac examination, should be systematic, and starts with the vital signs to include height, weight, and an assessment of body habitus. This is followed by a detailed examination of the head and neck. Particularly, one should note the presence of xanthelasma, conjuctival pallor, thyroid enlargement, and elevated jugular venous pulsations [5, 6] and assess the carotid upstroke. Additionally, the carotid artery can be auscultated for the presence of bruits or radiation of a murmur, and the upstroke palpated for fullness (pulsus parvus if lessened) and timing (pulsus tardus if delayed) [3, 7].

The precordial examination starts with inspection, followed by percussion, palpation, and finally auscultation. It is important to balance exposure of the patient, which is essential to an adequate examination, versus the privacy of the patient. The majority of female athletes will be adolescents or teenagers and should be examined in the presence of a chaperone. The examination should be performed on the patient's right side [6].

Rarely will any of the patients have had previous cardiac surgeries, but inspection may identify the presence of any chest wall abnormalities such as pectus excavatum or carinatum (each is a major criterion of the skeletal system in the diagnosis of Marfan's syndrome). One should pay close attention to the body habitus of the patient. The tall and thinner body habitus athletes will have a more vertical heart position, whereas the athletes with an obese midsection will have a more horizontal heart. The heart's position will affect where you will auscultate the athlete's murmur. Next, the precordium is percussed in a lateral-to-medial fashion starting at the level of the diaphragm and working superiorly to outline the border of the heart and hence to assess for cardiomegaly. This is followed by palpation of the left ventricle (LV) and right ventricle (RV) with the base of the right hand. The LV apex can be appreciated in either a supine position or more easily in the left lateral decubitus position. The apical impulse should be brisk and firm and about the size of a dime. Patients with a cardiomyopathy will generally have a laterally displaced, widened, and diffusely hypokinetic apex. The RV is next palpated along the right and left parasternal borders at the fourth and fifth intercostal (note change from inner costal) spaces. Normally, the RV should be silent and not appreciated when the pulmonary artery (PA) pressures are <30 mmHg. As PA pressures increase, the RV impulse becomes greater and is appreciated as a heave or a lift [6–8].

Next, we move to auscultation. This, as with all parts of a detailed physical examination, needs to be performed in a systematic manner. Starting with the patient sitting upright, the diaphragm of the stethoscope is placed in the right parasternal second intercostal space and is then moved in an "inching" manner to the left, and then inferiorly to the level of the xiphoid, before moving leftward around the apex, and if necessary to the axilla or to the back to determine if there is any radiation of a murmur. At the apex, the diaphragm is switched to the bell which will better allow the examiner to hear lower pitched sounds such as a S3 or a diastolic rumble. The bell is "inched" back retracing the movements from the apex to the right parasternal border. This is repeated with the patient lying supine. Important to note is the examiner must apply their understanding of the patient's body habitus and positioning of the heart to their strategy for auscultation. Therefore, the examination may require more auscultation of the right parasternal border and inferiorly if a patient has a more vertical heart or conversely more of the left lateral border if the patient has a more horizontal heart. Additional maneuvers or positions should be performed if a murmur is identified [3, 7].

With particular attention to the focus of this chapter, a brief review of the description of cardiac murmurs is presented. Laminar blood flow is considered the normal state of blood flow as it moves easily through the major blood vessels and is not audible through a stethoscope. Structural changes and/or hemodynamic changes in the heart produce turbulent blood flow, which in turn causes an audible noise. Once a murmur has been identified on the exam, specific descriptive characteristics detected on auscultation can be applied to help determine the etiology of the murmur. The descriptive characteristics are (1) *timing*, (2) *intensity*, (3) *pitch*, (4) *shape*, (5) *location*, (6) *radiation*, and (7) *response to maneuvers. Timing* describes where in the cardiac cycle the murmur is audible: systolic, diastolic, or continuous. *Intensity* is subjective but can be somewhat quantified using the grading system in Table 11.2. *Pitch* relates to the frequency of tone, described as high-pitched to low-pitched murmurs. High-pitched murmurs are generally better heard with the diaphragm, whereas low-pitch murmurs are best heard with the bell piece of the stethoscope. *Shape* relates to changes in intensity from the audible start of murmur to the end. Common terms used to describe shape include crescendo–decrescendo (diamond shaped), decrescendo, and uniform (the intensity is constant). Additionally, murmurs should be described in their relationship to the cardiac cycle. A crescendo–decrescendo murmur of aortic stenosis (AS) would also be referred to as a mid-systolic murmur, whereas the murmur of atrioventricular (mitral or tricuspid) valvular insufficiency or a ventricular septal defect would be referred to as either a holo-(aka pan) systolic murmur versus a uniform murmur. Semilunar (aortic or pulmonic) valvular insufficiency murmurs are referred to as diastolic decrescendo murmurs. Please refer to Figs. 11.2 and 11.3 [7]. *Location* describes where on the chest the

Table 11.2 Grading intensity of systolic and diastolic murmurs

Systolic murmurs	Diastolic murmurs
Grade 1/6: barely audible	Grade 1/4: barely audible
Grade 2/6: faint, but immediately audible	Grade 2/4: faint but immediately audible
Grade 3/6: easily heard	Grade 3/4: easily heard
Grade 4/6: easily heard and associated with a palpable thrill	Grade 4/4: very loud
Grade 5/6: very loud; heard with a stethoscope lightly on chest	
Grade 6/6: audible without the stethoscope directly on the chest wall	

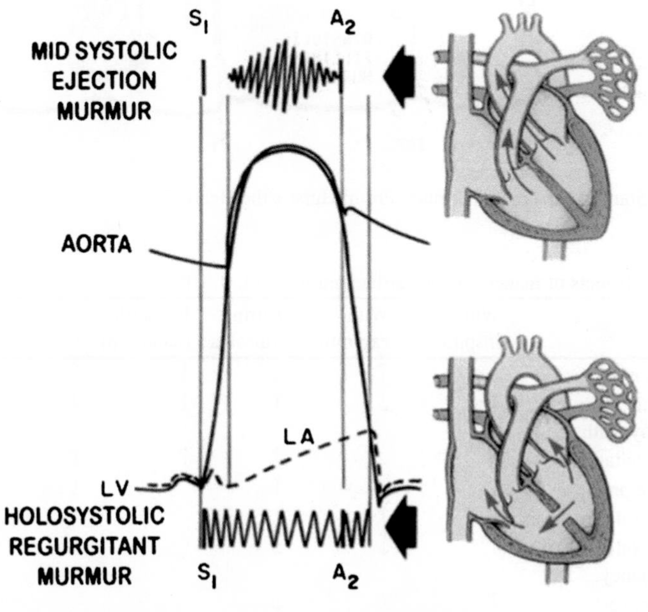

Fig. 11.2 Standard systolic murmurs. From: Hurst's the Heart [7]

murmur's maximum intensity is best heard. These locations are generally described as aortic (second intercostal space at right sternal border), pulmonic (second intercostal space, left sternal border), tricuspid (lower left sternal border), and mitral (cardiac apex). The sound of the primary murmur may be heard in other locations on the chest or neck and therefore are said to *radiate*, and this is usually in the direction of the turbulent flow. Finally, response to specific *maneuvers* may differentiate between similar murmurs. Common maneuvers include standing upright, squatting down, and performing a Valsalva (forced expiration against a closed glottis). These maneuvers and the effects on specific valvular conditions are described in Table 11.3. It is of particular importance to perform these maneuvers on athletes in whom a cardiac murmur has been identified, where the goal of the examiner should be to identify what valvular lesion the murmur most likely represents: aortic stenosis, hypertrophic obstructive cardiomyopathy, mitral valve prolapse, etc. [3, 7].

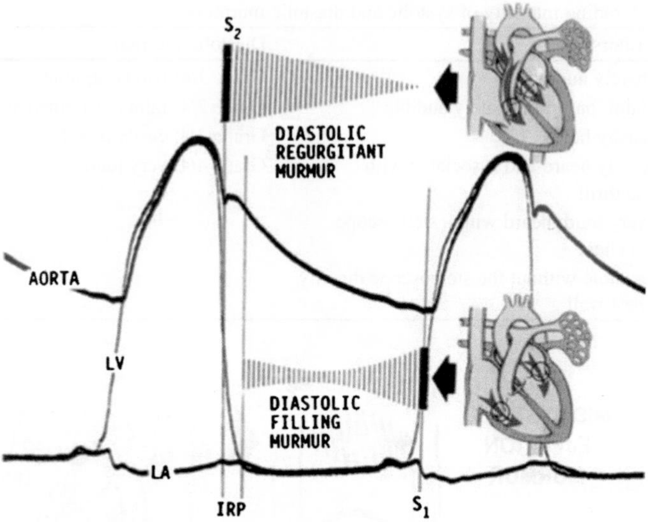

Fig. 11.3 Standard diastolic murmurs. From: Hurst's the Heart [7]

Table 11.3 Effects of maneuvers on cardiac murmurs [3, 9, 10]

	With inspiration	With expiration	During Valsalva	Isometric (handgrip)	Squatting	Standing
Aortic stenosis	↓	↑	↓	↓	↑	↓
Hypertrophic obstructive cardiomyopathy	↑	↓	↑	↓	↓	↑
Mitral regurgitation			↑	↑	↑	↓
Mitral valve prolapse	↑	↓	↑		↓	↑
Pulmonary valve stenosis	↑	↑	↓			
Pulmonary valve insufficiency	↑	↓	↓			
Tricuspid valve insufficiency	↑	↓	↓			

↑ = Intensity of the murmur increases (accentuates)
↓ = Intensity of the murmur decreases (diminishes)

A study published in the New England Journal of Medicine in 1988 looked at the sensitivity and specificity of different maneuvers and their diagnostic accuracy [11]. Notably, distinguishing hypertrophic obstructive cardiomyopathy (HOCM) by using the Valsalva maneuver, for which the murmur would intensify, had a 65% sensitivity with a 96% specificity, while the squatting-to-standing maneuver (murmur intensifies) had a 95% sensitivity with a 84% specificity. The diagnosis of HOCM by standing-to-squatting maneuver (murmur lessens) showed a 95% sensitivity with an 85% specificity; while a hand-grip maneuver (murmur lessens) had an 85% sensitivity with a 75% specificity.

Approach to Murmurs

An easy approach to murmurs is to first distinguish if the murmur is systolic, diastolic, or continuous and then if it is left-sided or right-sided. It is not uncommon to encounter a benign systolic murmur; however, every diastolic murmur is pathologic. Left-sided systolic murmurs can be better identified by relating the murmur to the predominant effect of the maneuver: increase or decrease of the preload or after load to afterload. The two low-preload-dependent murmurs are mitral valve prolapse (MVP) and hypertrophic obstructive cardiomyopathy (HOCM). These murmurs need to be evaluated for both timing and intensity [3, 4].

MVP and HOCM murmurs will augment (combination of increasing intensity and earlier onset) with decreasing preload. In the setting of HOCM, decreased intracavitary volumes allow for a greater degree of subaortic obstruction and earlier onset of obstruction. This can be accomplished with a variety of maneuvers, most notably standing upright after squatting or the strain phase of Valsalva. The systolic murmur's intensity will increase more with upright standing from a combination of decreasing preload and increasing the gradient across the left ventricular outflow tract (decreasing afterload) in comparison to the Valsalva maneuver which actually increases afterload mildly, but not enough to negate the predominant effect, which is decreasing preload. Additionally, the apex should be listened to because as the dynamic obstruction occurs, the mitral valve will become audibly regurgitant in mid to late systole. This is related to the anterior leaflet of the mitral valve that is sucked anteriorly into the left ventricular outflow track midway through systole due to the forces created by the gradient across the hypertrophied and hyperkinetic septum. This systolic anterior motion of the mitral valve leads to mid to late systolic mitral regurgitation (MR). Therefore, in patients with HOCM, they will have augmentation of their outflow murmur and their mitral insufficiency murmur. Additionally, the presence of premature ventricular contractions (PVC's) will aid in the diagnosis. The pause following the PVC will result in increased catecholamines, leading to increased contractility, with a net result of an increased dynamic gradient across the outflow track. This will intensify the murmur and cause it to occur earlier in systole [4, 7].

The murmur of MVP is very similar. The regurgitant murmur is caused by redundant and sclerotic myxomatous mitral valve leaflets causing incomplete coaptation. During initial systole, when ventricular volume is still elevated, the leaflets coapt appropriately. As further contraction occurs, the LV volume decreases. This decrement in volume causes the myxomatous and sclerotic leaflets to stop coapting normally and essentially fold-in on themselves, thus causing the mitral insufficiency. Maneuvers that increase the preload of the LV will lessen the midsystolic mitral regurgitant murmur. Conversely, reducing the preload will facilitate this poor coaptation, leading to an earlier onset and a louder regurgitant murmur. The strain phase of the Valsalva is the preferred technique to demonstrate this physiology. As discussed previously, preload is reduced and afterload increased with the Valsalva maneuver. While the change in afterload is not the predominant effect, it helps further augment this murmur. In severe cases, the murmur will intensify with normal respiration, as during inspiration the normal drop in left ventricular preload is enough to accentuate the murmur, but it will augment with rapid standing from a squatting position, where the predominant mechanism is reducing preload causing an earlier onset of the murmur, but it may not be as intense as that maneuver also reduces afterload. The MR murmur of MVP is preceded by a mid-systolic click which may or may not be appreciated and is generally a higher pitched sound that may sound extrathoracic [3, 4, 7].

Valvular aortic stenosis is a mid-systolic murmur intensified by increasing left ventricular preload or by reducing afterload. Hence, squatting will intensify the murmur, while it will be diminished by rapid standing or the strain phase of the Valsalva maneuver (the contrary to HOCM). Non-MVP mitral regurgitation is generally intensified with increasing afterload and lessened with decreasing afterload. This pan-systolic murmur will increase with squatting or isometric exercise and will lessen with rapid standing or with the use of amyl nitrate [3, 11].

The benign systolic murmur of the young, otherwise known as a Still's murmur, will be a mid-systolic murmur and is related to a more forceful ejection of blood causing the flow to be nonlaminar, and is not related to any pathologic obstruction or regurgitation. This occurs because the patient is well conditioned and bradycardiac (HR ~ 50 bpm), and the increase force is related to simply greater stroke volumes from the bradycardia. Occasionally, you may encounter an anxious patient who has a benign murmur related to increased forceful ejection from simply the increase catecholamines related to their anxiety. Benign murmurs will be grade 1–2 out of 6, but never higher, and are generally heard in the Aortic (second right intercostal space and sometimes the Pulmonic (second left intercostal space) positions. Additionally, a benign s (heard after S2) can sometimes be appreciated in the bradycardiac patients related to the volume of blood moving from the left atrium into the left ventricle during early diastole. S3's are rarely heard with higher heart rates, and S4's are always pathologic. And finally, exercise will cause a systolic murmur through the left ventricular outflow tract and possibly the right as well due to the rapidity and forcefulness of systolic ejection. This underscores the necessity of examining patients in the resting state in a calm environment [12, 13].

Right-sided systolic murmurs are related to either tricuspid insufficiency (holo systolic), which occurs quite frequently in heart failure patients, or pulmonic stenosis (mid-systolic), which is a rare finding. Pulmonic stenosis (PS) is a crescendo–decrescendo murmur heard best in the left upper sternal border, whereas tricuspid insufficiency is heard more inferiorly and is a decrescendo murmur. PS will actually lessen with inspiration as the driving pressures through the valve drop with decreases in intrathoracic pressure. TR will intensify with inspiration, and this augmentation is given the eponym "Carvallo's sign." [3].

Diastolic murmurs are pathologic, but their presence does not necessarily portend a bad prognosis. Left-sided diastolic murmurs include aortic insufficiency (AI) and mitral stenosis (MS). AI is heard best along the left lower sternal border, with patient leaning forward against the diaphragm of the stethoscope and exhaling. This will be a decrescendo murmur. In the setting of chronic severe AI, transmitral flow is obstructed by the anterior leaflet being pushed posteriorly from the force of the aortic insufficiency jet. This diastolic inflow obstruction causes a late diastolic murmur known as the Austin Flint murmur. Mitral stenosis is most commonly related to rheumatic heart disease. There is an opening snap related to the forceful opening of the mitral valve to allow diastolic flow into ventricle. The more severe the stenosis, the later the opening snap occurs, and paradoxically, the less intense the opening snap. The snap is followed by a diastolic rumble best heard with the bell of the stethoscope. Right-sided diastolic murmurs include tricuspid stenosis, which is extremely rare, and would give a right-sided opening snap and diastolic rumble. The other is pulmonic insufficiency, which can be difficult to hear, but is auscultated in the same fashion as AI and is decrescendo in nature [3, 7].

Continuous murmurs are always pathologic and most likely represent a patent ductus arteriosus or more rare etiologies such as arteriovenous fistulas, anomalous left coronary arteries arising from the pulmonary artery, or fistulas arising from the sinuses of Valsalva.

Other congenital heart anomalies include Atrial Septal Defect (ASD) and Ventricular Septal Defect (VSD). When direct communication between the left and right atria fails to close shortly after birth, an ASD is present. ASD accounts for around 35% of congenital heart diseases in adults and 10% of all congenital heart diseases. It is rarely of consequence in the infant/toddler population with symptoms generally presenting in the fourth of fifth decade of life. The most commonly reported symptoms are dyspnea on exertion and easy fatigability. ASD is associated with a fixed splitting of the second heart sound (S2). Generally speaking, a moderately large left-to-right shunt produces a pulmonary outflow murmur that begins shortly after the S1 heart sound, peaks in early to mid systole, and ends before S2. Atrial septal defects can produce various murmur patterns depending on the size of the shunt and include a crescendo-decrescendo grade 2–3 murmur at the second intercostal space, left sternal border as one example. Ventricular Septal defects are classified into three major categories: muscular, membranous, or doubly committed. Some VSD lesions will close spontaneously in childhood. Small VSD lesions pose a risk for endocarditis. However, the majority of adults with small restrictive VSD are asymptomatic. The associated murmur is generally described as harsh or high-frequency and pan-systolic. The grade is usually 3–4 out of 6, and heard at maximal intensity at the left sternal border in the third or fourth intercostal space. A moderately restrictive VSD usually presents with dyspnea in adult life. Other examination findings of a VSD include apical diastolic rumble and third heart sound as well as central cyanosis and clubbing of the nail beds. In either case, previously undiagnosed congenital heart disease murmurs can present to a primary-care physician office as a new patient looking to start an exercise program or an individual having symptoms with exercise [3, 7, 11].

Complex congenital heart conditions such as repaired Tetralogy of Fallot and d-Transposition of the Great Vessels are beyond the scope of this chapter. These patients should be followed in an adult congenital heart disease clinic by a specialist. It would be rare and unlikely for a primary-care physician to encounter a previously undiagnosed complex cyanotic congenital heart defect.

Aids to Physical Examination

Recent advances in the development of detailed algorithms and computer-assisted analysis (CAA) of heart sounds has led to a number of studies showing benefits of using CAA to assist the physician in making confident decisions on when a murmur is a pathologic versus innocent murmur. In 2004, Watrous and colleagues of Zargis Medical Corporation published a pilot study that compared the interpretations of an experienced cardiologist listening to recorded heart sounds to the murmur detection algorithm results [14]. The study included 12 subjects, 11 of which had known hypertrophic cardiomyopathy. The computer program analysis was reported to have a sensitivity of 90.7% and a positive predictive value of 93%. CAA detected 36 murmurs, one of which was a false positive, giving specificity of 97.6%. The algorithm was more accurate in detecting high-grade (louder) murmurs with 100% of grade 2–3 and grade 3 murmurs but only 50% of grade 1 murmurs. The authors concluded that the CAA showed promise for use in larger applications for assisting practitioners in preparticipation sports physicals. A subsequent [15] study found that computer-assisted auscultation improved sensitivity of correct identification of pathological murmurs and improved the specificity of identifying benign cases (innocent or no murmurs). In regard to referrals to pediatric cardiologists, the sensitivity and specificity also improved and was statistically significant. The study conclusion was that CAA appears to be a promising new technology for informing the referral decisions of primary-care physicians. More research will be needed to evaluate these claims on a large population-based screening scope, and questions regarding the cost, availability, and insurance reimbursement will need to be answered.

Training Tools

Currently, there are various training tools available for the practicing physicians and physicians in training to improve their ability to recognize and distinguish cardiac murmurs and extra heart sounds (Table 11.4). Most are commercialized products, and there

Table 11.4 Selected websites with cardiac auscultation sounds (as of September 1, 2008)

http://www.blaufuss.org/ Ears On Cardiac Auscultation Teaching Program	For profit organization developing teaching tools for physicians	limited free tutorials; 300+ heart sounds for $149 on CD-Rom
http://www.cardiosource.com/heartsounds/index.asp "Heart Songs" audio product	American College of Cardiology	A few free audio files available; 3 CD + 1 CD-ROM – $130 nonmember price
http://www.usmlehelp.com//learn_cardiac_auscultation/heart_auscultation.html USMLE Help: Cardiac Auscultation	USMLE Help	text and audio comprehensive review; 1 month online subscription for $17.95

are too many of them to be objectively reviewed. One, called Teach and Learn Heart Auscultation, has been referenced in a few studies and has been shown to improve diagnostic skills [16–18]. Other studies have demonstrated efficacy in teaching and improving cardiac auscultation skills [16], and with the availability of MP3 players increasing, the ability to conveniently listen to examples of cardiac murmurs and extra heart sounds repetitively is easily accomplished. Using an iPod to teach cardiac examination skills to residents, Barrett [19] found that repetition in the order of 500 times is necessary to train the ear to pick up the differences in the various valvular conditions.

Diagnostic Evaluation

The *Electrocardiogram* (ECG) is an easy and essential first step in evaluating an athlete who presents with symptoms suggesting a cardiovascular etiology. The specifics of the ECG as they pertain to the athlete are covered elsewhere in the text. In light of a normal or equivocal ECG, additional investigation is likely necessary.

A standard *chest X-ray*, consisting of P–A and Lateral views, is used to investigate the mediastinum, lungs, and heart. The chest X-ray is of special importance in an athlete that has additional associated symptoms of cough, fever, peripheral edema, and/or fatigue. X-ray allows for a quick determination of cardiac size, presence of pneumonia or other potential infectious cause, or findings suggestive of heart failure such as Kerley-B lines.

Echocardiography is a valuable tool which provides both anatomic and physiologic information. In particular, when dealing with an athlete that has a new or chronic cardiac murmur, or symptoms to suggest a murmur, the echocardiogram will be the most important diagnostic tool. Data obtained includes the size of the cardiac chambers, presence of valvular disease and the severity of these conditions, septal wall thickness, the presence of abnormal communications between the heart chambers, and an estimate of systolic function (ejection fraction percentage). Specific results which aid in the disposition and management of athletes with a murmur include the following: (1) Left ventricular wall thickness – of primary concern due to its role in causing left ventricular outflow obstruction in hypertrophic cardiomyopathy (HOCM). A left ventricular wall thickness of greater than 15 mm is considered abnormal, and consistent with HOCM in the adult athletic population. (2) Transvalvular pressure gradient across stenotic valves – for example, a peak trans-valvular gradient in Pulmonic stenosis of less than 50 mmHg denotes mild to moderate disease, where severe PS is defined by a valve area smaller than 0.5 cm^2 and a peak transvalvular gradient of greater than 75 mmHg. In most cases, a standard echocardiogram (with Doppler) is usually sufficient to gather all the needed information – unless there is high suspicion for cardiac ischemia affecting left ventricular function. Additional details of the echocardiogram are covered elsewhere in this text.

Stress Testing is commonly used to evaluate symptoms and conditions in athletes, since it is a mode of reproducing similar exercise conditions in which their symptoms generally arise. The Bruce protocol for exercise stress testing is often insufficient for producing adequate cardiac stress in high-caliber athletes (as measured by VO_2 max and/or peak heart rate). Specific findings of greatest interest include evidence of myocardial ischemia on the ECG, abnormal blood pressure response, and the presence of abnormalities of rhythm and conduction (PVCs, nonsustained ventricular-tachycardia) that are new or changed from baseline. In terms of diagnosis or management, stress testing does not provide much information directly pertaining to the status of a known or suspected murmur.

In selected patients, additional workup may include *cardiac MRI/MRA*, *tilt table testing*, *electrophysiologic* (EP) testing, and *cardiac catheterization*. Details of some of these tests are covered in other chapters of this text and are obtained in conjunction with cardiology consultation. In an individual suspected to have Marfan's syndrome, a dilated eye exam is necessary as well. Laboratory evaluation may include complete blood count, sedimentation rate, viral titers, and thyroid studies based on information gathered in the history and physical exam [3, 7, 11].

Management of Specific Valvular Conditions

The details of some specific cardiovascular conditions causing valvular abnormalities are covered in other chapters of this book. However, The 36th Bethesda Conference provides eligibility recommendations for competitive athletes with cardiovascular abnormalities, including specific valvular abnormalities [20]. It is important to remember that these are guidelines not steadfast, and specific recommendations are to be individualized to each athlete's situation by his or her own physician. Task Force 3 of the 36th Bethesda Conference contains specific recommendations for the sports participation of athletes as it relates to ten separate valvular pathologies. They are Mitral Stenosis (MS), Mitral Regurgitation (MR), Aortic Stenosis (AS), Aortic Regurgitation (AR), Bicuspid Aortic Valves with Aortic Root Dilatation, Tricuspid Regurgitation (TR), Tricuspid Stenosis (TS), Multivalvular disease, Prosthetic Heart Valves, and Valve Repair/Percutaneous Mitral Balloon Valvotomy. Tables 11.5–11.14 summarize the specific recommendations on six of these ten conditions, plus three congenital cardiac abnormalities causing murmur (Pulmonic Stenosis, Atrial Septal Defect, and Ventricular Septal Defect), and finally Mitral Valve Prolapse – covered by Task Force 4. These are some of the more common valvular conditions that a primary-care physician may encounter in the athletic population. The tables include references to the classification of sports (based on the degree of static and dynamic components required), and this is provided in Fig. 11.4.

Case 1

Patient History

A 20-year-old female collegiate varsity swimmer presents to the training room with diminished exercise tolerance and inability to maintain her usual times in the pool. She states that she feels more tired than usual halfway into her training, which

Table 11.5 Guidelines from the 36th Bethesda Conference for specific valvular abnormalities: mitral stenosis

Diagnosis	Qualifier	Recommendation
Mild MS	• Sinus rhythm • Peak pulmonary artery systolic pressure during exercise of <50 mmHg	• Can participate in all sports
Moderate MS	• Sinus rhythm or atrial fibrillation • Peak pulmonary artery systolic pressure during exercise of <50 mmHg	• Low & moderate static sports • Low and moderate dynamic sports • (Class IA, IB, IIA, IIB – see Fig. 11.4)
Severe MS	• Sinus rhythm or atrial fibrillation • Peak pulmonary artery systolic pressure greater than 50 mmHg	• Should not participate in competitive sports
MS any severity	• Concurrent anticoagulation therapy	• Should not participate in competitive sports involving the risk of bodily injury or trauma

Table 11.6 Guidelines from the 36th Bethesda Conference for specific valvular abnormalities: mitral regurgitation

Diagnosis	Qualifier	Recommendation
Mild to Moderate MR	• Sinus rhythm • Normal LV size and function • Normal pulmonary artery pressures	• Can participate in all sports
Mild to Moderate MR	• Sinus rhythm • Nomal LV systolic function at rest • Mild LV enlargement (<60 mm – which may be explained by athletic training alone)	• Some low and moderate static sports • Low and moderate dynamic sports • (Class IA, IB, IC, IIA, IIB, IIC – see Fig. 11.4)
Severe MR	• And… • Definite LV enlargement (greater than 60 mm), OR • Pulmonary hypertension, OR • LV dysfunction at rest	• Should not participate in competitive sports
MR any severity	• In atrial fibrillation • Or, history of atrial fibrillation on long-term anticoagulation therapy	• Should not participate in competitive sports involving the risk of bodily injury or trauma

currently consists of a morning 5,000 m session and an afternoon 2,500 m session. She has had fatigue only with exercise now for about 2 weeks. Her daily activities do not seem to be affected. She has only had to stop swimming once in the preceding 2 weeks but otherwise notices that her times are a full 5–10 s behind her usual pace. Only once or twice she reports coughing when getting out of the pool.

Table 11.7 Guidelines from the 36th Bethesda Conference for specific valvular abnormalities: aortic stenosis

Diagnosis	Qualifier	Recommendation
Mild AS	• Should have serial evaluations of AS severity on at least an annual basis	• Can participate in all sports
Moderate AS	• All athletes	• Low intensity sports (Class IA)
	• In athletes who have had exercise tolerance testing to at least the level of activity achieved in competition without the demonstration of: symptoms, ST-segment depression, or ventricular tachyarrhythmias, and with a normal blood pressure response	• Low and moderate static sports • Low and moderate dynamic sports • (Class IA, IB, IIA)
	• Athletes with supraventricular tachycardia or multiple or complex ventricular tachyarrhythmias at rest or with exercise	• Low intensity sports (Class IA)
Severe AS or moderate AS w/symptoms		• Should not participate in competitive sports

Table 11.8 Guidelines from the 36th Bethesda Conference for specific valvular abnormalities: aortic regurgitation

Diagnosis	Qualifier	Recommendation
Mild or Moderate AR	• LV end-diastolic volume that is normal or only mildly increased, consistent with that resulting solely from athletic training	• Can participate in all sports
	• Moderate LV enlargement (60–65 mm) if exercise tolerance testing to the level of activity achieved in competition demonstrates no symptoms or ventricular arrhythmias	• Low and moderate static • Low, moderate, and high dynamic sports • Class IA, IB, IC, IIA, IIB, IIC
	• Asymptomatic nonsustained ventricular tachycardia at rest or with exertion	• Low intensity sports (Class IA)
Severe AR	• LV diastolic diameter greater than 65 mm • Or mild-moderate AR with symptoms (regardless of LV size)	• Should not participate in competitive sports
AR (not associated with Marfan's Syndrome)	• And significant dilatation of the proximal ascending aorta (greater than 45 mm)	• Low intensity sports (Class IA)

Table 11.9 Guidelines from the 36th Bethesda Conference for specific valvular abnormalities: bicuspid aortic valves

Diagnosis	Qualifier	Recommendation
Bicuspid aortic valves	• No aortic dilatation • Dilatation less than 40 mm, or • The equivalent according to body surface area in children and adolescents	• Can participate in all competitive sports
Bicuspid aortic valves	• Dilated aortic roots between 40 and 45 mm	• Low and moderate static sports • Low and moderate dynamic sports • (Classes IA, IB, IIA, IIB) • Avoid any sports that involve potential for bodily collision or trauma
Bicuspid aortic valves	• Dilated aortic roots greater than 45 mm	• Only low intensity sports (Class IA)

Table 11.10 Guidelines from the 36th Bethesda Conference for specific valvular abnormalities: prosthetic heart valves

Diagnosis	Qualifier	Recommendation
Bioprosthetic mitral valve	• Not taking anticoagulants • Normal valvular function • Normal or near-normal LV function	• Low and moderate dynamic competitive sports • Classes IA, IB, IIA, IIB
Bioprosthetic aortic valve	• Normal valve function • Normal LV function	• Low and moderate static competitive sports • Low and moderate dynamic competitive sports • Classes IA, IB, IIA
	• Athletes participating in greater than low intensity sports (Class IA) should undergo exercise testing to at least the level of activity in competition to evaluate exercise tolerance and symptomatic and hemodynamic responses	
Mechanical or Bioprosthetic mitral or aortic valves	• Currently taking anticoagulants	• Should not participate in sports that involve the risk of bodily contact or trauma

Past Medical History

She is otherwise healthy with no significant past medical history. Three months prior, she was diagnosed with acute sinusitis and was put on a decongestant, expectorant, and

Table 11.11 Guidelines from the 36th Bethesda Conference for specific valvular abnormalities: mitral valve prolapse (Task Force 4)

Diagnosis	Qualifier	Recommendation
MVP *without* any of the following	• Prior syncope, judged probably to be arrhythmogenic in origin • Sustained or repetitive and non-sustained supraventricular tachycardia or frequent and/or complex ventricular tachyarrhythmias on ambulatory Holter monitoring • Severe mitral regurgitation assessed with color-flow imaging • LV systolic dysfunction (ejection fraction less than 50%) • Prior embolic event • Family history of MVP-related sudden death	• Can engage in all competitive sports
MVP	• *with* any of the following disease features listed above	• Low-intensity competitive sports only • Class IA
MVP with significant mitral regurgitation	See Table11.6	

Table 11.12 Guidelines from the 36th Bethesda Conference for specific valvular abnormalities: pulmonary valve stenosis (from Task Force 2)

Diagnosis	Qualifier	Recommendation
Mild PS untreated	• A Doppler peak instantaneous gradient less than 40 mmHg • Normal right ventricular function • No symptoms	• Can engage in all competitive sports • Annual re-evaluation is recommended
Moderate PS untreated	• Peak systolic gradient greater than 40 mmHg	• Low-intensity competitive sports only • Class IA, IB • Often referred for balloon valvuloplasty or operative valvotomy before sports participation

antibiotics and recovered without residual symptoms. The remainder of her review of systems is negative. Her family history is significant for an uncle that died of a heart attack at age 55. The social history reveals that she is a binge alcohol user and consumes six to eight beers in a given night, two or three times a month. She denies recreational drug use, nutritional and herbal supplement use and does not smoke.

Table 11.13 Guidelines from the 36th Bethesda Conference for specific valvular abnormalities: atrial septal defect (Task Force 2)

Diagnosis	Qualifier	Recommendation
Atrial septal defect – untreated	• Small defects • Normal right heart volume • No pulmonary hypertension	• *ECG and echocardiogram are required for evaluation. • Can engage in all competitive sports
	• large defect, and • normal pulmonary artery pressure	• Can participate in all competitive sports
	• Mild pulmonary hypertension	• Low-intensity competitive sports (Class IA)
	• Those with associated pulmonary vascular obstructive disease with cyanosis and large left-to-right shunt.	• Cannot participate in sports
	• Symptomatic atrial or ventricular tachyarrhythmia or moderate-to-severe mitral regurgitation	• Refer to recommendations in Task Force 1 and Task Force 6
Atrial septal defect – closed via surgery or catheterization	• 3–6 months after surgery/intervention, patients can participate in all sports unless one of the following is present	• Evidence of pulmonary HTN • Symptomatic atrial or ventricular tachyarrhythmias/ or 2nd–3rd degree heart block • Evidence of myocardial dysfunction
	• Patients with any of the above abnormalities should have an exercise evaluation and an individualized exercise prescription with respect to competitive sports	• Specific recommendations are available in Task Force 7 and the separate section titled Elevated Pulmonary Resistance and Ventricular Dysfunction After Cardiac Surgery

*=ECG/Echo applies in all above situations

Physical Exam

Her initial exam was performed in the aquatic center training room. At rest, the athlete was in no distress, was breathing easily and appeared well. A brief cardiopulmonary exam was performed. Her lungs were clear without rales, rhonchi, or wheezing. The cardiac examination revealed no parasternal heave or displaced PMI. Auscultation revealed a regular rhythm and a soft blowing grade 2/6, mid-systolic murmur preceded by an ejection click, heard best at the apex without radiation to other regions of the chest. It was accentuated by rapid standing or the strain phase of the Valsalva maneuver and lessened with squatting. There was no jugular venous distension. Peripheral pulses were strong and regular, and there was no peripheral edema of the lower extremities.

Table 11.14 Guidelines from the 36th Bethesda Conference for specific valvular abnormalities: ventricular septal defect (Task Force 2)

Diagnosis	Qualifier	Recommendation
VSD untreated	• Normal pulmonary artery pressure • Large VSD • No marked elevation of pulmonary resistance • Candidates for repair	• Can engage in all competitive sports • Full participation in all sports following successful closure
VSD treated by operation or catheterization	• 3–6 months after repair • Asymptomatic athletes with no or small residual defect • No evidence of: pulmonary artery HTN • Ventricular or atrial tachyarrhythmias • Myocardial dysfunction	• Can participate in all competitive sports
	• Patients with any of the above abnormalities should have an exercise evaluation and an individualized exercise prescription with respect to competitive sports	• Specific recommendations are available in Task Force 7 and the separate section titled Elevated Pulmonary Resistance and Ventricular Dysfunction After Cardiac Surgery
	• Persistent, severe pulmonary HTN	• Cannot participate in competitive sports.

Diagnostic Tests

Echocardiography revealed classic Mitral Valve Prolapse with moderate to moderately severe MR at rest.

Treatment

The patient underwent successful open surgical mitral valve repair and annuloplasty.

Outcome

The patient missed the remainder of the swimming season as she recovered from the operation. She presented to the sports medicine clinic for consultation regarding her ability to return to the swimming team and compete again in the pool. After a negative review of symptoms, and unremarkable physical exam, the 36th Bethesda Conference guidelines are reviewed for participation recommendations. Task Force 3 recommends athletes that have had mitral valve repair for MR not participate in sports involving bodily contact or risk of trauma. Athletes may participate in class

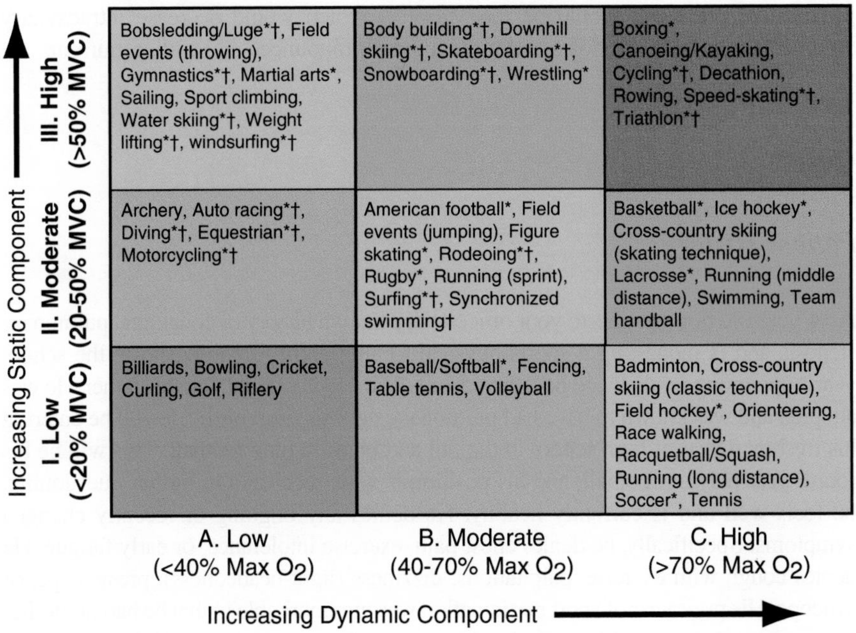
Increasing Static Component
III. High (>50% MVC)
II. Moderate (20-50% MVC)
I. Low (<20% MVC)
Bobsledding/Luge*†, Field events (throwing), Gymnastics*†, Martial arts*, Sailing, Sport climbing, Water skiing*†, Weight lifting*†, windsurfing*†
Body building*†, Downhill skiing*†, Skateboarding*†, Snowboarding*†, Wrestling*
Boxing*, Canoeing/Kayaking, Cycling*†, Decathlon, Rowing, Speed-skating*†, Triathlon*†
Archery, Auto racing*†, Diving*†, Equestrian*†, Motorcycling*†
American football*, Field events (jumping), Figure skating*, Rodeoing*†, Rugby*, Running (sprint), Surfing*†, Synchronized swimming†
Basketball*, Ice hockey*, Cross-country skiing (skating technique), Lacrosse*, Running (middle distance), Swimming, Team handball
Billiards, Bowling, Cricket, Curling, Golf, Riflery
Baseball/Softball*, Fencing, Table tennis, Volleyball
Badminton, Cross-country skiing (classic technique), Field hockey*, Orienteering, Race walking, Racquetball/Squash, Running (long distance), Soccer*, Tennis
A. Low (<40% Max O2)
B. Moderate (40-70% Max O2)
C. High (>70% Max O2)
Increasing Dynamic Component

Fig. 11.4 Classification of sports [20]. This classification is based on peak static and dynamic components achieved during competition. It should be noted, however, that higher values may be reached during training. The increasing dynamic component is defined in terms of the estimated percent of maximal oxygen uptake (Max O_2) achieved and results in an increasing cardiac output. The increasing static component is related to the estimated percent of maximal voluntary contraction (MVC) reached and results in an increasing blood pressure load. The lowest total cardiovascular demands (cardiac output and blood pressure) are shown in *green* and the highest in *red*. *Blue*, *yellow*, and *orange* depict low moderate, moderate, and high moderate total cardiovascular demands. *Asterisks* indicate danger of bodily collision. *Daggers* indicate increased risk if syncope occurs. Jere H. Mitchell, William Haskell, Peter Snell, Steven P. Van Camp, 36th Bethesda Conference: Eligibility Recommendations for Competitive Athletes With Cardiovascular Abnormalities/Task Force 8: Classification of sports, Copyright 2005, with permission from Elsevier

IA (low dynamic, low static) and in selected cases, class IA, IB, and IIA sports. Swimming is classified as a class IIC sport due to the high dynamic (VO_2 Max > 70%) component of the sport. Therefore, the athlete was not cleared to participate in swimming events, thereby ending her collegiate swimming career.

Discussion

MR related to a myxomatous mitral valve and subsequent prolapse is the most likely etiology in this patient. Other causes of MR would be unlikely and more likely to occur in a patient with rheumatic heart disease, coronary disease-related papillary muscle dysfunction, dilated cardiomyopathy, or endocarditis of the mitral valve. The ideal provocative maneuver would be the Valsalva, which would decrease intracavitary volume and increase afterload leading to a more pronounced and earlier murmur.

Case 2

Patient History

A 14-year-old boy presents to your office with a known history of congenital pulmonary stenosis and is requesting a sports physical to allow him to participate in the school year's upcoming football and hockey seasons. The boy is present with his father. He was adopted and was known to have had pulmonary stenosis from birth. He will be entering his freshman year of high school in the fall and plans to play football. This will be his fourth year playing football, and his position is wide receiver. On further questioning, he feels well and is currently healthy. He denies any ongoing or recently changed symptoms. Specifically, he denies chest pain, exercise intolerance, or early fatigue. He denies cough with exercise, palpitations, dizziness (light-headedness), presyncope, or syncope. His prior year of sport participation was unremarkable in that he had no limitations, symptoms, or problems during his season. The year prior, he had undergone a routine 2D-Echocardiogram that showed "mild" impairment of the valve.

Past Medical History

His medical history is only significant for the pulmonic stenosis. He has had one catheterization at the age of 5 for balloon valvuloplasty. He currently takes no medications and has no allergies. His social history is unremarkable for substance use, and he is a good student. His family history is not attainable as he was adopted.

Physical Examination

The athlete is noted to be a young adolescent in no distress. His blood pressure is 106/60, heart rate of 84 bpm, and respirations of 12 bpm. He is of thin build. Pulmonary exam is within normal limits. Cardiovascular examination reveals flat neck veins with a normal carotid upstroke without any bruits. The point of maximal impulse is normal, but a mild RV heave was noted. The rhythm and rate are both regular, with a normal S1 with a split S2 that widens with inspiration. S2 is heard best in the left ICS 3 area and a grade 2 crescendo–decrescendo murmur that lessens in intensity with inspiration. There is no associated diastolic murmur. Otherwise, peripheral pulses are normal in caliber. The remainder of his examination is unremarkable.

Diagnostic Tests

An ECG is performed in the office and shows sinus rhythm with diffusely increased voltage of the QRS and changing to plural complexes. The axis is shifted rightward. Afterwards, an echocardiogram is obtained. The patient returns to review the results, which show a transvalvular gradient of 30 mmHg, normal RV and LV systolic function, with an estimated LV ejection fraction of 55%. There was trivial tricuspid insufficiency.

Treatment/Disposition

The history and physical are reassuring in that he has had no symptoms or difficulties related to his pulmonary stenosis in the preceding year. His prior success in football and hockey are also reassuring in that he has been able to handle the physical demands of the sports so far. The echo also appears to indicate no worsening of the valvular pressure gradient. To determine sport participation/clearance at this point, a review of the 36th Bethesda Guidelines is performed. The guidelines state an athlete with a peak systolic transvalvular gradient of less than 50 mmHg and normal systolic function is safe to participate. The good news is discussed with the patient and his father, with the additional recommendation of annual reevaluation prior to each sporting year (also per the Bethesda guidelines). The patient is referred to a congenital heart disease specialist for long-term follow-up. The patient will need to be followed on a yearly basis to assess for progression of the pulmonary valve stenosis and the status of RV size and systolic function.

References

1. Shaver JA: Cardiac auscultation: A cost-effective diagnostic skill. *Curr Probl Cardiol* 1995; 20:441.
2. American College of Cardiology/American Heart Association Task Force on Practice Guidelines; Society of Cardiovascular Anesthesiologists; Society for Cardiovascular Angiography and Interventions; Society of Thoracic Surgeons, Bonow RO, Carabello BA, Kanu C, de Leon AC Jr, Faxon DP, Freed MD, Gaasch WH, Lytle BW, Nishimura RA, O'Gara PT, O'Rourke RA, Otto CM, Shah PM, Shanewise JS, Smith SC Jr, Jacobs AK, Adams CD, Anderson JL, Antman EM, Faxon DP, Fuster V, Halperin JL, Hiratzka LF, Hunt SA, Lytle BW, Nishimura R, Page RL, Riegel B. ACC/AHA 2006 guidelines for the management of patients with valvular heart disease: A report of the American College of Cardiology/American Heart Association Task Force on Practice Guidelines (writing committee to revise the 1998 Guidelines for the Management of Patients With Valvular Heart Disease): Developed in collaboration with the Society of Cardiovascular Anesthesiologists: Endorsed by the Society for Cardiovascular Angiography and Interventions and the Society of Thoracic Surgeons. *Circulation* 2006;114(5):e84–e231.
3. O'Rourke RA, Braunwald E: Physical examination of the cardiovascular system. In: Kasper DL, et al eds. *Harrison's Principles of Internal Medicine*, 16th ed. New York: McGraw-Hill; 2005.

4. O'Rourke R: Approach to the patient with a heart murmur. In: Braunwald E, Goldman L, eds. *Primary Cardiology*, 2nd ed. Philadelphia: Elsevier; 2003:155–173.
5. Perloff JK: The jugular venous pulse and third heart sound in patients with heart failure. *N Engl J Med* 2001; 345:612.
6. Abrams J: Precordial palpation. In: Horwitz LD, Groves BM, eds. *Signs and Symptoms in Cardiology*, Philadelphia: JB Lippincott; 1985:156–177.
7. Valentin Fuster R, Alexander W, O'Rourke RA, Roberts R, King SB III, Nash IS, Prystowsky EN, eds. *Hurst's The Heart*, 11th Ed. New York: McGraw Hill; 2006.
8. Ellen SD, Crawford MH, O'Rourke RA: Accuracy of precordial palpation for detecting increased left ventricular volume. *Ann Intern Med* 1983; 99:628.
9. Bruanwald, E., Zipes, D, Libby, P. *Heart Disease*, 6th Ed. London: W.B. Saunders Company; 2001:76.
10. Chizner, M. *Classic Teachings in Clinical Cardiology*, Vol. 1. Cedar Grove, NJ: Laennec Publishing; 1996:192–195.
11. Lembo NJ, Dell'Italia JL, Crawford MH, O'Rourke RA: Bedside diagnosis of systolic murmurs. *N Engl J Med* 1988; 318:1572.
12. Joffe HS: Genesis of Still's innocent systolic murmur. *Br Heart J* 1992; 67:206.
13. Donnerstein RL, Thomsen VS: Hemodynamic and anatomic factors affecting the frequency content of Still's innocent murmur. *Am J Cardiol* 1994; 74:508.
14. Watrous RL, Bedynek J, Oskiper T, Grove DM. Computer-assisted detection of systolic murmurs associated with hypertrophic cardiomyopathy: A pilot study. *Tex Heart Inst J* 2004; 31(4):368–375.
15. Watrous RL, Thompson WR, Ackerman SJ. The impact of computer-assisted auscultation on physician referrals of asymptomatic patients with heart murmurs. *Clin Cardiol* 2008;31(2):79–83.
16. Roy D, Sargeant J, Gray J, Hoyt B, Allen M, Fleming M. Helping family physicians improve their cardiac auscultation skills with an interactive CD-ROM. *J Contin Educ Health Prof* 2002;22(3):152–159.
17. Finley JP, Sharratt GP, Nanton MA, Chen RP, Roy DL, Paterson G. Auscultation of the heart: A trial of classroom teaching versus computer-based independent learning. *Med Educ* 1998; 32(4):357–361.
18. Mahnke CB, Nowalk A, Hofkosh D, Zuberbuhler JR, Law YM. Comparison of two educational interventions on pediatric resident auscultation skills. *Pediatrics* 2004;113(5):1331–1335.
19. Barrett MJ, Kuzma MA, Seto TC, et al. The power of repetition in mastering cardiac auscultation. *Am J Med* 2006;119:73–75.
20. Maron BJ, Zipes DP. 36th Bethesda Conference:Eligibility recommendations for competitive athletes with cardiovascular abnormalities. *J Am Coll Cardiol* 2005;45:1312–1375.

Chapter 12
Management of Hypertension in Athletes

Shafeeq Ahmed and Paul D. Thompson

Introduction

Athletes have a lower incidence of high blood pressure than nonathletes, but the prevalence of hypertension among athletes is only 50% less than that in the general population [1]. Further, the risk of hypertension may actually be increased in some athletes and physically active individuals because of increased body mass. Indeed, hypertension is the most common cardiovascular problem in athletes.

Classification of Blood Pressure

According to the Seventh report of the Joint National Committee on Prevention, Detection, Evaluation, and Treatment of High Blood Pressure (JNC 7), hypertension is classified into prehypertension, stage 1 and stage 2 hypertension [2] (Table 12.1). Hypertension can also be classified as primary or secondary. Primary or idiopathic refers to hypertension with no identifiable cause, whereas secondary hypertension refers to hypertension "secondary" to some other disease process. Most athletes with hypertension have either prehypertension or stage 1 hypertension.

Case 1: A 37-year-old male was seen for an annual check up. He was 5′6″ tall and weighted 160 lb. His blood pressure(BP) by the nurse was 165/90 and 170/90 in the right and 165/90 in the left arm when repeated by the physician. Two weeks later, repeat measurement of his BP in the office showed nearly identical BP readings. Ambulatory BP monitoring demonstrated a mean 24-h BP of 118/65 and mean daytime BP of 122/70 confirming white coat hypertension.

P.D. Thompson (✉)
Cardiovascular Services Hospitalist, Hartford Hospital, Hartford, CT, USA
e-mail: Pthomps@harthosp.org

C.E. Lawless (ed.), *Sports Cardiology Essentials: Evaluation, Management and Case Studies*, DOI 10.1007/978-0-387-92775-6_12,

Table 12.1 Classification of blood pressure [2]

Category	SBP (mmHg)		DBP (mmHg)
Normal	<120	and	<80
Pre-hypertension	120–139	or	80–89
Hypertension			
Stage 1	140–159	or	90–99
Stage 2	≥160	or	≥100

JNC 7 7th Report of the Joint National Committee on Prevention, Detection, Evaluation, and Treatment of High Blood Pressure, *SBP* systolic blood pressure, *DBP* diastolic blood pressure

White Coat Hypertension

White coat hypertension (WCHT) is defined as an elevated blood pressure when taken in a medical setting such as a doctor's office, clinic, or hospital, but normal pressure when self-measured or measured by ambulatory devices. White coat hypertension is found in 20% of people with mild hypertension [3]. There have been no definitive outcome trials to demonstrate whether WCHT should be treated. As such, it is possible that individuals, who are hypertensive while recording a blood pressure measurement, may also be hypertensive at other stressful times. The possibility of WCHT should always be considered in athletes.

Secondary Hypertension in Athletes

Secondary hypertension is defined as hypertension that is a result of another medical condition and occurs in less than 5% of athletes and physically active people [4]. The diagnosis of secondary hypertension should be considered and investigated when hypertension occurs in younger patients, especially young female athletes at risk for fibromuscular dysplasia (FMD) [5], adults with severe hypertension, patients with the sudden onset of hypertension, and in patients who respond poorly to conventional medical treatment. The etiology of secondary hypertension can often be identified by a variety of readily available diagnostic tests (Table 12.2). The most common cause of secondary hypertension in the general population is parenchymal and vascular renal disease [4]. Drug use, including illicit such as cocaine and other stimulants, as well as nonprescription, nonsteroidal anti-inflammatory agents should always be considered as secondary causes of hypertension in athletes.

Case 2: An 18-year-old male was referred to the office after a BP of 182/105 was recorded in the left arm during a premilitary physical examination. He was totally asymptomatic, but on intense questioning did suggest that he occasionally develops leg cramping while running, but generally avoids this activity. Physical examination

Table 12.2 Screening tests for secondary hypertension [2]

Diagnosis	Diagnostic test
Chronic kidney disease	Estimated GFR
Coarctation of aorta	CT angiography
Cushing's syndrome and other glucocorticoid excess states including chronic steroid therapy	History, dexamethasone suppression test
Drug induced or drug related[a]	History, drug screening
Pheochromocytoma	24 h Urinary metanephrine and normetanephrine
Primary aldosteronism and other mineralocorticoid excess states	24 h Urinary aldosterone level or specific measurements of other mineralocorticoids
Renovascular hypertension including FMD in women	Doppler flow study; magnetic resonance angiography
Sleep apnea	Sleep study with O_2 saturation
Thyroid/parathyroid disease	TSH; serum PTH

[a]Drugs commonly associated with secondary hypertension in athletes are: Nonsteriodal anti-inflammatory drugs; cocaine, amphetamines; sympathomimetics (decongestants, anorectics); oral contraceptives hormones; anabolic steroids; adrenal steroid hormones; erythropoietin; licorice (including some licorice-flavored chewing tobacco); selected over-the-counter dietary supplements and medicines such as ephedra, ma huang, bitter orange.

confirmed hypertension. The femoral pulse was faintly present, but simultaneous palpation of the radial and femoral pulses demonstrated a distinctly late femoral pulse impulse. A magnetic resonance angiographic study revealed constriction of the aorta immediately distal to the left subclavian.

Clinical Evaluation

The clinical evaluation of athletes over the age of 18 years with hypertension should include blood pressure readings on at least two separate visits with an appropriately sized cuff. Table 12.3 shows guidelines for the measurement of BP. A frequent cause of "hypertension" in athletes is a cuff that is too small, falsely elevating the blood pressure. If at all possible, a mercury sphygmomanometer should be used, because aneroid devices generally require 6-month recalibrations, something that is rarely done in medical offices [6]. In athletes less than 18 years, it is recommended that three blood pressure readings be taken, and that the readings be compared with normative values based on height, age, and gender. The normative data may be found on the CDC (Center for Disease Control) website. A value in the 90th percentile or under is considered a normal reading in this age group.

The evaluation of athletes should also include a thorough medical history, physical examination, and limited laboratory tests. They should focus on detecting secondary causes of hypertension and to assess the target organ damage. The history should inquire about lifestyle habits that can increase blood pressure such as alcohol intake, ingestion of drugs such as cocaine, amphetamines, and anabolic steroids, and

Table 12.3 Guidelines for blood pressure measurement [23]

Posture

Blood pressure should be obtained after 5 min in the seated position, with the back supported by the chair, feet on the floor, and the arm supported at the level of the heart.

Circumstances

No caffeine during the hour preceding the reading. No smoking during the 30 min preceding the reading. The setting should be quiet and the room warm.

Equipment

Cuff size

The bladder should encircle at least 80% of the arm circumference. Small cuffs elevate the reading. Large cuffs reduce the reading.

Manometer: Use mercury, recently calibrated aneroid, or validated electronic device.

Technique

Number of readings

At least two readings (three readings in children and adolescents), separated by as much time as practical should be taken. If readings vary by >5 mmHg, additional readings are required. If the arm pressure is elevated, leg measurements should be obtained especially in individuals less than age 30 to detect coarctation.

Initial pressures should be obtained in both arms; if the pressures differ, use the arm with the higher pressure. If the initial values are elevated, obtain two other sets of readings at least 1-week apart.

Performance

The first step is to obtain a systolic measurement using palpation of the radial pulse. The bladder should then be quickly inflated to a pressure 20 mmHg greater than the palpated systolic pressure. The bladder is then deflated at 2 mmHg/s and the Korotkoff phase I (appearance) and phase V (disappearance) pressures recorded.

the use of dietary supplements (which often contain stimulants to boost energy or facilitate weight loss). Supplements may contain ma huang, ephedra, and guanara, which contain adrenergic compounds or caffeine-like stimulants [7]. Athletes with hypertension should also be asked about the use of nonsteroidal medications and cold remedies since both may increase blood pressure. In all of these instances, repeat blood pressure measurements should be recorded after discontinuation of the offending agent(s).

The physical exam of an athlete with hypertension should seek to detect end-organ damage and possible secondary causes of elevated blood pressure. The fundoscopic exam may reveal retinal changes such as A-V "knicking," "copper wires" arterioles, and rarely papilledema. Such findings suggest that the hypertension has been persistent or severe and that it warrants aggressive treatment. A critical physical examination maneuver is simultaneous palpation of the radial and femoral pulses. Detection of the radial and femoral pulses by palpation should be simultaneous. Delay in the appearance of the femoral pulses or a "radial–femoral pulse delay" is an important sign of aortic coarctation, which is an often-overlooked cause of secondary hypertension in young adults. Many clinicians think that the femoral pulse needs to be absent or nonpalpable and are unaware that the femoral pulse may be preserved because of collateral circulation that develops around the coarctation. Palpating for radial–femoral pulse delay detects coarctation of the aorta.

Cardiac auscultation should focus on detecting the murmurs of aortic valve. Aortic insufficiency is difficult to hear, but may cause isolated systolic hypertension in athletes. Aortic insufficiency is best heard listening at the cardiac base and over the sternum, with the patient sitting upright, leaning forward, and on exhalation.

In addition to cardiac auscultation, the abdomen should be examined for renal artery and femoral bruits. Renal artery stenosis can occur in young athletes, especially female athletes, with FMD [5]. The possibility of FMD with renal artery stenosis may first be suggested by the presence of bruits in other locations including the femoral arteries. It is important to detect FMD as a cause of hypertension, because the renal stenosis can be readily treated by angioplasty.

Routine laboratory testing should include a urinalysis, measurements of serum electrolytes, blood urea nitrogen, creatinine, and thyroid stimulating hormone. Hypokalemia in the absence of medications or a rapid reduction in potassium with diuretic therapy may indicate hyperaldosteronism. Hyperaldosteronism due to adrenal hyperplasia in the absence of a defined adenoma is increasingly recognized as a cause of difficult-to-treat hypertensive individuals and responds promptly to aldosterone antagonists such as spironolactone.

Treatment of Hypertension in Athletes

Nonpharmological therapy including lifestyle modification is the first step in managing hypertension in all patient groups. Weight loss, alcohol restriction, increasing aerobic exercise, and dietary adjustments all reduce blood pressure in nonathletic populations. Medications or drugs possibly contributing to the hypertension should be discontinued. The DASH (Dietary Approaches to stop Hypertension) diet reduces blood pressure in nonathletic populations [8]. It is rich in fruits, vegetables and incorporates low-fat dairy products; has reduced cholesterol as well as saturated and total fat; and is rich in calcium and potassium and low in sodium [8, 9].Although such measures are effective in the general population, their utility is often less in athletes. This is because athletes are already physically active and often lean, or because some, such as American football linemen, resist weight loss because of their athletic activity. Alcohol use, in contrast, is prevalent among college athletes and alcohol cessation may be effective in reducing hypertension in such patients. Nevertheless, most athletes with persistent hypertension will require pharmacologic therapy (Table 12.4).

Management of athletes with hypertension poses an even greater therapeutic challenge because some medications may impair exercise performance or not be allowed in certain sports. For example, beta blockers are prohibited in sports such as archery and shooting because they slow the heart rate [10–12]. A slower heart rate allows more time to aim between firings and reduces the possibility that a systolic surge in pressure will alter aim. Diuretics are also restricted in many sports because they dilute the urine and thereby mask the presence of other prohibited substances. These considerations apply only to drug testing in competitive sports. Table 12.5 shows the commonly used antihypertensives and their usual doses.

Table 12.4 Possible reductions in blood pressure with hygienic methods [2]

Modification[a]	Recommendation	Approximate SBP reduction
Weight reduction	Maintain normal body weight (body mass index 18.5–24.9 kg/m^2)	5–20 mmHg/10 kg
Adopt DASH eating plan	Consume a diet rich in fruits, vegetables, and low-fat dairy products with a reduced content of saturated and total fat	8–14 mmHg
Dietary sodium reduction	Reduce dietary sodium intake to no more than 100 mmol/day (2.4 g sodium or 6 g sodium chloride)	2–8 mmHg
Physical activity	Engage in regular aerobic physical activity such as brisk walking (at least 30 min/day, most days of the week)	4–9 mmHg
Moderation of alcohol consumption	Limit consumption to no more than two drinks (e.g. 24 oz beer, 10 oz wine, or 3 oz 80-proofwhiskey) per day in most men and to no more than one drink per day in women and lighter weight persons	2–4 mmHg

DASH Dietary Approaches to Stop Hypertension, *SBP* systolic blood pressure
[a] The effects of implementing these modifications are dose and time dependent and could be greater for some individuals

Diuretics

Thiazide and loop diuretics are the two major classes of diuretics available, each with its own advantage and side-effect profile. Thiazide and loop diuretics decrease plasma volume, cardiac output, and peripheral vascular resistance.

In numerous randomized controlled clinical trials, thiazide diuretics have demonstrated a significant cardiovascular mortality and morbidity benefit, with a favorable safety profile [13–17]. They are inexpensive and effective especially in black patients in whom hypertension is often salt-sensitive and responsive to volume depletion.

The adverse effects of thiazides include hypovolemia and othostatic hypotension, in addition to electrolyte imbalances such as hypokalemia and hypomagnesaemia. These side effects can increase the risk of muscle cramps, and even heat stroke and rhabdomyolysis in athletes engaged in intense exercise during warm weather. Consequently, their use in athletes routinely subjected to such conditions should be avoided, including American football players during warm weather workouts.

Table 12.5 Commonly used antihypertensive drugs and their usual doses [2]

Class	Drug (Trade name)	Usual dose range (mg/day)	Usual daily (frequency)
Diuretics			
	Chlorothiazide (Diuril)	125–500	1–2
	Chlorthalidone (generic)	12.5–25	1
	Hydrochlorothiazide (Microzide, HydroDIURIL)	12.5–50	1
	Polythiazide (Renese)	2–4	1
	Indapamide (Lozol)	1.25–2.5	1
	Metolazone (Mykrox)	0.5–1.0	1
	Metolazone (Zaroxolyn)	2.5–5	1
Beta blockers			
	Atenolol (Tenormin)	25–100	1
	Betaxolol (Kerlone)	5–20	1
	Bisoprolol (Zebeta)	2.5–10	1
	Metoprolol (Lopressor)	50–100	1–2
	Metoprolol extended release (Toprol XL)	50–100	1
	Nadolol (Corgard)	40–120	1
	Propranolol long-acting (Inderal LA)	60–180	1
Beta blockers with intrinsic sympathomimetic activity			
	Acebutolol (Sectral)	200–800	2
	Penbutolol (Levatol)	10–40	1
	Pindolol (generic)	10–40	2
Combined – alpha and beta blockers			
	Labetalol (Normodyne, Trandate)	200–800	2
ACE inhibitors			
	Benazepril (Lotensin)	10–40	1
	Captopril (Capoten)	25–100	2
	Enalapril (Vasotec)	5–40	1–2
	Fosinopril (Monopril)	10–40	1
	Lisinopril (Prinivil, Zestril)	10–40	1
	Moexipril (Univasc)	7.5–30	1
	Perindopril (Aceon)	4–8	1
	Quinapril (Accupril)	10–80	1
	Ramipril (Altace)	2.5–20	1
	Trandolapril (Mavik)	1–4	1
ARBs			
	Candesartan (Atacand)	8–32	1
	Eprosartan (Teveten)	400–800	1–2
	Irbesartan (Avapro)	150–300	1
	Losartan (Cozaar)	25–100	1–2
	Olmesartan (Benicar)	20–40	1
	Telmisartan (Micardis)	20–80	1
	Valsartan (Diovan)	80–320	1–2

(continued)

Table 12.5 (continued)

Class	Drug (Trade name)	Usual dose range (mg/day)	Usual daily (frequency)
Calcium channel blockers – NDHP			
	Diltiazem extended release (Cardizem CD, Dilacor XR, Tiazac)	180–420	1
	Diltiazem extended release (Cardizem LA)	120–540	1
	Verapamil immediate release (Calan, Isoptin)	80–320	2
	Verapamil long acting (Calan SR, Isoptin SR)	120–480	1–2
	Verapamil (Coer, Covera HS, Verelan PM)	120–360	1
Calcium channel blockers – DHP			
	Amlodipine (Norvasc)	2.5–10	1
	Felodipine (Plendil)	2.5–20	1
	Isradipine (Dynacirc CR)	2.5–10	2
	Nicardipine sustained release (Cardene SR)	60–120	2
	Nifedipine long-acting (Adalat CC, Procardia XL)	30–60	1
	Nisoldipine (Sular)	10–40	1
Alpha-1 blockers			
	Doxazosin (Cardura)	1–16	1
	Prazosin (Minipress)	2–20	2–3
	Terazosin (Hytrin)	1–20	1–2
Central alpha 2 agonists and other centrally acting drugs			
	Clonidine (Catapres)	0.1–0.8	2
	Clonidine patch (Catapres-TTS)	0.1–0.3	1 weekly
	Methyldopa (Aldomet)	250–1,000	2
	Reserpine (generic)	0.1–0.25	1
	Guanfacine (Tenex)	0.5–2	1
Direct vasodilators			
	Hydralazine (Apresoline)	25–100	2
	Minoxidil (Loniten)	2.5–80	1–2

Source: Physician's Desk Reference. 57th ed. Montvale, NJ: Thompson PDR, 2003

We also stop such medicines for 2 days prior to major competition in other athletes such as distance runners.

Loop diuretics such as furosemide and ethacrynic acid are more potent than thiazide diuretics, but because of a shorter duration of action are less useful than thiazides in long-term management of hypertension.

It must be stressed that diuretics cannot be used in athletes engaged in certain sports due to drug-testing regulations [10–12].

Angiotensin-Converting Enzyme Inhibitors

Angiotensin-converting enzyme (ACE) inhibitors are an excellent choice for managing hypertension in athletes because they do not diminish exercise performance, do not deplete electrolytes or reduce intravascular volume, and their use is not restricted by athletic association governing bodies. These agents block the conversion of angiotensin I to angiotensin II by inhibiting ACE. Angiotensin II is a potent vasoconstrictor and stimulates aldosterone release. ACE inhibitors have a more pronounced effect on lowering blood pressure when combined with a thiazide diuretic but can be used alone [10–12].

A dry hacking cough is the most common adverse effect with ACE inhibitors. The most serious and potentially life-threatening side effect of ACE inhibitors is angioedema. Cough and angioedema are both mediated by bradykinin, an effect not seen with angiotensin receptor blockers (ARBs) since ARBs do not increase bradykinin levels [18]. ACE and ARBs can produce hyperkalemia by reducing aldosterone production, but this is an unusual side effect in patients with normal renal function.

Administration of ACE inhibitors is contraindicated in pregnant women because they increase the risk of congenital anomalies [19]. Sexually active women should use contraception when taking ACE inhibitors. ACE inhibitors are our first choice for hypertensive treatment in athletes.

Angiotensin Receptor Blockers

ARBs have similar effects on hypertension to ACE inhibitors, but do not increase bradykinin and therefore do not induce cough. ARBs are an excellent choice for athletes who have had cough or angioedema during ACE-inhibitor treatment. The contraindications for ARBs are similar to those for ACE inhibitors.

Beta-Adrenergic Blockers

Beta-adrenergic blockers generally are not used when treating athletes, unless there is some other compelling indication for their use [20]. They are not highly effective in reducing blood pressure, especially when compared with other agents. They can reduce "performance anxiety" and heart rate and are therefore banned by the United States Olympic Committee for use in athletes participating in archery, shooting, diving, and figure skating [10–12].

Beta blockers can also cause fatigue, depression, and decrease exercise capacity when compared with ACE inhibitors. In addition, beta blockers can exacerbate reactive airways disease, including exercise-induced asthma which is frequent among athletes.

Calcium Channel Blockers

Calcium channel blockers decrease calcium concentrations in vascular smooth muscle thereby producing generalized vasodilatation, without affecting energy metabolism or reducing exercise performance [10, 20]. Calcium channel blockers are divided into the dihydropyridines (DHP) such as amlodipine, nifedipine, felodipine, and isradipine and the non-dihydropyridines (NDHP) such as verapamil and diltizem. All calcium channel blockers, however, are highly effective antihypertensive agents.

NDHP have the additional effects of decreasing heart rate and the force of cardiac contractility. The DHP are generally well tolerated in physically active patients and are a good selection for blood pressure treatment in black athletes, with or without a diuretic. The major adverse effect of calcium channel blockers is fluid retention. Therefore, depending on the sport and the mandates of the governing commission of the sport, combining a calcium channel blocker with a diuretic is a preferred regimen.

Alpha Blockers

These agents reduce blood pressure by decreasing peripheral vascular resistance by blocking alpha-1 receptor in arterial smooth muscle. They do not alter energy metabolism during exercise or reduce exercise capacity. Therefore, they have no major effect on training or athletic performance [10, 20]. Alpha-1 blocking agents such as terazosin and doxazosin are not frequently used to treat hypertension because alpha-1 blockers have been shown in the Antihypertensives and Lipid-Lowering Treatment to Prevent Heart Attack Trial (ALLHAT) to significanly increase the risk of heart failure compared to the diuretic chlorthalidone (8.1 versus 4.5% RR 2.04) [10, 21]. Nevertheless, alpha blockers may have occasional use in athletes.

Common adverse effects of alpha blockers are dizziness, headache, and weakness. They can also cause "first-dose syncope" because of their potent vasodilatation ability. Therefore, the first dose of any alpha blocker should be administered at bedtime to avoid postural hypotension. Dizziness can also occur with increasing doses. Alpha-1 blockers are commonly used to reduce the symptoms of prostatic hypertrophy in older men and may be considered for use in older hypertensive male athletes with this condition. Because of the ALLHAT results, however, all patients treated with an alpha blocker should also be treated with a diuretic.

Alpha Agonists

Alpha agonists, such as clonidine, act centrally and have no major effect on exercise or athletic performance. They frequently cause dry mouth, mild-to-moderate drowsiness, and impotence, making them useful only when blood pressure is refractory to other medications. Rebound hypertension can also occur if these drugs are stopped suddenly.

Combination Therapy

Most antihypertensive medicines except diuretics result in a plasma volume expansion, which reduces their effectiveness in reducing blood pressure. As such, the most effective medication for blood pressure reduction is often a combination therapy, with a diuretic at the core of this regimen. Again, this is predicated on the approval of the appropriate athletic oversight committee, and the avoidance of diuretics when the athlete is at risk of dehydration because of the sport or climate conditions. Diuretics should be avoided in athletes subjected to in- or out-of-competition testing, however, without clear, written permission from the governing body.

Recommendations for Athletic Participation in Hypertensive Athletes

The Hypertension Task Force (Task Force 5) of the 36 Bethesda Conference recommended that athletes should have their blood pressure monitored prior to competition [22]. Athletes with Stage 1 (systolic BP 140–159, diastolic BP 90–99) hypertension should undergo echocardiography. If they have left ventricular hypertrophy (LVH) by echocardiography, they should be restricted from competition until their pressure is controlled. Athletes with Stage 1 hypertension without LVH or other evidence of end-organ damage can participate in athletics without restriction. Their pressure should be monitored to evaluate the effect of exercise training. In contrast, patients with Stage 2 hypertension should be restricted from sports with a high static and/or isometric component, such as weight lifting or weight lifting in training, even if there is no evidence of target organ damage, until their pressure is controlled. Hypertensive athletes with other cardiac disease should follow the guidelines for athletic competition for their other heart disease. Any medication used by an athlete should be reported or registered with his/her sport's governing body, and if necessary, a medical exemption should be obtained [22].

References

1. Lehmann M, Durr H, Merkelbach H, Schmid A. Hypertension and sports activities: institutional experience. Clin Cardiol 1990;13(3):197–208.
2. Chobanian AV, Bakris GL, Black HR, Cushman WC, Green LA, Izzo JL Jr et al. Seventh report of the Joint National Committee on Prevention, Detection, Evaluation, and Treatment of High Blood Pressure. Hypertension 2003;42(6):1206–1252.

3. Pickering TG White coat hypertension. Curr Opin Nephrol Hypertens 1996;5(2):192–198.
4. Hanson P, Andrea BE. Treatment of hypertension in athletes. In:a DeLee J. Drez D. Starits ki CL, eds. Orthopaedic Sports Medicine: Principles and Practice. Philadelphia, Saunders, 1994:307–319.
5. Slovut DP, Olin JW. Fibromuscular dysplasia. N Engl J Med 2004;350(18):1862–1871.
6. Moore TA, Sorokin AV, Hirst C, Thornton-Thompson S, Thompson PD. The accuracy of aneroid sphygmomanometers in the ambulatory setting. Prev Cardiol 2008;11(2):90–94.
7. Samenuk D, Link MS, Homoud MK, Contreras R, Theoharides TC, Wang PJ et al. Adverse cardiovascular events temporally associated with ma huang, an herbal source of ephedrine. Mayo Clin Proc 2002;77(1):12–16.
8. Sacks FM, Svetkey LP, Vollmer WM, Appel LJ, Bray GA, Harsha D et al. Effects on blood pressure of reduced dietary sodium and the Dietary Approaches to Stop Hypertension (DASH) diet. DASH-Sodium Collaborative Research Group. N Engl J Med 2001;344(1):3–10.
9. Vollmer WM, Sacks FM, Ard J, Appel LJ, Bray GA, Simons-Morton DG et al. Effects of diet and sodium intake on blood pressure: subgroup analysis of the DASH-sodium trial. Ann Intern Med 2001;135(12):1019–1028.
10. USADA guide to prohibited classes of substances and prohibited methods of doping. www. 2008. 10-3-2001.
11. Fuentes RJ, Rosenberg JM. Athletic drug reference "99: complies with NCAA and USOC rules. Clean Data. Durhan, NC, Glaxco Wellcome. 2008:28–36, 52–54, 317–408.
12. IOC prohibited classes of substances and prohibited methods of doping. 10-2-2001.
13. SHEP Cooperative Research Group. Prevention of stroke by antihypertensive drug treatment in older persons with isolated systolic hypertension. Final results of the Systolic Hypertension in the Elderly Program (SHEP). JAMA 1991;265(24):3255–3264.
14. Curb JD, Pressel SL, Cutler JA, Savage PJ, Applegate WB, Black H et al. Effect of diuretic-based antihypertensive treatment on cardiovascular disease risk in older diabetic patients with isolated systolic hypertension. Systolic Hypertension in the Elderly Program Cooperative Research Group. JAMA 1996;276(23):1886–1892.
15. Philipp T, Anlauf M, Distler A, Holzgreve H, Michaelis J, Wellek S. Randomised, double blind, multicentre comparison of hydrochlorothiazide, atenolol, nitrendipine, and enalapril in antihypertensive treatment: results of the HANE study. HANE Trial Research Group. BMJ 1997;315(7101):154–159.
16. Amery A, Birkenhager W, Brixko P, Bulpitt C, Clement D, Deruyttere M et al. Mortality and morbidity results from the European Working Party on High Blood Pressure in the Elderly trial. Lancet 1985;1(8442):1349–1354.
17. Dahlof B, Lindholm LH, Hansson L, Schersten B, Ekbom T, Wester PO. Morbidity and mortality in the Swedish Trial in Old Patients with Hypertension (STOP-Hypertension). Lancet 1991;338(8778):1281–1285.
18. Nussberger J, Cugno M, Cicardi M. Bradykinin-mediated angioedema. N Engl J Med 2002;347(8):621–622.
19. Martin U, Foreman MA, Travis JC, Casson D, Coleman JJ (2008) Use of ACE inhibitors and ARBs in hypertensive women of childbearing age. J Clin Pharm Ther 33(5):507–511.
20. Chick TW, Halperin AK, Gacek EM. The effect of antihypertensive medications on exercise performance: a review. Med Sci Sports Exerc 1988;20(5):447–454.
21. ALLHAT Collaborative Research Group. Major cardiovascular events in hypertensive patients randomized to doxazosin vs chlorthalidone: the antihypertensive and lipid-lowering treatment to prevent heart attack trial (ALLHAT). JAMA 2000;283(15):1967–1975.
22. Kaplan NM, Gidding SS, Pickering TG, Wright JT Jr. Task Force 5: systemic hypertension. J Am Coll Cardiol 2005;45(8):1346–1348.
23. Pickering TG. Measurement of blood pressure in and out of the office. J Clin Hypertens (Greenwich) 2005;7(2):123–129.

Part III
Specific Cardiac Diseases and Return to Play Decisions in Athletes

Chapter 13
Hypertrophic Cardiomyopathy

Paul Sorajja and Steve R. Ommen

Case Vignette

A 22-year-old male college student who has been previously healthy presents with new symptoms of dyspnea. As a child and young adult, he had been told of a physiologic murmur but was never diagnosed with a heart condition. Until his symptoms began 4 months ago, he was a competitive athlete and was captain of his cross-country track team. Because of increasing symptoms, he visited his family physician, when an electrocardiogram was found to be abnormal (Fig. 13.1). He now has been referred to you for further evaluation.

On physical examination, he is 5′9″, weighs 155 lbs, and has a muscular athletic build. He is bradycardic (52 beats/min), and the blood pressure (100/70 mmHg) is normal. The lungs are clear. The carotid upstroke is rapid and bifid. The jugular venous pulse is normal. The apical impulse is localized, sustained, and nondisplaced. There is a loud first heart sound. A 3/6 systolic ejection murmur is heard over the left lower sternal border which radiates to the clavicles. The murmur increases with squat-to-stand maneuver.

A transthoracic echocardiogram demonstrates myocardial hypertrophy of the left ventricle with predominant involvement of the ventricular septum (20 mm thickness; Fig. 13.1). There is systolic anterior motion of the mitral valve and mitral regurgitation. A left ventricular outflow tract (LVOT) gradient of 36 mmHg is present at rest and increases to 80 mmHg during Valsalva strain.

The patient would like to have treatment for his dyspnea and return to his activities as a competitive runner. He also has been recently married and plans to begin a family following college graduation. The patient currently is on no medications.

P. Sorajja (✉)
Associate Professor of Medicine, Mayo Clinic College of Medicine,
Mayo Clinic, Rochester, MN, USA
e-mail: Sorajja.Paul@mayo.edu

C.E. Lawless (ed.), *Sports Cardiology Essentials: Evaluation, Management and Case Studies*, DOI 10.1007/978-0-387-92775-6_13,

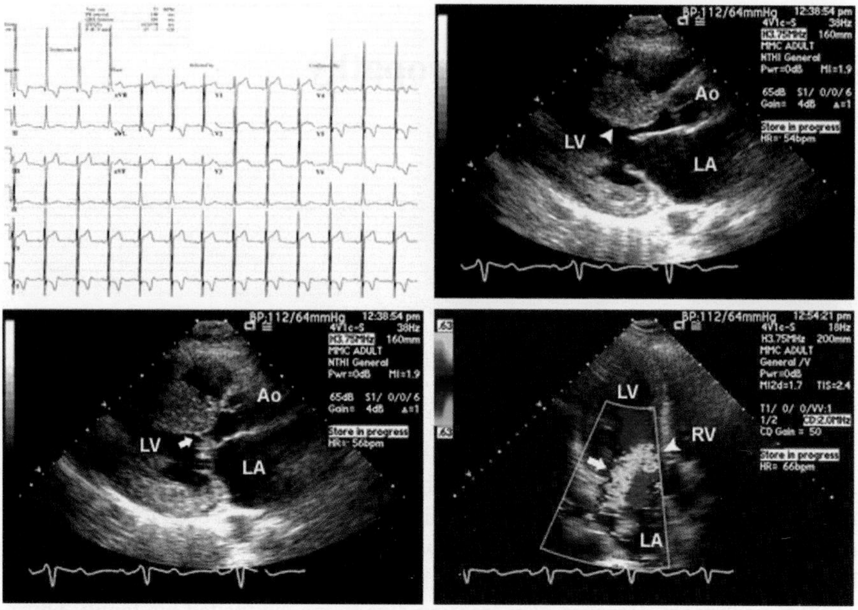

Fig. 13.1 A 21-year-old man with new-onset dyspnea. *Top left*, 12-lead electrocardiogram showing typical left ventricular hypertrophy and secondary ST-segment abnormalities. *Top right*, Echocardiographic parasternal long-axis view at end-diastole showing asymmetric septal hypertrophy (*arrowhead*). *Bottom left*, End-systolic frame demonstrating systolic anterior motion of the mitral valve (*arrow*). *Bottom right*, Apical long-axis view with color flow Doppler imaging showing high-velocity flow across the left ventricular outflow tract (*arrowhead*) and posteriorly directed mitral regurgitation (*arrow*). *Ao* ascending aorta; *LA* left atrium; *LV* left ventricle; *RA* right atrium; *RV* right ventricle

Introduction

Hypertrophic cardiomyopathy (HCM) is an autosomal dominant disease with a prevalence of 0.1–0.2% of the general population. While most patients with HCM can expect near-normal longevity with good quality of life, it is important to recognize that in North America, HCM is the most common cause of sudden death in young athletes [1, 2]. The catastrophic and highly visible nature of these events has led to increased awareness of the need to identify individuals with HCM either during preparticipation screening or among those already involved in competitive sports. Nevertheless, the diagnosis of the disorder in such individuals has proved to be challenging due to clinical features that overlap with those of physiological hypertrophy and the controversy about the most appropriate screening methods. This chapter reviews the clinical features and management of patients with HCM.

Definition and Etiology

Although HCM historically has been defined as myocardial hypertrophy without an underlying etiology, it is now known through molecular studies that sarcomeric genetic mutations give rise to the disease. Hundreds of mutations that affect genes encoding β-myosin heavy chain, myosin-binding protein C, α-tropomyosin, actin, titin, cardiac troponins T and I, and myosin light chains have been described thus far.

Severe gross myocardial hypertrophy is present in the majority of clinical cases of HCM, although mild hypertrophy and significant underlying histological abnormalities can occur in some patients (Fig. 13.2). The pathologic hallmark of HCM is myo-

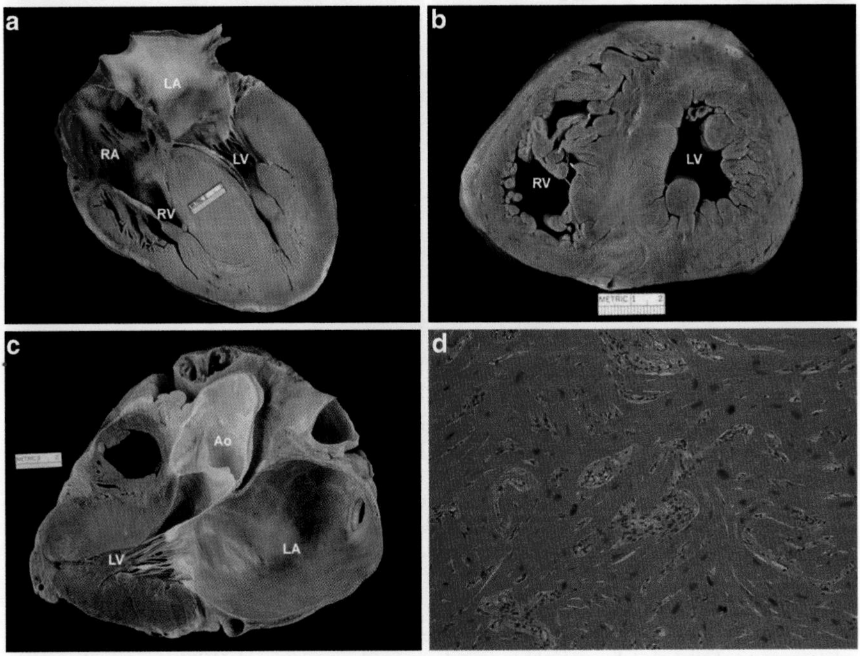

Fig. 13.2 Gross examination of hearts affected with hypertrophic cardiomyopathy. (**a**) Long-axis view of specimen from a 30-year-old person with hypertrophic cardiomyopathy who died of sudden cardiac death. (**b**) Short-axis view of specimen with predominantly septal hypertrophy. Septal/left ventricle wall thickness ratio = 1.8. Note the severe, concentric myocardial hypertrophy. (**c**) Long-axis view of specimen from a 43-year-old patient with apical variant of hypertrophic cardiomyopathy. (**d**) Myocyte disarray in hypertrophic cardiomyopathy. The pathological hallmark of hypertrophic cardiomyopathy is myocyte disarray, in which there is marked variation in cell shape, size, and arrangement. This patient also had severe left atrial dilatation. Photographs courtesy of Dr. William D. Edwards, Mayo Clinic, Rochester, Minnesota. Figure (**a**) is reproduced with permission from Sorajja and Nishimura. *Diagnosis and Management of Adult Congenital Heart Disease*, Hypertrophic cardiomyopathy, pp. 451–457, Copyright Elsevier 2003. *Ao* ascending aorta; *LA* left atrium; *LV* left ventricle; *RA* right atrium; *RV* right ventricle

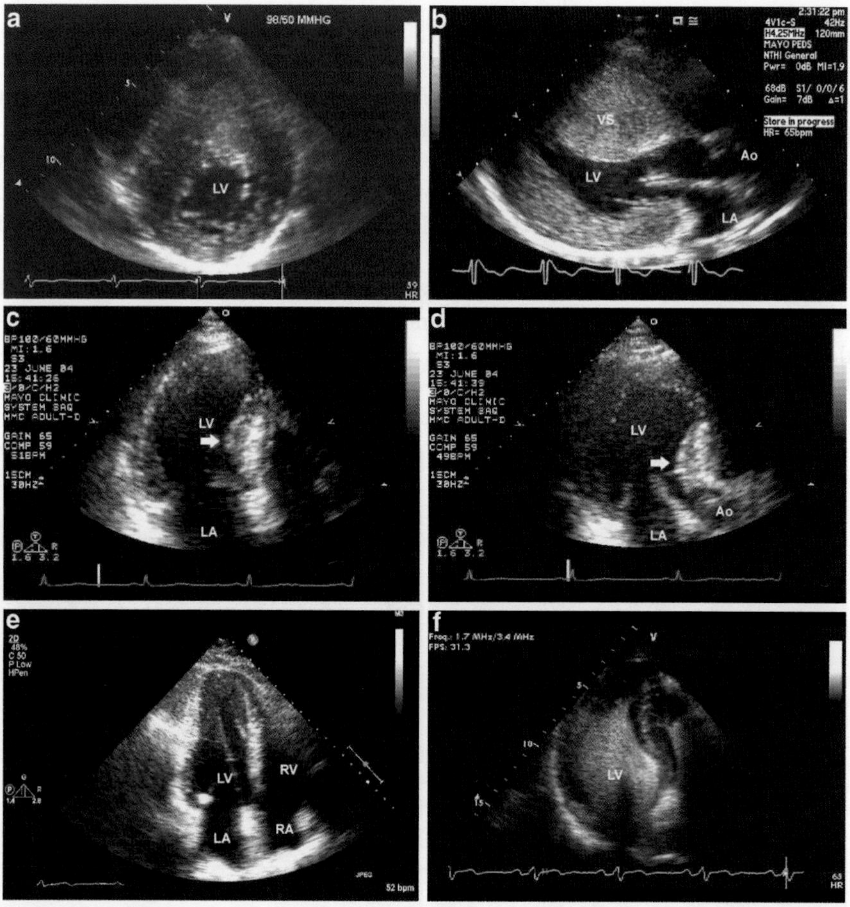

Fig. 13.3 Echocardiography in hypertrophic cardiomyopathy (HCM). In addition to concentric hypertrophy seen in Fig. 13.1, other patterns of myocardial hypertrophy can easily be seen on echocardiography. (**a**, **b**) Parasternal short-axis and long-axis views from two different patients showing severe myocardial hypertrophy of the left ventricle and ventricular septum. (**c**, **d**) Basal septal hypertrophy (*arrows*) seen respectively in an apical four-chamber view and apical long-axis view from a patient with HCM. (**e**) Apical myocardial hypertrophy in a patient with HCM. (**f**) Contrast-enhancement to better visualize apical hypertrophy in another patient with HCM. *Ao* ascending aorta, *LA* left atrium, *LV* left ventricle, *RA* right atrium, *RV* right ventricle, *VS* ventricular septum

cyte disarray, in which there is marked variation in cell shape, size, and arrangement (Fig. 13.3). Disarray may occur in other cardiac diseases, but not to the extent that it is present in HCM where it typically involves more than 5% of the myocardium. Both hypertrophied segments as well as segments of normal thickness can contain myocyte disarray. Structural and/or functional abnormalities of disarray potentially lead to inhomogeneous electrical conduction and provide the setting for micro-reentry pathways that may degenerate into lethal arrhythmias. Other histological abnormalities in HCM include myocardial fibrosis (replacement and/or interstitial types), coronary arteries with thickened walls and narrow lumens, and decreased arteriolar density.

Table 13.1 Proposed criteria for diagnosis of HCM in adult members of affected families

Major criteria	Minor criteria
Echocardiography	
LV wall thickness ≥13 mm in the anterior septum or posterior wall or ≥15 mm in the posterior septum or free wall	LV wall thickness ≥12 mm in the anterior septum or posterior wall or ≥14 mm in the posterior septum or free wall
Severe SAM	Moderate SAM
	Redundant mitral valve leaflets
Electrocardiography	
LVH with repolarization changes	Complete BBB or (minor) IVCD in LV leads
TWI in leads I and aVL (≥3 mm) (with QRS-T wave axis difference 30), V3–V6 (≥3 mm) or II and III and aVF (≥5 mm)	Minor repolarization changes in LV leads
Abnormal Q (>40 ms or >25% R wave) in at least two leads from II, III, aVF (in absence of left anterior hemiblock), V1–V4; or I, aV1, V5–V6	Deep S in lead V2 (≥25 mm)
	Unexplained chest pain, dyspnea, or syncope

Fulfillment of diagnosis requires one major criterion, or two minor echocardiographic criteria, or one minor echocardiographic plus two minor electrocardiographic criteria

Reproduced with permission from McKenna et al. [3]

BBB bundle branch block; *LV* left ventricular; *LVH* left ventricular hypertrophy based on Estes criteria; *SAM* systolic anterior motion of the mitral valve; *TWI* T wave inversion

Table 13.2 Clinical disorders that share morphologic features with hypertrophic cardiomyopathy

Genetic
Noonan's
Friedrich's ataxia
Lentiginosis
Mitochondrial disorders
Familial restrictive cardiomyopathy
Clinical mimics
Fabry's disease
Gaucher's disease
Infants of diabetic mothers
Amyloidosis
Exaggerated physiological response
Athlete's heart
Old-age hypertrophy
Afro-Caribbean hypertension

Gross myocardial hypertrophy in HCM may involve any segment, but three patterns commonly are described: asymmetric septal hypertrophy (~60%), concentric hypertrophy, and apical hypertrophy. Diagnostic criteria with a myocardial wall thickness of ≥15 mm (or ≥2 standard deviations above the mean in pediatric patients) in the absence of other local or systemic etiologies are routinely employed (Table 13.1) [3]. Studies have shown significant clinical consequences (e.g., sudden death) in patients with histologically-proven HCM, even though they had normal or only mildly increased myocardial hypertrophy. Other diseases that frequently share morphologic features with HCM also should be recognized and excluded (Table 13.2).

Screening for Hypertrophic Cardiomyopathy

The detection of HCM is a major objective of physicians who are asked to perform preparticipation screening of athletes. Among individuals in the general population who are less than 35 years of age, HCM accounts for 35% of sudden deaths and is the leading cause of sudden death in this age group [1].

Screening for Families with Known HCM

For family members of individuals affected with HCM, genetic counseling on the inheritable nature of the disorder and the importance of disease screening should be emphasized. Physical examination, electrocardiography, and comprehensive echocardiography of all first-degree relatives of the affected HCM patient should be performed, followed by repeated screening at regular intervals for those initially found to be free of the disease [4]. Increased frequency of family screening should be undertaken in the young, for patients during rapid physical growth, and for those participating in significant aerobic activities. Importantly, regular screening (i.e., every 3–5 years) should continue throughout adulthood because HCM can manifest at any age.

General Pre-Participation Screening

For individuals who are not relatives of patients with HCM, there is considerable controversy on the most appropriate screening methodology for the detection of HCM in athletes. In a study of nearly 34,000 athletes who underwent aggressive preparticipation screening over a 17-year period in the Veneto region of Italy, there was a lower incidence of sudden death due to HCM among the athletes (1 of 49 or 2.0%) in comparison to the nonathletes (16 of 220 or 7.3%) [5]. Moreover, none of the 22 athletes who were diagnosed with HCM and disqualified from sports participation died during follow-up. These observations have spurred great interest in the identification and disqualification of athletes with HCM. Both the European Society of Cardiology (ESC) and the International Olympic Committee (IOC) have recommended that all athletes undergo comprehensive preparticipation and periodic screening, including noninvasive testing – principally, a resting electrocardiogram – in addition to a history and physical examination (Table 13.3) [6, 7].

In 2007, the American Heart Association (AHA) guidelines endorsed a 12-step tool that encompasses a history and physical examination but excludes noninvasive testing (Table 13.4) [8]. There were multiple reasons that were cited that led to the exclusion of such testing in the AHA guidelines. These reasons included the considerable expense of implementing a nationwide screening program in the United States (estimated cost, >2 billion dollars per year), the relatively low

Table 13.3 Criteria for a positive 12-lead ECG

P wave
Left atrial enlargement: negative portion of the P wave in lead V1 $\geq$0.1 mV in depth and $\geq$ 0.04 s in duration; right atrial enlargement: peaked P wave in leads II and III or V1 $\geq$ 0.25 mV in amplitude
QRS complex
Frontal plane axis deviation: right $\geq$ + 120° or left −30° to −90°;increased voltage: amplitude of R or S wave in a standard lead $\geq$2 mV, S wave in lead V1 or V2 $\geq$3 mV, or R wave in lead V5 or V6 $\geq$3 mV; abnormal Q waves $\geq$0.04 s in duration or $\geq$25% of the height of the ensuing R wave or QS pattern in two or more leads; right or left bundle branch block with QRS duration $\geq$0.12 s; R or R′ wave in lead V1 $\geq$0.5 mV in amplitude and R/S ratio $\geq$1
ST-segment, T-waves, and QT interval
ST-segment depression or T-wave flattening or inversion in two or more leads; prolongation of heart rate corrected QT interval >0.44 s in males and >0.46 s in females
Rhythm and conduction abnormalities
Premature ventricular beats or more severe ventricular arrhythmias
Supraventricular tachycardias, atrial flutter, or atrial fibrillation
Short PR interval (<0.12 s) with or without: "delta" wave
Sinus bradycardia with resting heart rate $\leq$40 beats/min[a]
First (PR $\geq$ 0.21 s[b]), second or third degree atrioventricular block

[a] Increasing less than 100 beats/min during limited exercise test
[b] Not shortening with hyperventilation or limited exercise test
Reprinted with permission from Corrado et al. [5]

Table 13.4 American Heart Association 12-step tool for preparticipation cardiovascular screening

Medical history
Personal history
Exertional chest pain/discomfort
Unexplained syncope/near-syncope
Excessive exertional and unexplained dyspnea/fatigue, associated with exercise
Prior recognition of a heart murmur
Elevated systemic blood pressure
Family history
Premature death (sudden and unexpected, or otherwise) before age 50 years due to heart disease, in 1 relative
Disability from heart disease in a close relative <50 years of age
Specific knowledge of certain cardiac conditions in family members: hypertrophic or dilated cardiomyopathy, long-QT syndrome or other ion channelopathies, Marfan syndrome, or clinically important arrhythmias
Physical examination
Heart murmur
Femoral pulses to exclude aortic coarctation
Physical stigmata of Marfan syndrome
Brachial artery blood pressure (sitting position)

Reprinted with permission from Maron et al. [8]

incidence of deaths on the athletic field (1 in 200,000), the limited accuracy of the tests that could be widely utilized (i.e., electrocardiography and echocardiography), and the limited number of medical personnel who are appropriately trained in the interpretation of these tests.

The rationale for the routine use of electrocardiography in preparticipation screening programs stems from the high penetrance of HCM on the electrocardiogram, the significant false-negative detection rates of the history and physical examination, and the opportunity to identify other conduction abnormalities that could lead to sudden cardiac death (e.g., arrhythmogenic right ventricular dysplasia, long QT syndromes, preexcitation, Brugada syndrome). Implementation of routine electrocardiography may obviate the need for routine echocardiography in the detection of HCM in these programs [9]. In Italy, the law mandates the scope of cardiovascular screening, and physicians can be held criminally negligent for improperly clearing an athlete for sports participation [10]. Conversely, there is no similar mandate in the United States. Standards for the scope of preparticipation screening are left to the discretion of physicians and their collective medical judgment. Moreover, no federal or state laws require adoption of the ESC and IOC guidelines on the use of routine electrocardiography. In the United States, there are insufficient resources and no framework for the comprehensive screening of athletes on a national basis, particularly given the large and heterogeneous members in the population. Concerns about resource limitations also have been raised in other developed countries [11, 12]. Thus, current preparticipation screening methods for the detection of HCM in the United States will continue to be comprised mainly of a comprehensive history and physical examination, with further noninvasive testing reserved for those individuals with abnormalities found on this initial evaluation.

Differentiating Hypertrophic Cardiomyopathy from Physiologic Hypertrophy

Because myocardial hypertrophy in patients with HCM can be heterogeneous in both location and severity, the differentiation of HCM from physiologic left ventricular hypertrophy (i.e., athlete's heart) can be challenging. Physiologic hypertrophy has been observed in elite athletes, in whom accuracy in the proper diagnosis has profound implications.

Several clinical features can help reliably distinguish HCM from physiologic hypertrophy or athlete's heart. These include lack of a regression of myocardial hypertrophy following a period of detraining (e.g., >6 months), small left ventricular cavity size (end-diastolic diameter <45 mm), extreme or unusual patterns of myocardial hypertrophy, left atrial enlargement, bizarre patterns on the electrocardiogram, female gender, and a family history of HCM [13–16]. In elite athletes without HCM, there usually is left ventricular chamber dilatation (end-diastolic diameter >55 mm) in addition to the adaptive physiologic hypertrophy. Objective functional testing with measurement of peak myocardial oxygen consumption (VO_2) can also be used. Patients with HCM, even those with elite athletic training, rarely achieve a peak VO_2 of >50 ml/kg/min or >120% predicted [17]. Other clinical features that have been employed in distinguishing HCM from athlete's heart include regional abnormalities in myocardial function detected by Doppler tissue imaging, the presence of gadolinium hyperenhancement on contrast cardiac MRI, and impaired coronary flow reserve [18–21].

Clinical genetic testing is available to identify carriers with subclinical or equivocal findings of HCM. These testing programs accurately determine the presence of genetic variations in candidate loci. Nevertheless, an inherent limitation of these programs is the assumption that these detected variations are causative of disease. Furthermore, there are causative mutations that remain to be identified. Patients should be counseled on possibility of false-negative testing while participating in these programs.

Clinical Features and Management of Hypertrophic Cardiomyopathy

Pathophysiology of HCM

The pathophysiology of HCM is a complex interplay of diastolic dysfunction, LVOT obstruction, myocardial ischemia, and mitral regurgitation. Diastolic dysfunction arises from multiple factors including ventricular nonuniformity, delayed sarcomeric inactivation, and altered loading conditions (i.e., LVOT obstruction). Impaired relaxation and increased chamber stiffness causes elevated ventricular filling pressures and pulmonary congestion, leading to dyspnea, which is the most frequent symptom in patients with HCM. Of importance, diastolic dysfunction commonly occurs in the absence of LVOT obstruction and may be present in cases of mild or localized hypertrophy. Symptoms, thus, are common in patients without evidence of LVOT obstruction.

LVOT obstruction may be present in up to two-thirds of patients. In the presence of LVOT obstruction, there is systolic anterior motion of the anterior or, less commonly, both mitral leaflets. Decreased mitral leaflet coaptation secondary to systolic anterior motion also leads to mitral regurgitation. Importantly, LVOT obstruction and secondary mitral regurgitation are highly dependent upon the ventricular preload, afterload, and the contractile state. Thus, provocative maneuvers (e.g., Valsalva strain, amyl nitrite inhalation) should be performed to determine the presence of latent LVOT obstruction in these patients.

Myocardial ischemia is evident in approximately one-fourth of HCM patients during regular daily activity and in ~40% during exercise. Myocardial ischemia results from a combination of increased oxygen demand of the hypertrophied segments, abnormalities in coronary artery and small vessel architecture, and impairment in coronary flow reserve. Symptoms of myocardial ischemia due to HCM frequently are similar to those due to coronary atherosclerosis but also can be atypical in nature.

Clinical Evaluation of Patients with HCM

The clinical manifestations of HCM characteristically are heterogeneous. The vast majority of patients live without significant morbidity [22]. However, others are afflicted with incapacitating symptoms such as dyspnea or heart failure, presyncope and syncope, and angina. Classically, individuals with HCM have been identified in the third and fourth decades, but clinical presentations now have been observed in neonates as well as octogenarians. Approximately one-fourth of patients have a family history of the disease. Increased awareness of the inheritable nature of HCM and the availability of noninvasive diagnostic modalities both have contributed to the identification of a growing number of patients who are either asymptomatic or mildly symptomatic.

Physical Examination in HCM

The hyperdynamic nature of the disease characteristically leads to a rapid upstroke in the carotid contour, which also may be bifid in the presence of LVOT obstruction. A heightened atrial wave may be present in the jugular venous pulse when there is significant infundibular hypertrophy. The apical impulse is usually localized, sustained and may be bifid or even trifid. A fourth heart sound is usually present, and in younger patients, an early diastolic filling sound is frequently heard. Significant LVOT obstruction may cause paradoxical splitting of the second heart sound, a systolic ejection murmur, and a concomitant apical murmur of mitral regurgitation. Augmentation of the ejection murmur during Valsalva strain characterizes the murmur of LVOT obstruction, but is not a reliable sign in many patients due to inadequate lowering of preload during the maneuver. A more reliable sign of a murmur due to LVOT obstruction is a decrease in intensity from standing to squatting and a progressive increase in intensity from squatting to standing. In some patients, severe obstruction may become fixed, and the murmur does not change during these maneuvers.

Electrocardiography

Electrocardiographic abnormalities are present in ~90% of patients with HCM [23]. These findings consist of left ventricular hypertrophy, secondary ST-segment and T-wave abnormalities, interventricular conduction defects, left atrial abnormality, and left axis deviation as seen in the case vignette. Pathologic Q waves also are common, especially in the inferior and precordial leads. Although these Q waves do not appear to follow the pattern of underlying hypertrophy, their presence may help to differentiate physiologic hypertrophy from that due to HCM. Giant T-wave inversions (negativity ≥10 mV) were first reported in apical HCM, but these abnormalities also have been observed in patients with other patterns of myocardial hypertrophy (Fig. 13.4). Clinically significant conduction defects are rarely present.

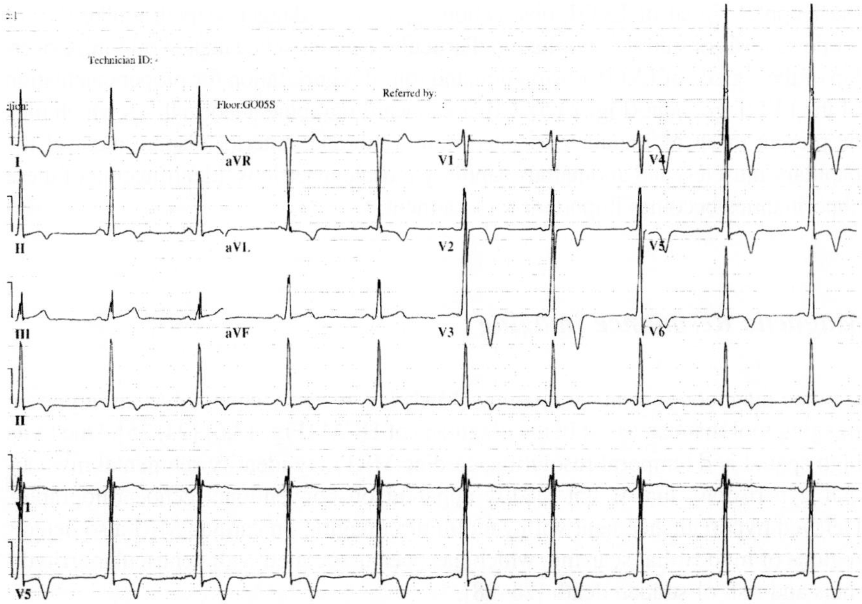

Fig. 13.4 Electrocardiogram from a patient with apical hypertrophic cardiomyopathy. Note the deep T-wave inversions in the precordial leads. These findings frequently are not only found in patients with apical hypertrophic cardiomyopathy but also have been observed in patients with other hypertrophy patterns

In ~25% of HCM patients, nonsustained ventricular tachycardia is evident on ambulatory electrocardiography. Sustained monomorphic ventricular tachycardia is rare in HCM but is usually associated with ventricular aneurysms. These aneurysms may arise from midcavity systolic obliteration and resultant high apical intracavitary pressures. Atrial fibrillation occurs in ~20% of patients with HCM. In addition to embolic risk, atrial fibrillation can precipitate hemodynamic deterioration because of underlying diastolic dysfunction that is present in HCM.

Echocardiography

Due to its noninvasive nature and established techniques, echocardiography is the standard method for assessing cardiac morphology and function in patients with HCM. Echocardiography also is the most widely used imaging modality for the screening of relatives of HCM patients in conjunction with electrocardiography. Two-dimensional, color Doppler echocardiography allows visualization of hypertrophied myocardium, LVOT obstruction, and secondary mitral regurgitation. The onset and duration of systolic anterior motion of the mitral valve correlate with the severity of the gradient across the LVOT. Using peak LVOT velocity (v), the LVOT gradient is calculated using the modified Bernoulli equation: $LVOT\ gradient = 4v^2$. Of note, the Doppler signal of LVOT obstruction typically is dagger-shaped, unlike that of aortic stenosis or mitral regurgitation. Particular care must be taken to minimize overlap of the signals of LVOT obstruction and mitral regurgitation for proper calculation of the LVOT gradient (Fig. 13.5). Other echocardiographic abnormalities which may be present in HCM include elongated mitral chordae, anterior displacement of the papillary muscles, and anomalous papillary muscle insertions. Identification of these abnormalities becomes important for treatment.

Magnetic Resonance Imaging

Cardiac magnetic resonance imaging (MRI) has recently emerged as an important imaging tool that can assist in the diagnosis of HCM (Fig. 13.6) [24, 25]. Due to its high spatial and temporal resolution, cardiac MRI may identify segmental myocardial hypertrophy that is not readily apparent on conventional echocardiography. Delayed hyperenhancement with gadolinium imaging on cardiac MRI also detects regions of myocardial scarring, which has been associated with ventricular arrhythmias and risk of sudden death [26–28].

Risk Stratification for Sudden Cardiac Death

The most important challenge in the management of HCM is the identification of those patients at increased risk of sudden cardiac death. The inheritable nature of the disease, the relative ease with which affected individuals can be identified, and the known efficacy of implantable cardioverter-defibrillators warrant the cardiac screening of at least all first-degree relatives of HCM patients [4, 29]. The major risk factors for sudden cardiac death in HCM are prior cardiac arrest, ventricular tachycardia, family history of sudden cardiac death due to HCM, a hypotensive or flat blood pressure response during exercise, massive myocardial hypertrophy (wall thickness ≥30 mm), and recurrent, unexplained syncope [4]. Youth at clinical presentation classically has been cited as a risk factor, but differentiation of those patients undergoing uncomplicated family screening from those who present on their own accord (i.e., due to symptoms) is necessary. Some genetic mutations have been shown to carry an increased risk of sudden death, but considerable heterogeneity in such an attributable risk has been demonstrated in several studies.

Specific challenges are evident in the risk stratification of patients with HCM. There is a low annual mortality rate in unselected patient populations (<0.5–1.0% per year). Given the sheer number of persons with HCM in the general population (1:500), the small cohorts studied thus far have brought forth relatively few high-risk patients. Moreover, prospective screening and genetic studies of index relatives have identified an increasing number of asymptomatic, healthy individuals with HCM who otherwise may have gone undiagnosed. The risk of disease complications

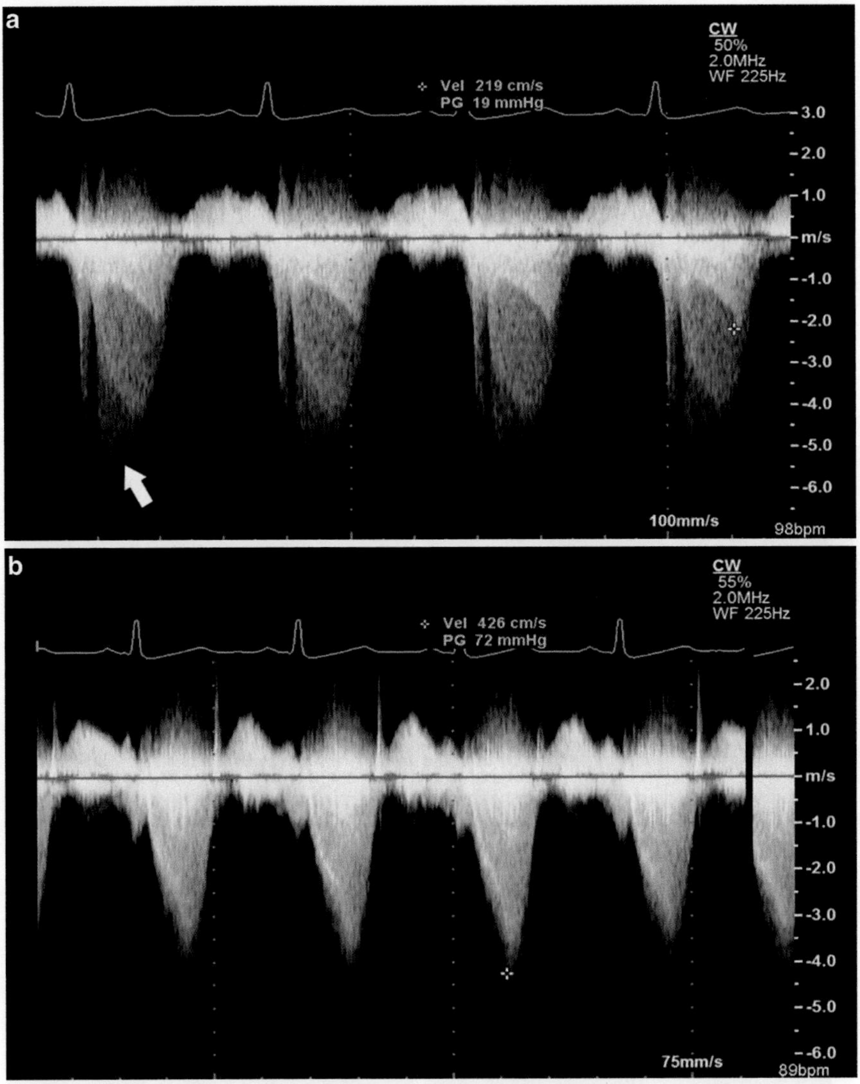

Fig. 13.5 Similarity of the left ventricular outflow tract signal to mitral regurgitation. In patients with hypertrophic cardiomyopathy, the peak velocity signal of the left ventricular outflow tract (*asterisk in bottom*, 4.2 m/s) must be carefully differentiated from the signal of mitral regurgitation (*arrow in top*, 5.5 m/s). These signals frequently overlap

in these individuals may be less than that of other patients, particularly those seen at referral institutions.

An important confounding factor is the characteristic heterogeneity of the disease. This heterogeneity limits the predictive power of each risk factor, making the broad application of strict management algorithms difficult. To overcome the low predictive accuracy of other risk factors, some experts have advocated that their addition

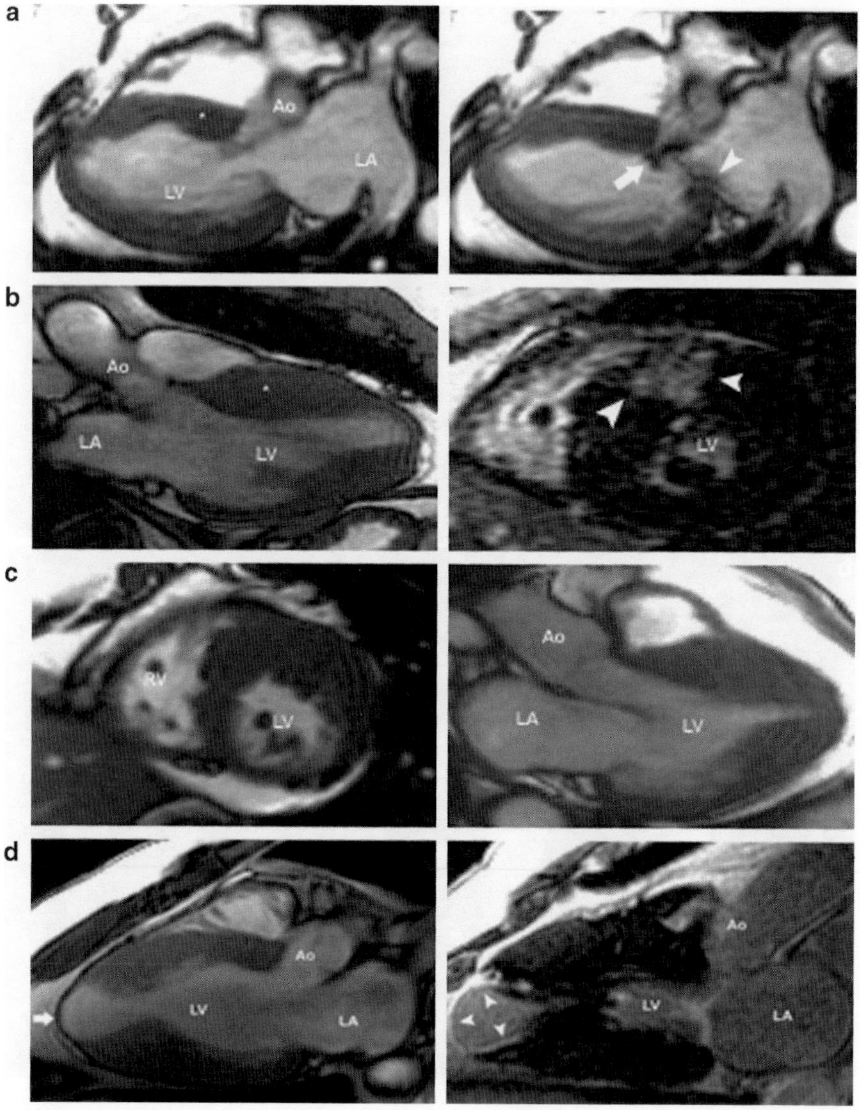

Fig. 13.6 Cardiac magnetic resonance imaging in four patients with hypertrophic cardiomyopathy (HCM). (**a**) Patient with HCM and basal septal hypertrophy at end-diastole (*left*) and left ventricular outflow tract obstruction during systole (*arrow, right*). There also is posteriorly directed mitral regurgitation (*arrowhead*). (**b**) HCM patient with severe anteroseptal hypertrophy (*asterisk*) and delayed gadolinium hyperenhancement in the area of septal hypertrophy (*arrowheads*). (**c**) Patient with HCM and severe nonobstructive hypertrophy of the left ventricular apex. (**d**) HCM patient with severe midcavitary hypertrophy and obstruction, and delayed gadolinium hyperenhancement of the left ventricular apex. Part (**d**) is reprinted with permission from Martinez MW, et al. Mid-cavitary obstruction in hypertrophic cardiomyopathy. Heart 2008;94:1287. *Ao* ascending aorta, *LA* left atrium, *LV* left ventricle, *RA* right atrium, *RV* right ventricle

signifies increased risk, and that the collective absence of the risk factors (due to their relatively high negative predictive values) suggests a favorable prognosis [30]. The approach at our institution is that any patient with either a history of prior cardiac arrest, sustained ventricular tachycardia, and/or a family history of sudden death due to HCM, should receive therapy aimed at sudden death prevention. For patients with other risk factors, an individualized approach is undertaken with full discussion of the therapeutic goals and the limitations of current predictive tools.

The principal therapy for the prevention of sudden cardiac death in HCM is implantation of a cardioverter-defibrillator. Several case series and a large retrospective study have demonstrated the efficacy of these devices in HCM patients at risk for sudden cardiac death [29]. For HCM patients with a prior history of cardiac arrest, the indication for these devices is evident. Among these patients, there is a high incidence of lethal arrhythmias (>11% per year), and the ability of implantable cardiac defibrillators to terminate such arrhythmias is known. Among HCM patients who undergo implantation for primary prevention, the annual rate of appropriate device therapy has been shown to be 4–5%, and the efficacy of these devices is no less than that in patients requiring secondary prevention. However, the precise clinical criteria that designate high risk have not been standardized. Further prospective investigation into the means of preemptive identification of such patients is still required.

Management of Patients with Hypertrophic Cardiomyopathy

Physical Exercise

Because significant aerobic physical exertion has been causally linked to sudden cardiac death in patients with HCM, activity restriction is advised in these patients. The 36th Bethesda Conference for Eligibility Recommendations for Competitive Athletes with Cardiovascular Abnormalities specifically recommends the exclusion of all patients with a probable or unequivocal clinical diagnosis of HCM from competitive sports, with the possible exception of those participating in sports with low intensity (<4 metabolic equivalents) [31]. For those participating in sports with moderate levels of intensity (e.g., jogging, doubles tennis, baseball, and surfing), the approach to activity restriction is individualized (Table 13.5) [32]. Factors to consider during individualization include the physical intensity imparted by the individual, psychological burden, potential effects of drugs, environmental conditions, and the unique clinical attributes of the individual. Of note, these recommendations apply to patients with clinically manifest HCM. For patients who are genotype-positive and phenotype-negative, there are no compelling data to disqualify these patients, especially in the absence of cardiac symptoms or a family history of sudden death. Specific guidelines on activity restriction for patients who have undergone defibrillator implantation are not available, but there is consensus

Table 13.5 Categorization of sports by intensity level and participation recommendation for patients with hypertrophic cardiomyopathy

Intensity level recommendation	
High	
Basketball	
Full court	0
Half court	0
Body building	1
Ice hockey	0
Racquetball/squash	0
Rock climbing	1
Running (sprinting)	0
Skiing (downhill)	2
Skiing (cross-country)	2
Soccer	0
Tennis (singles)	0
Touch (flag) football	1
Windsurfing	1
Moderate	
Baseball/softball	2
Biking	4
Modest hiking	4
Motorcycling	3
Jogging	3
Sailing	3
Surfing	2
Swimming (lap)	5
Tennis (doubles)	4
Treadmill/stationary bicycle	5
Weightlifting (free weights)	1
Hiking	3
Low	
Bowling	5
Golf	5
Horseback riding	3
Scuba diving	0
Skating	5
Snorkeling	5
Weights (nonfree weights)	4
Brisk walking	5

0–1, strongly advise against activity; 2–3, individualization recommended; 4–6, activity probably permitted
Modified with permission from Maron et al. [8]

that the antiarrhythmic protection afforded by the implanted defibrillator should not lead to explicit avocation of physical activity.

For all patients with HCM, a low level aerobic exercise program is recommended to improve or maintain overall cardiovascular fitness. Patients should always keep well hydrated and avoid circumstances where vasodilatation may occur, such as hot baths or saunas.

Medical Therapy

The most commonly used medications are β-adrenergic receptor antagonists and calcium-channel blockers (i.e., verapamil and diltiazem). These drugs depress contractility, thereby reducing intraventricular flow velocities that aggravate the development of LVOT obstruction and high intracavitary pressure, and improve the imbalance between myocardial oxygen supply and demand. In patients with significant diastolic dysfunction, the negative chronotropic properties of these agents allow more time for ventricular filling. Of note, verapamil must be used with caution, if at all, in patients with a severe LVOT obstruction, due to the potential for exacerbation of the gradient by its vasodilatory properties. Disopyramide, another negative inotrope with antiarrhythmic properties, also has been used successfully in HCM patients. Its use, however, is complicated by anticholinergic side effects and frequent tachyphylaxis. Concomitant β-adrenergic blockade also is recommended for those patients with atrial fibrillation because disopyramide may accelerate atrioventricular nodal conduction and lead to tachycardia. Peripheral vasodilators generally are avoided in HCM because they may exacerbate obstruction. In those patients whose disease has progressed to ventricular dilatation with systolic impairment, conventional heart failure medications (e.g., ACE-inhibitors, digoxin, diuretics, vasodilators, etc.) are employed.

Strategy in drug selection largely is based on the benefit perceived by the patient, as there is little data to suggest the superiority of either β-adrenergic antagonists or verapamil. As none of these drugs have been shown to prevent sudden death in HCM, their indication in patients without symptoms is not clear. For those patients with paroxysmal atrial fibrillation, amiodarone is helpful. Its initiation may help prevent acute hemodynamic deterioration and systemic embolization that may occur even with brief episodes of atrial fibrillation. Oral anticoagulation should be instituted in cases of either paroxysmal or chronic atrial fibrillation.

Septal Reduction Therapy

The two principal therapies for relief of LVOT obstruction in patients with HCM are surgical septal myectomy and percutaneous alcohol septal ablation. Surgical myectomy is the gold standard therapy that leads to durable relief of symptoms in >90% of patients with a low operative risk (<1%) when it is performed in experienced centers. Alcohol ablation is a relatively new alternative catheter-based therapy, in which a controlled infarction reduces septal thickening and thereby obstruction. Alcohol ablation results in symptom relief in ~80% of patients but can result in pacemaker dependency, and long-term effects remain unknown. Current guidelines recommend that consideration of septal reduction therapy be made in a tertiary center with expertise in comprehensive management of patients with HCM.

Natural History of Hypertrophic Cardiomyopathy

In the vast majority of patients with HCM, there is normal longevity with minimal cardiac morbidity. However, progression of the disease can vary. The degree of myocardial hypertrophy may increase in pediatric patients and occasionally young adults, especially during periods of rapid physical growth. Traditional screening recommendations have emphasized regular examinations until plateau of the individual's growth, but genetic investigations have demonstrated disease manifestation after the fifth decade of life. HCM may manifest as an inappropriate response to ventricular pressure overload in some patients. Progressive left ventricular dilatation and systolic dysfunction in HCM is uncommon (<5%), but there is a high morbidity and mortality in this patient subset.

Sudden death in HCM may occur without antecedent symptoms and be the first manifestation of the disease. Older studies from referral institutions historically estimated the annual incidence of sudden death to be ~4% in adolescents and young adults and 1–2% in older adults. However, more recent studies of less selected patient populations have demonstrated a lower incidence of sudden death (0.5–1% per year) and survival that appears to be comparable to non-HCM populations [6].

Patients with HCM have an increased susceptibility to age-related conditions. Atrial fibrillation occurs in ~20%of patients and is associated with increased risk of stroke (up to one-fifth of HCM patients with atrial fibrillation), severe functional impairment, and death due to heart failure [33]. In a large cohort study of 900 patients, the prevalence of stroke was 6% (0.8% per year) with events occurring almost exclusively in patients with atrial fibrillation [34]. For patients with HCM who develop coronary atherosclerosis, there is an adverse prognosis due to the combination of epicardial disease and the underlying inherent myocardial ischemia [35].

References

1. Maron BJ, Shirani J, Poliac LC, et al. Sudden death in young competitive athletes: clinical, demographic and pathological profiles. JAMA 1996;276;199–204.
2. Maron BJ, Gardin JM, Flack JM, Gidding SS, Kurosaki TT, Bild DE. Prevalence of hypertrophic cardiomyopathy in a general population of young adults: echocardiographic analysis of 4111 subjects in the CARDIA Study. Circulation 1995;92:785–789.
3. McKenna WJ, Spirito P, Desnos M, Dubourg O, Komajda M. Experience from clinical genetics in hypertrophic cardiomyopathy: proposal for new diagnostic criteria in adult members of affected families. Heart 1997;77:130–132.
4. Maron BJ, McKenna WJ, Danielson GK, et al., Task Force on Clinical Expert Consensus Documents, American College of Cardiology, Committee for Practice Guidelines, European Society of Cardiology, American College of Cardiology/European Society of Cardiology clinical expert consensus document on hypertrophic cardiomyopathy. A report of the American College of Cardiology Foundation Task Force on Clinical Expert Consensus Documents and the European Society of Cardiology Committee for Practice Guidelines. J Am Coll Cardiol 2003;42:1687–1713.
5. Corrado D, Basso C, Schiavon M, Thiene G. Screening for hypertrophic cardiomyopathy in young athletes. N Engl J Med 1998;339:364–369.

6. Corrado D, Pelliccia, A, Bjornstad HH, et al. Cardiovascular pre-participation screening of young competitive athletes for prevention of sudden death: proposal for a common European protocol. Consensus Statement of the Study group of Sport Cardiology of the Working Group of Cardiac Rehabilitation and Exercise Physiology and the Working Group of Myocardial and Pericardial Diseases of the European Society of Cardiology. Eur Heart J 2005;26:516–524.
7. IOC Medical Commission, International Olympic Committee. Sudden Cardiovascular Death in Sport: Lausanne Recommendations: Preparticipation Cardiovascular Screening. December 10, 2004. Available at http://multimedia.olympic.org/pdf/en_report_886.pdf Accessed January 23, 2008.
8. Maron BJ, Thompson PD, Ackerman MJ, et al. Recommendations and considerations related to preparticipation screening for cardiovascular abnormalities in competitive athletes: 2007 update: a scientific statement from the American Heart Association Council on Nutrition, Physical Activity, and Metabolism. Circulation 2007;115:1643–455.
9. Pelliccia A, Di Paolo FM, Corrado D, et al. Evidence for efficacy of the Italian national pre-participation screening programme for identification of hypertrophic cardiomyopathy in competitive athletes. Eur Heart J 2006;27:2196–2200.
10. Colucci M. Part I: organization of sport (Italy), §2,IV (Sports Doctors). In: Hendrickx F (ed) International Encyclopaedia of Laws: Sports Law. New York, NY: Aspen Publishers; 2004; 29–31.
11. Prescott E. Cardiovascular pre-participation screening of young competitive athletes for prevention of sudden death: proposal for a common European protocol. Eur Heart J 2006;27:2904–2905.
12. Hanson JR. Screening is inefficient and too expensive for the NHS. BMJ 2008;337:a906.
13. Maron BJ, Pelliccia A, Spirito P. Cardiac disease in young trained athletes: insights into methods for distinguishing athlete's heart from structural heart disease with particular emphasis on hypertrophic cardiomyopathy. Circulation 1995;91:1596–1601.
14. Sharma S, Maron BJ, Whyte G, et al. Physiologic limits of left ventricular hypertrophy in elite junior athletes: relevance to differential diagnosis of athlete's heart and hypertrophic cardiomyopathy. J Am Coll Cardiol 2002;40:1431–1436.
15. Pelliccia A, Maron BJ, De Luca R, et al. Remodeling of left ventricular hypertrophy in elite athletes after long-term deconditioning. Circulation 2002;105:944–949.
16. Basavarajaiah S, Wilson M, Junagde S, et al. Physiological left ventricular hypertrophy or hypertrophic cardiomyopathy in an elite adolescent athlete: role of detraining in resolving the clinical dilemma. Br J Sports Med 2006;40:727–729.
17. Sharma S, Elliott PM, Whyte G, et al. Utility of metabolic exercise testing in distinguishing hypertrophic cardiomyopathy from physiologic left ventricular hypertrophy in athletes. J Am Coll Cardiol 2000;36:864–870.
18. Radvan J, Choudhury L, Sheridan DJ, Camici PG. Comparison of coronary vasodilator reserve in elite rowing athletes versus hypertrophic cardiomyopathy. Am J Cardiol 1997;80:1621–1623.
19. Vinereanu D, Florescu N, Sculthorpe N, et al. Differentiation between pathologic and physiologic left ventricular hypertrophy by tissue Doppler assessment of long-axis function in patients with hypertrophic cardiomyopathy or systemic hypertension and in athletes. Am J Cardiol 2001;88:53–58.
20. Cardim N, Oliveira AG, Longo S, et al. Doppler tissue imaging: regional myocardial function in hypertrophic cardiomyopathy and in athlete's heart. J Am Soc Echocardiogr 2003;16:223–232.
21. Saghir M, Areces M, Makan M. Strain rate imaging differentiates hypertensive cardiac hypertrophy from physiologic cardiac hypertrophy. J Am Soc Echocardiogr 2007;20:151–157.
22. Spirito P, Chiarella F, Carratino L, Berisso MZ, Bellotti P, Vecchio C. Clinical course and prognosis of hypertrophic cardiomyopathy in an outpatient population. N Engl J Med 1989; 320:749–755.
23. Montgomery JV, Harris KM, Casey SA, Zenovich AG, Maron BJ. Relation of electrocardiographic patterns to phenotypic expression and clinical outcome in hypertrophic cardiomyopathy. Am J Cardiol 2005;96:270–275.
24. Hansen MW, Merchant N. MRI of hypertrophic cardiomyopathy: part I, MRI appearances. Am J Roentgenol 2007;189:1335–1343.

25. Rickers C, Wilke NM, Jerosch-Herold M, Casey SA, Panse P, Panse N, Weil J, Zenovich AG, Maron BJ. Utility of cardiac magnetic resonance imaging in the diagnosis of hypertrophic cardiomyopathy. Circulation 2005;112:855–861.
26. Moon JC, Reed E, Shephard MN, et al. The histologic basis of late gadolinium enhancement cardiovascular magnetic resonance in hypertrophic cardiomyopathy. J Am Coll Cardiol 2004;43:2260–2264.
27. Choudhury L, Mahrholdt H, Wagner A, et al. Myocardial scarring in asymptomatic or mildly symptomatic patients with hypertrophic cardiomyopathy. J Am Coll Cardiol 2002;40:2156–2164.
28. Adabag AS, Maron BJ, Appelbaum E, et al. Occurrence and frequency of arrhythmias in hypertrophic cardiomyopathy in relation to delayed enhancement on cardiovascular magnetic resonance. J Am Coll Cardiol 2008;51:1369–1374.
29. Maron BJ, Shen W-K, Link MS, et al. Efficacy of implantable cardioverter-defibrillators for the prevention of sudden death in patients with hypertrophic cardiomyopathy. N Engl J Med 2000;342:365–373.
30. Elliott PM, Poloniecki J, Dickie S, et al. Sudden death in hypertrophic cardiomyopathy: identification of high risk patients. J Am Coll Cardiol 2000;36:2212–2218.
31. Maron BJ, Ackerman MJ, Nishimura RA, Pyeritz RE, Towbin JA, Udelson JA. Task Force 4: HCM and other cardiomyopathies, mitral valve prolapse, myocarditis, and Marfan syndrome. J Am Coll Cardiol 2005;45:1340–1345.
32. Maron BJ, Chaitman BR, Ackerman MJ, et al. Recommendations for physical activity and recreational sports participation for young patients with genetic cardiovascular diseases. Circulation 2004;109:2807–2816.
33. Olivotto I, Cecchi F, Casey SA, et al. Impact of atrial fibrillation on the clinical course of hypertrophic cardiomyopathy. Circulation 2001;104:2517–2524.
34. Maron BJ, Olivotto I, Bellone P, et al. Clinical profile of stroke in 900 patients with hypertrophic cardiomyopathy. J Am Coll Cardiol 2002;39:301–307.
35. Sorajja P, Ommen SR, Nishimura RA, et al. Adverse prognosis of patients with hypertrophic cardiomyopathy and epicardial coronary artery disease. Circulation 2003;108:2342–2348.

Chapter 14
Commotio Cordis: Practical Aspects in Sports

Mark S. Link

Commotio cordis has achieved markedly increased attention because of the increased awareness of sudden death that occurs during sports in the playing field [1, 2]. The rising popularity of lacrosse and the widespread media attention to several prominent lacrosse deaths due to commotio cordis have also put this phenomenon in the forefront of sports safety. Commotio cordis is defined as sudden death secondary to relatively innocent chest wall impact. In the nineteenth century, commotio cordis occurred predominantly in occupational activities, but in the latter half of the twentieth century, the epidemiologic pattern has switched to commotio cordis in sports. Before 1995, the knowledge of commotio cordis was patchwork, from a number of case reports. In 1995, however, a systematic collection of commotio cordis cases was reported by Barry Maron in the NEJM [3]. It is only after the publication of these 25 cases and the subsequent development of an animal model [4] that the entity known as commotio cordis has received widespread attention. Indeed, commotio cordis is currently the second leading cause of sudden cardiac death in youth sports in America; up to 20 events a year are reported to the US Commotio Cordis Registry [5].

Commotio Cordis-Clinical Characteristics

Individuals succumbing to commotio cordis are typically adolescents with a mean age of 14 and an age range from 1 to 50 years (Fig. 14.1) [1]. It is thought that the relative pliability of the chest wall predisposes adolescents to commotio cordis. However, there may be other contributing factors such as a higher likelihood of getting hit in the chest due to more frequent sporting activities and a decreased skill in catching the ball. Commotio cordis most commonly occurs in sports in which a hard object is thrown, such as baseball, lacrosse, and hockey (Fig. 14.2). In other

M.S. Link (✉)
Tufts University School of Medicine, Boston, MA, USA
e-mail: mlink@tuftsmedicalcenter.org

C.E. Lawless (ed.), *Sports Cardiology Essentials: Evaluation, Management and Case Studies*, DOI 10.1007/978-0-387-92775-6_14,

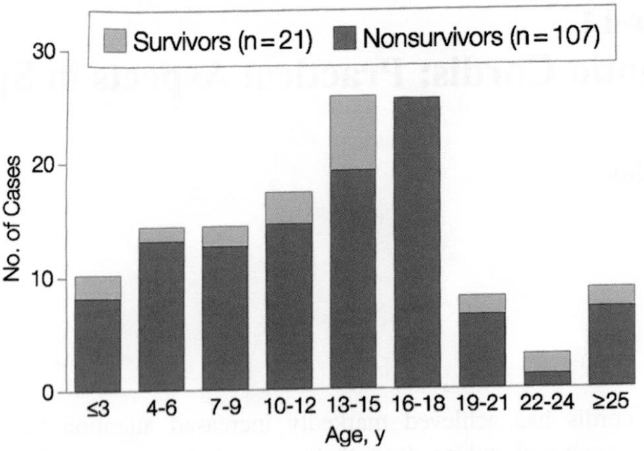

Fig. 14.1 Individuals succumbing to commotio cordis are typically adolescents with a mean age of 14 and an age range from 1 to 50 years. Reprinted with permission from JAMA [1]

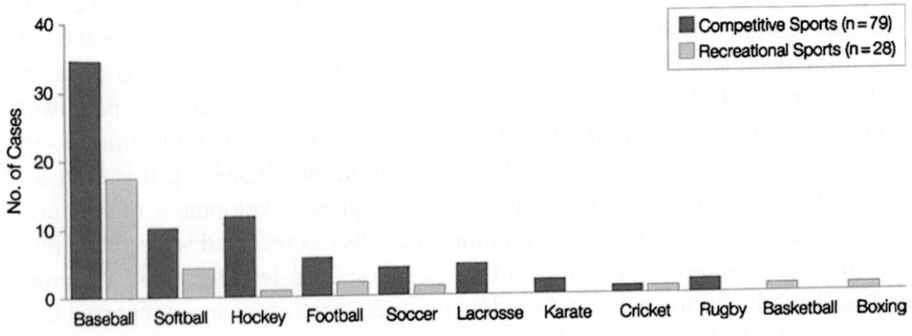

Fig. 14.2 Commotio cordis most commonly occurs in sports in which a hard object impacts the chest, such as baseball, lacrosse, and hockey. Reprinted with permission from JAMA [1]

sports with pneumatic balls, commotio cordis can also occur but is generally due to being struck in the chest by elbows or fists. Approximately 60% of commotio cordis victims are participating in competitive or league sports, while 40% occur around the home. In competitive activities, increased sympathetic tone and adrenergic activity may increase vulnerability to traumatic chest wall-induced sudden death. Of the individuals in competitive or league sports, approximately one-third have been wearing a chest protector [6]. In sports such as hockey, the chest protector has been lifted from the chest and the hockey puck has thus struck the individual directly over the heart. In other sports such as baseball and lacrosse, the chest protector has remained anterior to the cardiac silhouette, yet despite this appropriately placed chest protector, sudden death has resulted from a direct blow.

Initial arrhythmias in the victims at resuscitation have been ventricular fibrillation (Fig. 14.3). Resuscitation can be successful if CPR and defibrillation are prompt; however, even prompt defibrillation does not guarantee a successful outcome [7].

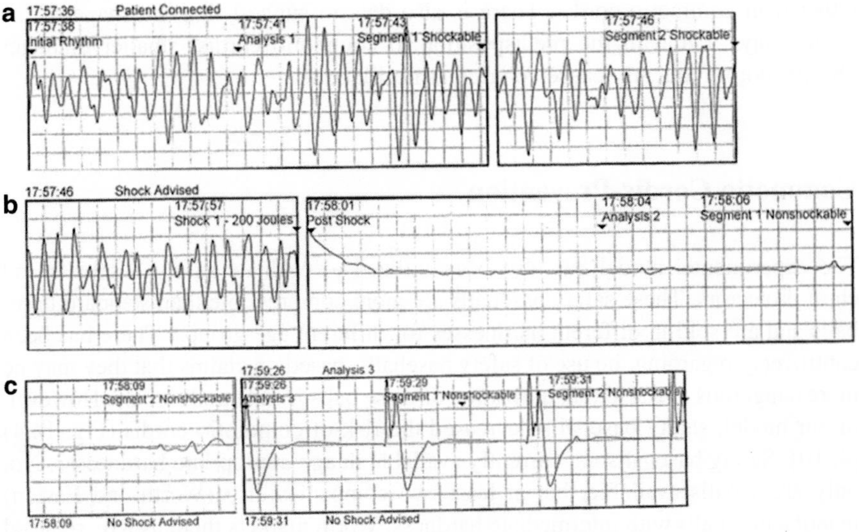

Fig. 14.3 AED tracing from a 22-year-old male struck in the chest by a ball during a lacrosse match [7]. The tracing demonstrates ventricular fibrillation that is terminated by the AED

Defibrillation may be followed by asystole, as in other causes of sudden cardiac death. Survival in commotio cordis approaches 15–20% with rapid resuscitation efforts. Electrocardiograms after resuscitation nearly always demonstrate ST segment elevation.

Experimental Models of Commotio Cordis

An animal model developed at Tufts University has allowed us to explore the mechanism, prevention, and treatment for commotio cordis [4]. Commotio cordis appears to be a primary electrical event; ventricular fibrillation occurs immediately upon chest wall impact, and thus, cannot be secondary to myocardial ischemia, ventricular tachycardia, or asystole.

A confluence of critical variables appear to be necessary for commotio cordis to occur. Perhaps the most important variable is the time window of impact relative to the cardiac cycle. Only impacts on the upslope of the T-wave will cause VF. In our animal model, this time window of vulnerability is 1–2% of the cardiac cycle [2, 4]. The site of impact is also critical, and only impacts which directly overlie the cardiac silhouette will cause VF [8]. Interestingly, as energy of impact increases to 40-miles-per-hour balls, the incidence of VF increases to 70%; however, at impact velocities greater than that, the probability of VF decreased, while the frequency of structural damage including myocardial rupture and contusions increased [9]. It is thus likely that at these velocities, our model becomes one of cardiac contusion rather than commotio cordis. There is also data to suggest that the shape of the object plays a role in the predisposition to commotio cordis; smaller diameter objects more frequently cause ventricular fibrillation.

Commotio Cordis-Prevention

The experimental model has also been utilized to evaluate safety baseballs and chest protectors. These safety baseballs are more compressible than standard baseballs and are sold in different hardnesses for different age groups. There has been controversy regarding the use of safety baseballs, based on claims that they may be more dangerous and also that utilization of these balls is not "traditional". However, in our model, safety baseballs decreased the risk of commotio cordis (Fig. 14.4) [4, 10]. Safety baseballs are currently available in age-appropriate hardnesses. Not only are T-balls available, but at least two companies also (Worth and Easton) manufacture balls with intermediate hardness. Worth markets them as RIF, reduced injury factor; I include this datum in Fig. 14.4 legend below. These balls are judged playable by age-appropriate youths and can be effective in reducing not only the risk of commotio cordis but also head and soft-tissue injury.

However, commercially available chest wall protectors have not been shown to be effective in preventing commotio cordis both in the clinical arena and in our laboratory (Figs. 14.5 and 14.6) [6, 11]. In our laboratory, even models that appeared robust

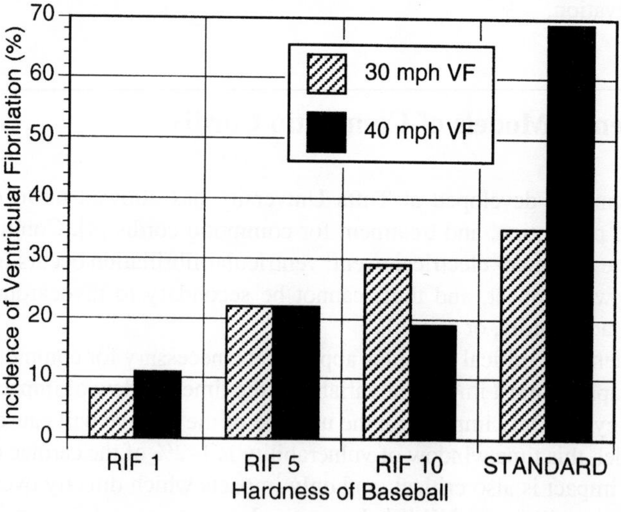

Fig. 14.4 Safety baseballs are marketed in different hardnesses for use in age-appropriate athletes. Softer balls are less likely to cause commotio cordis in an experimental model. Balls in this experiment were manufactured by Worth. Reduced injury factor (RIF) 1 are marketed for T-ball use, while RIF 5 are marketed for 8–10 year olds and RIF 10 for 11–13 year olds. Reprinted with permission from Pediatrics [10]

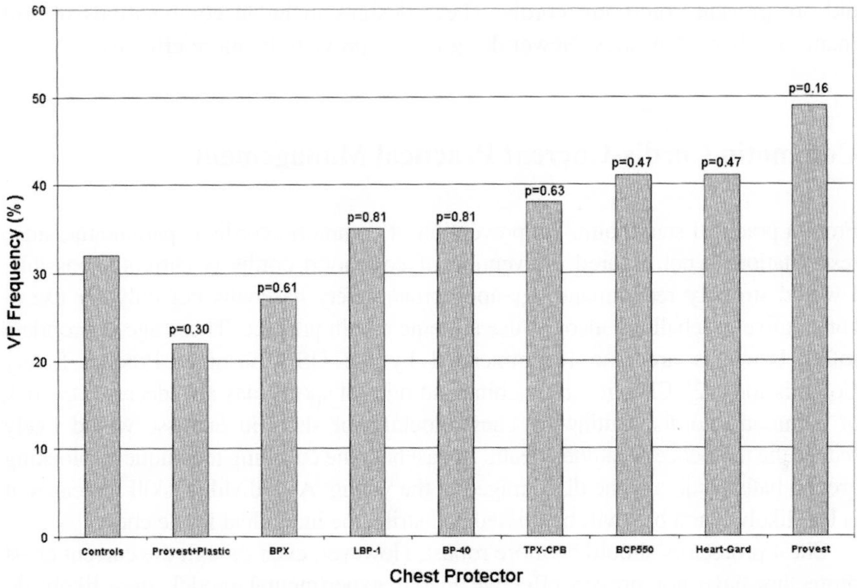

Fig. 14.5 Chest protectors marketed for use in baseball did not significantly decrease the risk of ventricular fibrillation. Reprinted with permission from Pediatrics [11]

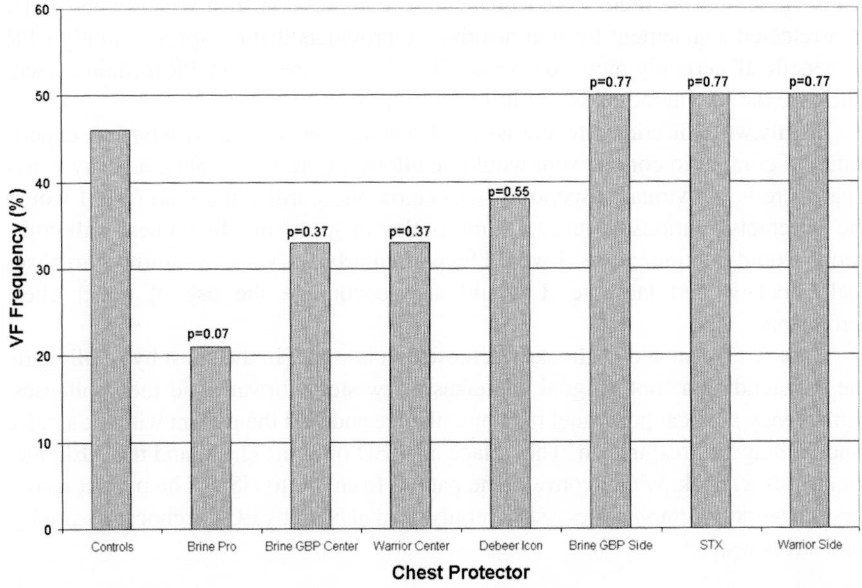

Fig. 14.6 Chest protectors marketed for use in lacrosse did not significantly decrease the risk of ventricular fibrillation. Reprinted with permission from Pediatrics [11]

did not prevent commotio cordis. These designs included combinations of soft foams and harder plastics. Newer designs may prove to be more effective.

Commotio Cordis-Current Practical Management

From a practical standpoint, the prevention of commotio cordis is paramount, since resuscitation is not assured. Prevention of commotio cordis is currently possible. I would strongly recommend age-appropriate safety baseballs not only for use in competitive baseball but also for use at home and in practice. These age-appropriate safety baseballs are also recommended by the US Consumer Product Safety Commission [12]. Changes in coaching and rules of sports may also decrease the risk of commotio cordis. Outlawing chest blocking of shots in lacrosse would likely reduce the incidence of sudden death. In baseball, the coaching technique of blocking ground balls could also be discouraged in the young. As individual skill increases, it is less likely that a ball will be missed and strike the individual in the chest.

Chest protectors should be more robust. However, even though the current chest protectors have not proven effective in our experimental model, they likely do reduce the risk of soft-tissue injury.

Resuscitation must not only be prompt but also complete and include CPR and defibrillation. The more universal placement of AEDs will save the lives of athletes and their parents and grandparents. However, excellent quality CPR must not take a back seat to AEDs. I believe that coaches, trainers, and even athletes should know CPR, including the focus on adequate chest compression. Just recently, the AHA has released a statement for non-health-care providers that compression only CPR is beneficial, certainly more so than no CPR. Improvements in CPR techniques will increase the likelihood of successful resuscitation.

Finally,when it comes to the issue of whether an individual who has experienced a commotio cordis event would be allowed to return to play, it is my belief that there is individual susceptibility to commotio cordis, and therefore, I would be extremely cautious about returning to play in sports in which chest wall collisions would continue; thus, I would be particularly wary about returning to baseball, hockey, and lacrosse. I would also encourage the use of better chest protectors.

Case A 17-year-old ice hockey defenseman is struck in the chest by a ball while he is defending a shot on goal. He takes a few steps forward and then collapses. Emergency medical personnel rush onto the ice and find the patient without a pulse and with agonal respiration. They place an AED onto his chest, and the AED recommends a shock, which converts the patient from VF to NSR. The patient recovers and workup demonstrates a structurally normal heart by ECG, echocardiography, and stress test.

Questions:

1. Should he receive an ICD?
2. Can he return to play hockey?

Discussion:

1. This appears like a relatively standard commotio cordis incident. The type of impact, clinical scenario, and subsequent workup are classic for commotio cordis. Importantly, a normal ECG, echocardiogram, and stress test effectively rule out hypertrophic cardiomyopathy, arrhythmogenic right ventricular dysplasia, anomalous coronary arteries (although this one can be difficult to absolutely rule out), Brugada Syndrome, Long QT Syndrome, catecholiminergic polymorphic ventricular tachycardia, dilated cardiomyopathies, and myocarditis. Thus, in general, these individuals diagnosed with commotio cordis do not need an ICD.
2. I remain suspicious that individuals with commotio cordis are more susceptible to chest-wall-impact-induced VF. There are thousands of chest impacts daily, yet commotio cordis is uncommon. Thus, I would not favor return to any sport in which chest impact is common (i.e., not only hockey but also baseball, softball, lacrosse, and football). An implanted ICD would not change my opinion, and according to the Bethesda Guidelines, athletes with ICDs should not return to competitive sports [13].

Conclusion

Commotio cordis is the second leading cause of cardiac death in youth sports. An athlete losing consciousness after being hit in the chest should be assumed to be in ventricular fibrillation, and CPR should be immediately begun, along with calls for an AED. Use of age-appropriate safety baseballs should be encouraged and more robust chest protectors should be tested and utilized.

References

1. Maron BJ, Gohman TE, Kyle SB, Estes NA, 3rd, Link MS: Clinical profile and spectrum of commotio cordis. JAMA 2002; 287:1142–1146.
2. Madias C, Maron BJ, Weinstock J, Estes NA, 3rd, Link MS: Commotio cordis – sudden cardiac death with chest wall impact. J Cardiovasc Electrophysiol 2007; 18:115–122.
3. Maron BJ, Poliac LC, Kaplan JA, Mueller FO: Blunt impact to the chest leading to sudden death from cardiac arrest during sports activities. N Engl J Med 1995; 333:337–342.
4. Link MS, Wang PJ, Pandian NG, Bharati S, Udelson JE, Lee MY, Vecchiotti MA, VanderBrink BA, Mirra G, Maron BJ, Estes NA, 3rd: An experimental model of sudden death due to low-energy chest-wall impact (commotio cordis). N Engl J Med 1998; 338:1805–1811.
5. Maron BJ: Sudden death in young athletes. N Engl J Med 2003; 349:1064–1075.
6. Doerer JJ, Haas TS, Estes NA, 3rd, Link MS, Maron BJ: Evaluation of chest barriers for protection against sudden death due to commotio cordis. Am J Cardiol 2007; 99:857–859.
7. Maron BJ, Wentzel DC, Zenovich AG, Estes NA, 3rd, Link MS: Death in a young athlete due to commotio cordis despite prompt external defibrillation. Heart Rhythm 2005; 2:991–993.
8. Link MS, Maron BJ, VanderBrink BA, Takeuchi M, Pandian NG, Wang PJ, Estes NA, 3rd: Impact directly over the cardiac silhouette is necessary to produce ventricular fibrillation in an experimental model of commotio cordis. J Am Coll Cardiol 2001; 37:649–654.

9. Link MS, Maron BJ, Wang PJ, VanderBrink BA, Zhu W, Estes NA, 3rd: Upper and lower limits of vulnerability to sudden arrhythmic death with chest-wall impact (commotio cordis). J Am Coll Cardiol 2003; 41:99–104.
10. Link MS, Maron BJ, Wang PJ, Pandian NG, VanderBrink BA, Estes NA, 3rd: Reduced risk of sudden death from chest wall blows (commotio cordis) with safety baseballs. Pediatrics 2002; 109:873–877.
11. Weinstock J, Maron BJ, Song C, Mane PP, Estes NA, 3rd, Link MS: Failure of commercially available chest wall protectors to prevent sudden cardiac death induced by chest wall blows in an experimental model of commotio cordis. Pediatrics 2006; 117:e656–e662.
12. Adler P, Monticone RCJ: Injuries and deaths related to baseball. In Kyle SB, ed: Youth Baseball Protective Equipment Project Final Report. Washington, DC: United States Consumer Product Safety Commission, 1996, pp. 1–43.
13. Zipes DP, Ackerman MJ, Estes III NAM, Grant AO, Myerburg RJ, Van Hare G: Task Force 7: Arrhythmias. 36th Bethesda Conference: Eligibility recommendations for competitive athletes with cardiovascular abnormalities. J Am Coll Cardiol 2005; 45:43–52.

Chapter 15
Coronary Artery Anomalies and Sports Activities

Paolo Angelini

Your vision will become clear only when you can look into your heart.
Who looks outside, dreams; who looks inside, awakes.
(Carl Jung)

Introduction: Three Stories

Case 1: Sudden Cardiac Death in a Top High-School Athlete

A 19-year-old African-American male basketball player had trained and competed intensively for at least 5 years without having cardiovascular signs or symptoms. He excelled at this sport and was the star of his high-school basketball team. He had passed multiple annual preparticipation examinations without showing any evidence of disease. At the end of the first half of a citywide championship game, he was the top-scoring player. After completing a successful offensive play, he switched to a defensive position and became suddenly confused. A few seconds later, he fell onto his back, hit his head, and became unconscious. He remained motionless on the floor while the coaching staff attended to him. When emergency medical personnel arrived, 10 min later, the electrocardiographic monitor showed a straight line. Resuscitation efforts were initiated and continued until hospital admission. Despite intravenous infusion of epinephrine, repeated external defibrillation, and hour-long cardiopulmonary resuscitation, the patient never regained a spontaneous, stable pulse. At autopsy, he was found to have a structurally normal, moderately hypertrophied heart, with anomalous origin of the right coronary artery (RCA), which arose from the left sinus of Valsalva, just a few millimeters to the left of the anterior aortic commissure (Fig. 15.1a, b). The dominant RCA penetrated into the aortic wall and pursued a tangential proximal course, remaining within the

P. Angelini (✉)
Texas Heart Institute at St. Luke's Episcopal Hospital, Houston, TX, USA

C.E. Lawless (ed.), *Sports Cardiology Essentials: Evaluation, Management and Case Studies*, DOI 10.1007/978-0-387-92775-6_15,

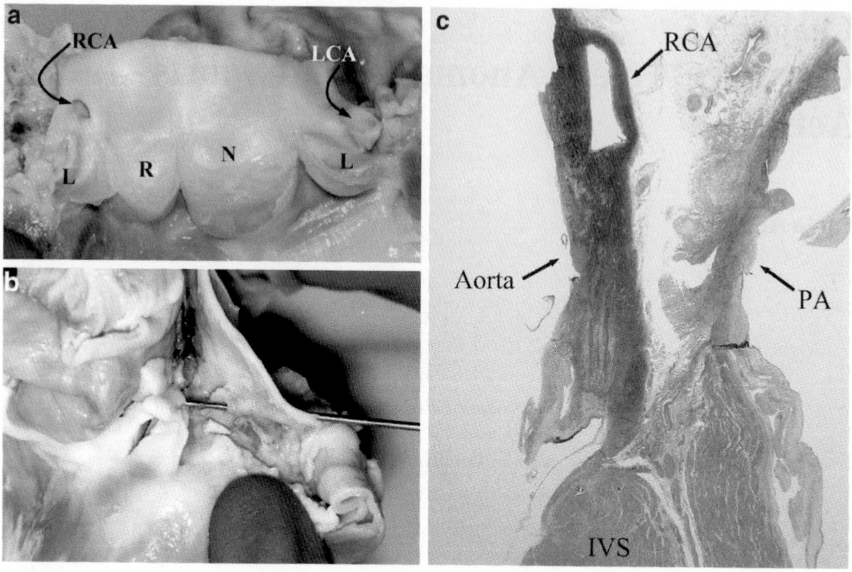

Fig. 15.1 Autopsy results, Case 1: (**a**) Internal view of the aortic root, showing the anomalous location of the orifice of the right coronary artery (RCA), which is positioned to the left of the anterior commissure of the aortic valve at the left sinus of Valsalva (L), next to the normally located left ostium (LCA). Notice the tangential origin of the ectopic RCA, which has a slit-like appearance. *N* noncoronary sinus; *R* right sinus. (**b**) External view of the aortic root, showing the intramural course of a probe, which is introduced into the ostium and is brought out through the transected extramural coronary artery, at its exit from the aortic wall. (**c**) Histologic cross-section of the aortic and pulmonary (PA) trunks, showing the intramural course of the RCA. The RCA shows the same lateral compression as seen on intravascular ultrasonography (see Fig. 15.6) and lacks a proper media and adventitia (the RCA intima is free of atherosclerotic buildup and is surrounded by the aortic media). *IVS* interventricular septum (courtesy of Dwayne A. Wolf, PhD, Office of the Medical Examiner of Harris County, Texas). Part (**c**) is reprinted from Angelini et al. [57] with permission

aortic wall for 5 mm. Figure 15.1c shows a cross-section of the intramural segment. Detailed examination revealed no histologic changes characteristic of focal necrosis. Figure 15.2 provides a further description of this anomaly by means of radiologic methods.

Case 2: Sudden Crib Death in an Infant

Thirty minutes after being seen by his grandparents in his normal healthy state, a 2-month-old boy was found motionless in his crib. He could not be resuscitated by the emergency medical team, which arrived 15 min later. An autopsy showed only an abnormal coronary pattern, characterized by anomalous origination of the RCA from the left sinus of Valsalva with an intramural proximal course (Fig. 15.3). Histologic examination revealed no signs of a myocardial infarction.

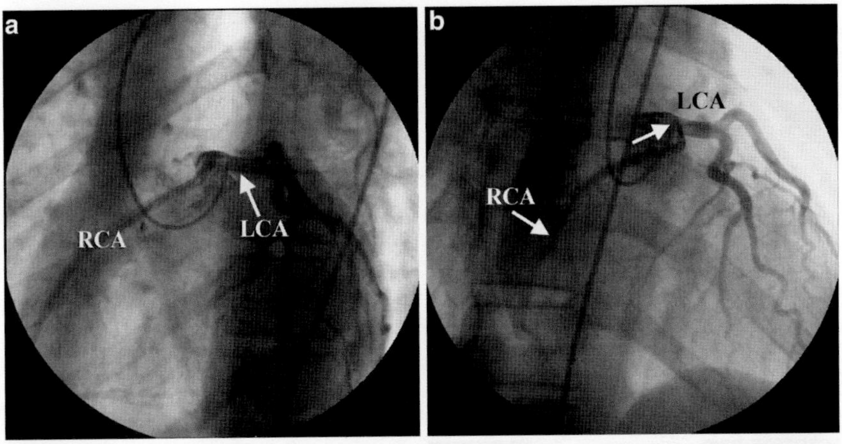

Fig. 15.2 Angiographic appearance of an anomalous right coronary artery arising from the opposite sinus, in the left anterior oblique (**a**) and right anterior cranial oblique (**b**) projections. In this case (which differs from the ACAOS case seen in Fig. 15.1), the right coronary artery (RCA, with an *arrow* at its ostium) arises ectopically, next to the left coronary artery (LCA), and both arteries are visualized simultaneously. In (**b**), the RCA clearly has an ostial narrowing, unlike in view (**a**). See Fig. 15.6 for the intravascular ultrasonographic appearance of the same RCA

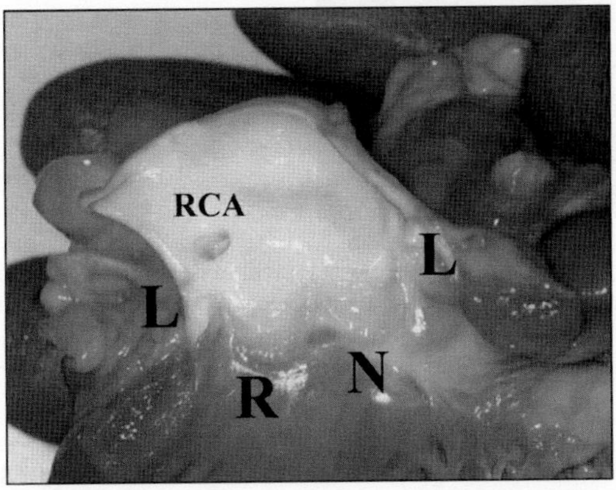

Fig. 15.3 Autopsy results, Case 2: View from the internal aortic root, showing high origination of the right coronary artery (RCA), above the left sinus of Valsalva, with a slit-like ostium, in a case of sudden crib death involving a newborn boy. Abbreviations as in Fig. 15.1 (courtesy of Dwayne A. Wolf, PhD, Office of the Medical Examiner of Harris County, Texas)

Case 3: A Surprising Accidental Finding in an 83-Year-Old Woman

An 83-year-old asymptomatic, physically active woman underwent heart catheterization because a routine nuclear pharmacologic stress test had shown probable reversible ischemia of the inferior wall. On coronary angiography, the left coronary

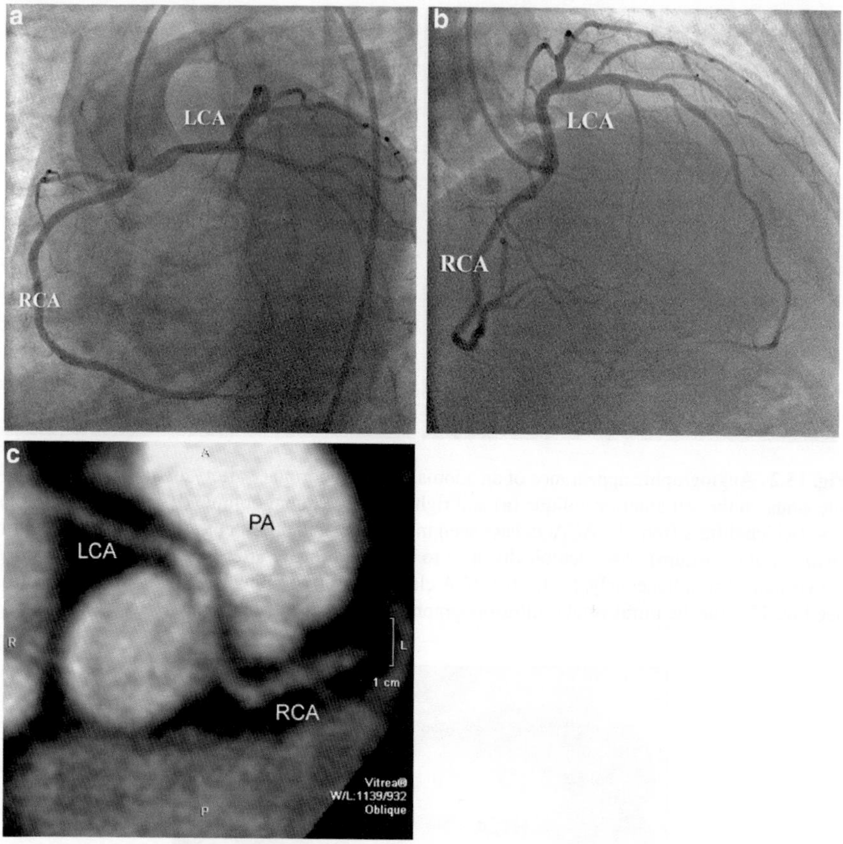

Fig. 15.4 (**a**, **b**) Angiographic appearance of a typical case of anomalous origin of the left coronary artery from the right sinus of Valsalva, with an intramural course (between the aorta and pulmonary artery), in the left anterior oblique (**a**) and the right anterior oblique (**b**) projections. (**c**) Computed tomographic angiogram of the same case. *LCA* left coronary artery; *RCA* right coronary artery

artery (LCA) was found to originate from the RCA at the right sinus of Valsalva. The LCA had an intramural course, which crossed from right to left between the aorta and pulmonary artery, as confirmed by magnetic resonance imaging (MRI). No atherosclerotic stenosis was observed. The patient refused to undergo further testing. Figure 15.4 shows a typical angiographic image of this anomaly.

Comment

These three case histories illustrate the spectrum of clinical manifestations that may be seen in patients with coronary artery anomalies (CAAs). In the first case, an ectopic RCA was associated with sudden cardiac death (SCD) in a star athlete who had previously been asymptomatic. In the second case, an apparently healthy infant died suddenly and unexpectedly in his crib. In the third case, an asymptomatic elderly woman was incidentally found to have the anomaly generally considered to be the most lethal CAA (LCA originating from the right sinus of Valsalva with an intramural course). The patient had had a long, cardiologically uneventful life until the diagnosis was accidentally made, as a consequence of what was probably a false-positive nuclear stress test.

This chapter focuses on current anatomic, physiologic, and clinical concepts regarding CAAs in the context of sports activities. The author discusses some newly defined principles and urges a structured approach to this confusing area of cardiology and sports medicine.

Coronary Artery Anomalies: A Brief Appraisal of a Complex Entity

For some 40 years, the medical literature has reported a worrisome association between competitive sports activities and CAA-related SCD [1–7]. Cheitlin et al. [7] initially raised this issue in 1974 when they reported a limited series. Since then, the belief has become widely pervasive in the medical community, as well as in the public at large, that any kind of CAA entails an increased risk of SCD, especially during sports activities. This belief was underscored by the guidelines published in 1994 by the 26th Bethesda Conference for determining eligibility for competition in athletes with cardiovascular abnormalities [8]. The authors alluded to "coronary anomalies" as a generic label and stated that 19% of deaths in athletes were due to CAAs (not including 5% due to muscular bridging, which is also a CAA but was listed separately in that document). Recent, more advanced studies have clarified that only a few types of CAAs, by means of specific, plausible, and possibly quantifiable mechanisms, have a high risk of severity in individual cases; these few CAAs can indeed cause transient ischemic symptoms and – only rarely – SCD [9–11], typically in the context of extreme exertion [12, 13] (Capsule 15.1).

> **Capsule 15.1** There are many kinds of coronary anomalies, and each kind is variable in severity. The current challenge is to differentiate the severe anomalies from the clinically insignificant ones

Today, CAAs are increasingly being recognized by clinical screening techniques such as standard coronary angiography or computed tomographic angiography (CTA). Although our understanding of these anomalies continues to evolve, our current knowledge is far from satisfactory or comprehensive, mainly because the medical community has not yet fully understood the involved pathophysiologic mechanisms or established definite severity criteria for identifying individual risk.

Table 15.1 and Fig. 15.5 present most of the known CAAs. Several recent comprehensive reviews [14, 15] give a more complete description of these anomalies, which may be considered to involve a congenital defect in coronary origination,

Table 15.1 Classification of coronary anomalies in human hearts[a]

1. Anomalies of origination and course
   - (a) Absent left main trunk (split origination of LCA)
   - (b) Anomalous location of coronary ostium within aortic root or near proper aortic sinus of Valsalva (for each artery):
     - High
     - Low
     - Commissural
   - (c) Anomalous location of coronary ostium outside normal "coronary" aortic sinuses
     - Right posterior aortic sinus
     - Ascending aorta
     - Left ventricle
     - Right ventricle
     - Pulmonary artery. Variants:
       - LCA arising from posterior facing sinus
       - Cx arising from posterior facing sinus
       - LAD arising from posterior facing sinus
       - RCA arising from anterior right facing sinus
       - Ectopic location (outside facing sinuses) of any coronary artery from pulmonary artery
         - * From anterior left sinus
         - * From pulmonary trunk
         - * From pulmonary branch
     - Aortic arch
     - Innominate artery
     - Right carotid artery
     - Internal mammary artery
     - Bronchial artery
     - Subclavian artery
     - Descending thoracic aorta
   - (d) Anomalous location of coronary ostium at improper sinus (which may involve joint origination or "single" coronary pattern). Variants:
     - RCA arising from left anterior sinus, with anomalous course:
       - Posterior atrioventricular groove or retrocardiac
       - Retroaortic
       - Between aorta and pulmonary artery (intramural)
       - Intraseptal
       - Anterior to pulmonary outflow
       - Posteroanterior interventricular groove (wraparound)
     - LAD arising from right anterior sinus, with anomalous course:
       - Between aorta and pulmonary artery (intramural)
       - Intraseptal
       - Anterior to pulmonary outflow
       - Posteroanterior interventricular groove (wraparound)
     - Cx arising from right anterior sinus, with anomalous course:
       - Posterior atrioventricular groove
       - Retroaortic

(continued)

Table 15.1 (continued)

- LCA arising from right anterior sinus, with anomalous course:
  - Posterior atrioventricular groove
  - Retroaortic
  - Between aorta and pulmonary artery
  - Intraseptal
  - Anterior to pulmonary outflow
  - Posteroanterior interventricular groove

(e) Single coronary artery (see point d)

2. Anomalies of intrinsic coronary arterial anatomy
   (a) Congenital ostial stenosis or atresia (LCA, LAD, RCA, Cx)
   (b) Coronary ostial dimple
   (c) Coronary ectasia or aneurysm
   (d) Absent coronary artery
   (e) Coronary hypoplasia
   (f) Intramural coronary artery (muscular bridge)
   (g) Subendocardial coronary course
   (h) Coronary crossing
   (i) Anomalous origination of posterior descending artery from the anterior descending branch or a septal penetrating branch
   (j) Split RCA. Variants:
   - Proximal + distal PDs, both arising from RCA
   - Proximal PD arising from RCA, distal PD arising from LAD
   - Parallel PDs ×2 (arising from RCA, Cx) or "codominant"

   (k) Split LAD. Variants:
   - LAD + first large septal branch
   - LAD, double (parallel LADs)

   (l) Ectopic origination of first septal branch. Variants:
   - RCA
   - Right sinus
   - Diagonal
   - Ramus
   - Cx
3. Anomalies of coronary termination
   (a) Inadequate arteriolar/capillary ramifications?
   (b) Fistulas from RCA, LCA, or infundibular artery to:
   - Right ventricle
   - Right atrium
   - Coronary sinus
   - Superior vena cava
   - Pulmonary artery
   - Pulmonary vein
   - Left atrium
   - Left ventricle
   - Multiple, right + left ventricles
4. Anomalous anastomotic vessels

Cx circumflex; *LAD* left anterior descending coronary artery; *LCA* left coronary artery; *PD* posterior descending branch; *RCA* right coronary artery

[a] Modified from Angelini et al. [15]. Copyright 1999, Lippincott Williams & Wilkins

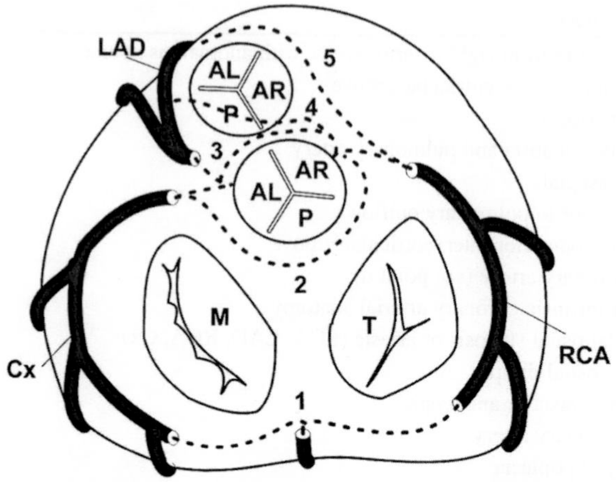

Fig. 15.5 Diagrammatic summary of all possible cases of anomalous origin of the coronary arteries from the aortic root (coronal view). The five alternative courses by which an ectopic coronary artery can cross to the normal dependent myocardial area are represented by *dotted lines*: (1) prepulmonic; (2) intraseptal; (3) intramural, aortic (or "between the aorta and pulmonary artery"); (4) retroaortic; (5) retrocardiac. *AL* anterolateral cusp; *AR* anterior-right cusp; *Cx* circumflex artery; *LAD* left anterior descending artery; *M* mitral valve; *P* posterior cusp; *RCA* right coronary artery; *T* tricuspid valve Reprinted from Angelini et al. [15] with permission

course, and/or termination (Capsule 15.2). All CAAs are due to a defect in embryologic development that occurs during the first trimester of human gestation. The ultimate cause of such defects can occasionally be traced to a genetic disorder; most CAAs are due to biologic variations in a complex process that is influenced by multiple, redundant, morphogenetic factors [16].

Capsule 15.2 Coronary artery anomalies include a wide spectrum of variants that are related to abnormalities in coronary origin, course, or termination. Each kind of anomaly has a different potential mechanism for restricting coronary flow

Table 15.2 lists various postulated or proven pathophysiologic mechanisms capable of impairing the function (i.e., supplying blood flow to the dependent myocardium) of an abnormally shaped coronary artery [15]. The only anomaly that has an intrinsic consistent pathophysiologic mechanism capable of causing ischemia is number 3, in Fig. 15.5 (see also Figs. 15.4, 15.6, and 15.7), which features anomalous origin and crossing of the ectopic vessel in a preaortic course ("between the aorta and pulmonary artery"). This anomaly is a case of "anomalous origin of a coronary artery from the opposite sinus of Valsalva" with an intramural course in the aortic wall (ACAOS). Recent experience, as reflected in the medical literature, has shown that ACAOS is the culprit in most cases of SCD in athletes and other persons who undergo extreme exertion (Capsule 15.3) [9, 10, 12–15, 17–19]. As shown in Figs. 15.1–15.4, the peculiar, insidious, and only recently recognized mechanism of ischemia in ACAOS is related to the abnormal vessel's ectopic proximal course inside the aortic wall.

Table 15.2 Pathophysiologic mechanisms and coronary anomalies (functional classification)[a]

		Proof of action		
Pathophysiologic mechanism	Coronary anomaly	Certain	Possible	Unlikely
Misdiagnosis	"Missing" coronary artery	+		
	"Hypoplastic" coronary artery		+	
Myocardial ischemia, primary (fixed and/or episodic)	Ostial atresia	+		
	Ostial stenosis	+		
	Coronary fistula		+	
	ALCAPA	+		
	Muscular bridge			+
Myocardial ischemia, secondary (episodic)	Tangential origin (ACAOS) intramural course	+		
	Myocardial bridge, plus spasm and/or clot	+		
	Coronary ectasia (plus mural clot)	+		
	Coronary fistula (plus mural clot)	+		
Increased risk of fixed coronary atherosclerotic disease	Coronary fistula	+		
	ALCAPA	+		
	Coronary ectasia	+		
	Muscular bridge (proximal to)	+		
Secondary aortic valve disease	Coronary aneurysm (ostial)		+	
	Coronary fistula		+	
	ALCAPA		+	
Increased risk of bacterial endocarditis	Coronary fistula		+	
Ischemic cardiomyopathy (hibernation)	ALCAPA	+		
Volume overload	Coronary fistula	+		
	ALCAPA	+		
Unusual technical difficulties during coronary angiography or angioplasty	Ectopic ostia (tangential)	+		
	Split left coronary artery		+	
	Coronary fistula		+	
Complications during cardiac surgery	Ectopic ostia and proximal course	+		
	Muscular bridge	+		

ACAOS anomalous coronary artery originating from the opposite sinus; *ALCAPA* anomalous origination of the left coronary artery from the pulmonary artery

[a]Modified from Angelini et al. [15]. Copyright 1999, Lippincott Williams & Wilkins

Capsule 15.3 Coronary anomalies have recently been linked to sudden cardiac death in athletes. Ectopic origination of a coronary artery with an intramural course (inside the aortic wall) is the main culprit in sudden death during maximal exertion. Symptoms of this anomaly may also include shortness of breath, chest pain, and dizziness/syncope

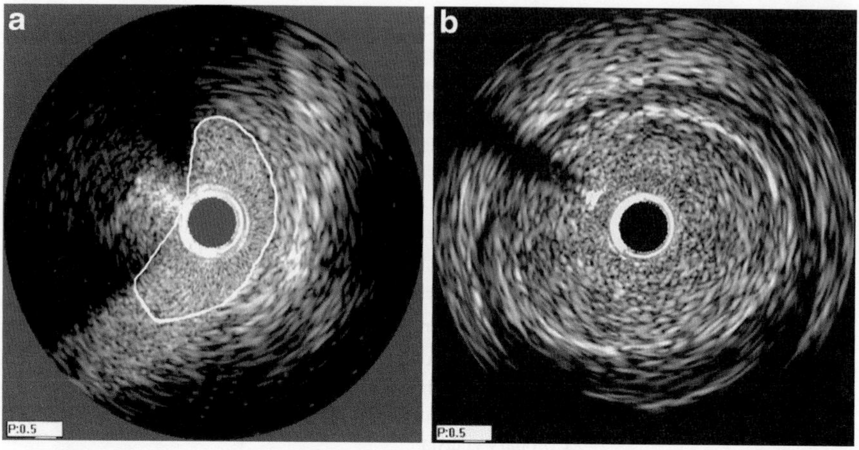

Fig. 15.6 Intravascular ultrasonographic images of the ostium (**a**) and distal artery (**b**), in cross-section in a case of anomalous right coronary artery arising from the opposite sinus. Only with this method can the investigator evaluate cross-sectional area stenosis: in this case of anomalous right coronary artery arising from the opposite sinus, the stenosis was 63% in diastole. Note the similarity of (**a**) to Fig. 15.1c, which shows the corresponding histologic features

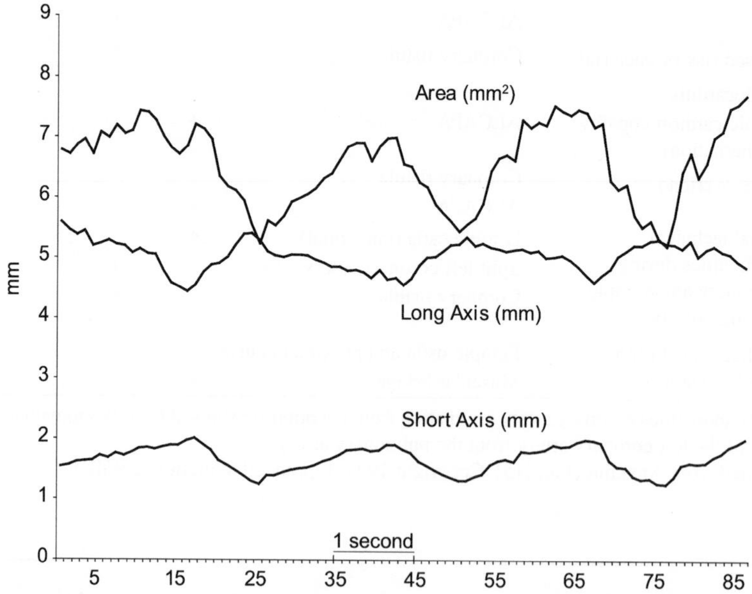

Fig. 15.7 Diagrammatic reconstruction of the systolic and diastolic dimensions of the cross-sectional area (30 frames/s), as seen on intravascular ultrasonography in a case of anomalous right coronary artery arising from the opposite sinus. Note the important phasic variations in these parameters: the cross-sectional area decreases by some 40% in systole (from 7.6 to 5.2 mm^2) (measurements courtesy of Jonathan Aliota, MD, Texas Heart Institute)

The basic mechanisms of stenosis in ACAOS (Figs. 15.6 and 15.7) are: (1) hypoplasia of the proximal lumen with respect to the distal vessel, (2) lateral compression of the intramural segment, which runs inside the aortic media, and (3) further compression of the same segment during systole (Fig. 15.7) and tachycardia [17].

At baseline, only occasional cases of ACAOS involve critical stenosis (Fig. 15.4), but severe stenosis can develop during extreme exertion or a hypertensive crisis, resulting in an increased stroke volume, systolic pressure, and/or "systolic time/minute" (as in severe tachycardia) [17]. Unfortunately, the methods typically used to establish the severity of coronary stenosis – even stress nuclear scintigraphy or measurement of the pressure decrease at the coronary ectopic origin [19] – usually fail to provide objective evidence of significant ischemia.

A major limitation of the literature (especially the early literature) concerning the clinical implications of CAAs is related to the fact that necropsy case series were initially the basis for generalized statements about these disorders and that the "denominator" of the reported cases (involving the same anomalies) was not available or taken into account [10, 15]. Additionally, in cases of otherwise unexplained death, the "mere presence" of a CAA was automatically assumed to be the "cause" of death. More recently, clinicians have realized that most CAAs are quite benign and compatible with a normal, and even an active lifestyle [10, 15, 18].

The recent pursuit of large population-based studies has enabled researchers to evaluate the real risk of SCD in the context of a definite exercise program. Thus far, the most significant study has been one by Eckart et al. [19], who studied 6.35 million US Army recruits over 25 years. The recruits underwent an initial 2-month period of boot-camp training, which included running long distances and lifting or carrying heavy weights. These activities entailed some degree of dehydration in addition to maximal physical exertion. Two hundred sixty-three recruits died of nontraumatic causes. At necropsy, a third of these deaths were found to be related to the presence of a CAA – specifically ACAOS of the LCA (L-ACAOS) in all cases. No other type of CAAs was responsible for the lethal events. Nevertheless, one cannot conclude that all other CAAs may be considered benign because they cannot cause exercise-related death. Coronary anomalies have been claimed to be the cause of some 20% of death in athletes [1–7] (Capsule 15.4). Other studies (unfortunately without a denominator) have shown that ACAOS of the RCA (R-ACAOS) and anomalous origination of the LCA from the pulmonary artery are additional culprits [2, 5, 12, 13, 20]. Most studies, though, do not describe the population at risk, in terms of either the total population from which the target patients were derived [20] or the expected incidence of CAAs, especially ACAOS.

Capsule 15.4 The mortality due to coronary anomalies has been clearly related to maximal exertion in athletes and military recruits. One third of "medical deaths" in military recruits and one quarter of such deaths in athletes are due to coronary artery anomalies

In addition to SCD, other symptoms may be seen during exertion or even at rest in patients with some CAAs (see section "Screening, Diagnosis, and Counseling," below). The clinically important concept that has resulted from recent CAA series is not only that each type of CAA has fundamentally different clinical implications but also that each individual patient with a given type of CAA may have a different severity of the disorder, depending on the mechanism responsible for ischemic events [17]. As a consequence, the popular concept that CAAs generically pose a high risk of ischemic consequences during exertion should, in fact, be qualified by asking the questions "what type of anomalies?" and "what level of severity?" Unfortunately, the subclassification of each anomaly, and especially of the markers of severity in individual cases, is still subject to guesswork and speculation [9, 17–19, 21, 22].

With regard to athletics, it is largely unknown whether the most serious forms of CAAs cause physical limitations and, if so, whether they automatically imply preclusion from involvement in competitive sports. Both of these possibilities are likely and warrant investigation.

Sports Activities and Coronary Anomalies

Sports activities are intrinsically competitive, involving a need for maximal physical performance. During training and especially during the competition itself, athletes exceed their usual level of physical activity, going well beyond that reached during submaximal clinical stress testing. The following three facts are well established: (1) Of persons who have a "potentially lethal" CAA variant, nonathletes have a much lower probability of SCD than do athletes with the same condition [3, 13, 18, 23]; (2) most CAA-related deaths occur during or immediately after exertion [2, 3, 4, 7, 12, 13, 16, 23–25]; and (3) older patients with ACAOS do not have a clearly increased incidence of either SCD or myocardial infarction [2, 10, 12, 18].

What sports-related factors increase the likelihood that a CAA will have catastrophic consequences? In general, with any CAA that has an intrinsic ischemic potential, the chance of clinical manifestations may be expected to increase when the myocardial oxygen demand is maximal and the oxygen supply limited. Additionally, peak exercise conditions (characterized by a cardiac output and workload up to five times baseline levels), emotion-related catecholamine surges, and dehydration can extend the intrinsic ischemic burden and risk of complications beyond tolerable limits. In this setting, ACAOS-related functional changes that occur during or early after peak exertion, or both, may be related to the unique mechanism of (unexpected) ischemia.

The basic pathophysiologic mechanism in ACAOS seems to be related to lateral compression of the intramural aortic segment: the ectopic artery originates tangentially, and the initial segment is embedded in the aortic media (see Figs. 15.1–15.5). At baseline, intravascular ultrasonography (IVUS) shows a variable amount of cross-sectional narrowing that may be compatible with a lack of symptoms during physical training. However, maximal physical exertion may cause critical worsening of the stenosis because of (1) an increased cardiac output and, more especially, an increased stroke volume (leading to increased pulsatility and systolic expansion of the aortic root), (2) increased systolic compression of the intramural ectopic artery (Figs. 15.6 and 15.7), and (3) extreme tachycardia (frequently >200 beats/min), which increases the systolic time with respect to the diastolic time to an exceptional degree. Interestingly, in the above-mentioned military recruits, 86% of the SCDs occurred during or soon after exercise [24] (Capsule 15.5).

Capsule 15.5 Maximal exertion may induce critical ischemia, even in cases with only mild coronary dysfunction at baseline, due to worsening of stenosis, and/or increased oxygen demand, and/or catecholamine discharge

Other, more frequent coronary anatomic variants such as myocardial bridges or small coronary fistulas are occasionally reported to cause symptoms or even SCD during exertion [2, 3, 23, 25]. Speculation about the cause/effect of these events is ongoing. Even in the military recruits [19], for example, about 25% of the SCDs were unexplained by necropsy findings; any such case involving a minor CAA could give rise to an unjustified association between that anomaly and SCD.

It is not clear whether any particular sports activity is specifically associated with an increased risk of SCD in individuals who have a given type of CAA. It has long been suspected that the aorta may be unusually elastic or distensible in persons with Marfanoid phenotypes, especially tall basketball players [17]. In the presence of an intramural ectopic coronary artery, such an association might have specific repercussions (possibly resulting in increased systolic compression). Heavy weight lifting, which is transiently associated with an extremely high intrathoracic pressure, may be associated with similar levels of aortic root dilatation during exertion. In itself, regular training can lead, over time, to dilatation of both the left ventricle and the aortic root [26].

In addition to SCD, the clinical manifestations of myocardial ischemia normally seen in ischemic heart disease have also been observed in ACAOS and should be detectable during preparticipation screening: unusual dyspnea on exertion, with or without chest pain or pressure, and/or dizziness or syncope [27]. These symptoms should be properly evaluated because they are frequently the only ones an athlete reports before succumbing to SCD in the context of ACAOS. Recently, the popularization of CTA screening for coronary artery disease in adults has resulted in the fortuitous detection of a growing number of CAAs, causing anxiety and uncertainty for both patients and physicians [28].

The few reports of ACAOS-related SCD that have included clinical details [29, 30] suggest that in athletes with CAAs, SCD has the following specific functional and electrocardiographic features: (1) initially, hypotension and bradycardia, (2) later, asystole (primary ventricular fibrillation is probably unusual under such conditions) (Capsule 15.6), and (3) finally, reperfusion-related rapid ventricular arrhythmias (ventricular fibrillation), usually after resuscitative treatment [10, 31]. These features are relevant to the planning of effective resuscitative efforts (see section "Prevention and Treatment of Sudden Cardiac Death in Athletes," below).

Capsule 15.6 In coronary anomalies, asystole seems to be a more common initial mechanism of syncope with respect to ventricular tachycardia/fibrillation

Screening, Diagnosis, and Counseling

Whereas ACAOS is relatively rare in the general population, it must be similarly rare [5] or even more so in trained athletes, because of a spontaneous selection bias due to symptoms or physical limitations. Maron et al. [6, 32] estimated that the incidence of SCD risk factors is about 1/10,000 in marathon runners older than age 45 years (mostly because of atherosclerotic coronary artery disease) but is only 1/200,000 in runners below that age. Crawford and coauthors [33] indicated that the incidence of SCD is 1–2/100,000 per year in high-school athletes, 1/50,000 in marathon runners, and 1/15,000 in recreational joggers of any age. If the health-care system could (or would) support generalized screening by means of echocardiography, coronary magnetic resonance angiography (MRA), or CTA [28, 34–37] (Figs. 15.4 and 15.8), at least in athletes, it should be technically easy to reliably diagnose serious CAAs (essentially, ACAOS). The cost-effectiveness of such a policy can be grossly based on the fact that probably close to 1% of the general population has ACAOS [14]. If young athletes in the United States number 5 million per year [6, 38], about 50,000 of these athletes would be expected to have a CAA. Moreover, because experience in the catheterization laboratory [15] has shown that 0.1% of the general population has L-ACAOS, 5,000 young athletes would be at the

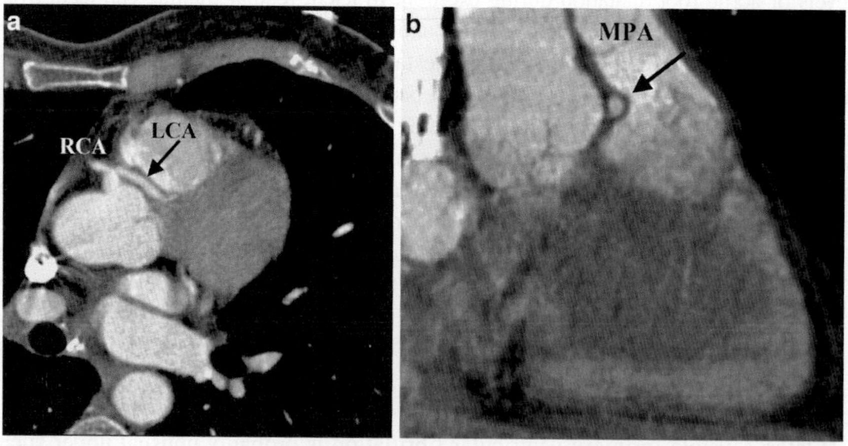

Fig. 15.8 Computed tomographic images of an anomalous intraseptal left coronary artery arising from the right sinus of Valsalva. The proximal left coronary artery (LCA) is directed inferiorly, below the aortic root (view **a**), passing into the crista supraventricularis (view **b**, *black arrow*) and finally into the ventricular septum. For comparison, see Fig. 15.4c, which involves an intramural aortic course. The prognosis is quite different in these two cases, as discussed in the text. *MPA* main pulmonary artery; *RCA* right coronary artery

highest risk in any given year. About 0.9% of the general US population is estimated to have the other significant variant, R-ACAOS, accounting for 45,000 cases.

As discussed above, the mortality rate during maximum physical exertion has been only approximately established. The best available evidence for L-ACAOS has been provided by the US Army Recruits study [24] and by a database established in Veneto, Italy [23, 39]. Specifically, of the 6,350,000 recruits, about 6,300 would have been expected to have L-ACAOS, of whom, 36 (4/1,000) died during the 2-month exposure to an unusually high level of physical exertion; therefore, we may conclude that SCD affects about 1.4/100,000 recruits during the 2-month exposure period, or 8.4/100,000 recruits per year. In the same population, there were 263 "nontraumatic deaths," for a mortality of 25/100,000 over the 2-month period [24]. In comparison, in the state of Minnesota, the general risk of SCD in high-school athletes was reported to be about 0.5/100,000 per year, while the CAA-related risk was 20% of the total or 0.1/100,000 athletes [38]. In a similar study performed in Washington state, the estimated annual incidence of cardiac arrest was 1.8/100,000 [40]. Evidently, the risk of CAA-related SCD in army recruits would be about 16.8 times higher (or more frequently diagnosed) than in athletes of an equivalent age. In professional athletes, the reported incidence of SCD is 1/3,500 (or 30/100,000) per year [41].

If policy guidelines were instituted regarding CAAs, screening would initially apply only to athletes. Sedentary persons with ACAOS have a lower probability of SCD (although their risk – and that associated with less aggressive sports activities – has not been evaluated in reasonable detail). This selection policy would greatly improve the cost-efficiency of screening. In athletes and possibly military recruits, one could further restrict the use of expensive and possibly risky (in the context of a large population study) screening, by subselecting candidates who have clinical symptoms such as unusual shortness of breath, dizziness, syncope, or chest pain. Unfortunately, however, when retrospectively studied, only about 20% of SCD victims who had ACAOS with an intramural course were found to have reported suspicious symptoms that could have warranted such screening (Capsule 15.7).

Capsule 15.7 Only about 20% of the victims of sudden cardiac death due to coronary anomalies have reported effort-related chest pain, syncope, or other prodromal symptoms that would had indicated the need for further testing. None of these coronary anomalies were diagnosed before the reported lethal event. Otherwise, the involved athletes would have been routinely discouraged from continuing their sports activities

In general, athletes are highly motivated, aggressive individuals who tend to underappreciate or underreport symptoms. To be useful, a history-taking session would need to be highly structured and informative [6, 8, 22, 33, 39]. Therefore, athletes and their coaches should be made generally aware of the current thinking about CAAs and other causes of SCD during sports activities and should necessarily be included in relevant discussions.

Electrocardiography, both at rest and during treadmill exercise, is a relatively inexpensive screening method that is frequently used to identify cardiomyopathies and coronary artery disease. Unfortunately, however, electrocardiography is not a sensitive method for identifying ACAOS [12, 16, 27, 38, 42–44]. Similarly, in this setting, nuclear stress testing is of dubious utility, yielding an unacceptably high level of false-positive and false-negative data [10]. A dedicated, prospective echocardiographic study of ACAOS patients has not yet been carried out; however, preliminary testing [34] suggests that echocardiography can reliably diagnose L-ACAOS (without determining the specific course of the ectopic artery) in non-obese young individuals. Likely, the positive predictive value would be near 90% in L-ACAOS [34, 37] but 50–70% in R-ACAOS [27, 45].

Currently, we prefer to use cardiac MRA, CTA, or traditional coronary angiography to identify the presence of CAAs [27]. Although coronary angiography is almost 100% successful in expert hands, it has three main limitations:

1. The diagnosis of ACAOS implies that the ectopic proximal coronary artery courses inside the anterior wall of the aorta. Selective catheter cannulation for angiography may be difficult, because of the tangential proximal course of the ectopic artery. Additionally, a similar anatomic variant, ectopic LCA with an intraseptal course, is frequently mistaken for L-ACAOS (with an intramural aortic course) by nonexpert interpreters of CTA or MRA studies [27]. Unlike true L-ACAOS, this variant does not involve a clear mechanism of ischemia; its prognosis is generally benign, so no intervention is required, and no physical restrictions are indicated.
2. Mere recognition of ACAOS is inadequate to identify the specific risk incurred by a given patient, especially during sports activities. As discussed above, a fundamental issue involves determining the severity of the anomaly in each individual case, which basic screening methods do not allow.
3. The diagnosis of ACAOS (or some other CAA) may negatively affect an athlete's emotional outlook if he or she has to abandon sports activities. Therefore, referral to an expert center for disease subclassification and counseling is advised.

Criteria for increased risk in L-ACAOS patients are still being defined. Our group has suggested that high-risk criteria should include both specific symptoms (reproducible exercise-related chest pain, dyspnea, objective signs of ischemia, and especially syncope or a history of SCD) and also features that are quantifiable on IVUS examination (>50% baseline cross-sectional area stenosis, with further phasic systolic worsening of >10% during simulated exercise testing [17)]. Until validated recommendations are issued, as approved by a representative professional organization, many authors [6, 21, 22, 42] suggest that all L-ACAOS patients should be strongly discouraged from participating in maximal sports activities and should be referred to a specialized center. In contrast, R-ACAOS apparently has a more benign prognosis with respect to SCD [10, 12, 13, 18, 21, 22, 24], but this prognosis varies in individual patients, probably depending on the clinical history [27], coronary dominance pattern, and IVUS findings [17]. Multicenter investigations are underway to establish reliable guidelines based on general principles. At specialized centers dedicated to CAAs, current efforts are concentrated on establishing solid criteria by which to judge the severity of individual cases [17].

Prevention and Treatment of Sudden Cardiac Death in Athletes

On the sports field, SCD is a tragic experience, not only for the victim but also for the witnesses, while survival in that setting is much less likely than in a hospital environment. Society has come to recognize that it has a moral duty both to prevent such incidents and to facilitate rescue efforts when SCD occurs. Several specific considerations apply to the rescue of athletes affected by a CAA: (1) These individuals generally have a healthy heart, so expeditious resuscitation should result in a good chance of recovery (Capsule 15.8)

> **Capsule 15.8** Sudden cardiac death in athletes with coronary anomalies occurs in the absence of early anatomic changes in the coronary arteries (thrombosis) or myocardium (necrosis). Therefore, the chances of recovery are unusually favorable if specific and effective resuscitative efforts are quickly enacted

[46]. (2) Unlike older patients who have a coronary event caused by atherothrombotic disease, these patients are unlikely to have had an anatomic event that would necessitate recanalization. (3) In patients with L-ACAOS (and in the few with R-ACAOS), the mechanism of SCD probably depends on a specific, unique behavior that, though still unclear, seems initially to involve hypotension and bradycardia more than ventricular fibrillation. Likely, a critical hemodynamic overload and increased compression of the intramural, ectopic artery leads to a dramatic ("suicidal") negative spiral of events, whereby bradycardia leads to hypotension, and hypotension to bradycardia, as observed in patients with acquired >50% stenosis of the left main coronary artery [47, 48]. Whereas some of these episodes result in SCD, others abort, usually due to the cessation of exertion, resulting only in syncope and spontaneous recovery, as in L-ACAOS patients who have a sudden cardiac arrest followed by successful recovery. Early recovery from a sudden cardiac arrest in L-ACAOS patients is likely if early resuscitation is aggressively instituted, especially with rapid external cardiac massage (Capsule 15.9) [49–51].

> **Capsule 15.9** At the time of sudden cardiac death on the sports field, rescuers should perform early, rapid external cardiac massage while awaiting the arrival of an automated external defibrillator (which should ideally be available within 5 minutes after the onset of the event)

If resuscitation efforts are delayed or inadequate, SCD frequently results in secondary complications: (1) Ventricular tachycardia and fibrillation (as a likely manifestation of myocardial reperfusion arrhythmias, which may be potentiated by high levels of circulating catecholamines), (2) refractory, persistent hypotension or a low cardiac output that is poorly responsive to vasopressors, and (3) ischemic brain damage caused by head trauma, the initial syncopal fall, or the cardiac arrest itself. In such cases, resuscitation may necessitate more aggressive support than medical treatment alone. An easily implantable ventricular assist device, such as the TandemHeart (Cardiac Assist Inc., Pittsburgh, Pa.) or the Impella pump (Abiomed, Danvers, Mass.) [52, 53], may stabilize the patient's condition, allowing myocardial unloading and eventual recovery. In this context, the diagnosis of L-ACAOS is generally established by echocardiography in the emergency room and confirmed by traditional angiography, CTA, or MRA in the catheterization laboratory [16, 17].

After recovery from SCD, the causes of the event should be quickly ascertained insofar as possible because secondary prevention is mandatory and may be not only lifesaving but also quite cost-effective. Clearly, in the absence of effective correction, syncope or SCD resulting from L-ACAOS is likely to recur. Both echocardiography and CTA are urgently indicated for survivors of a sudden cardiac arrest. Counseling about interventions and/or discontinuation of sports activities should be pursued at specialized centers (Capsule 15.10). Most experts believe that such activities should be routinely curtailed unless the causative problem is effectively treated, for example, with surgical correction of L-ACAOS followed by a negative appropriate follow-up study [18, 21].

> **Capsule 15.10** Coronary anomalies should be evaluated at a specialized, dedicated center not only after the occurrence of major symptoms but also when anxiety/uncertainty necessitates objective, test-based counseling or credentialing (such as certification for participation in competitive sports)

In the absence of established, evidence-based guidelines concerning CAAs [6, 22, 27, 41, 54, 55], we can only make reasonable temporary and tentative recommendations while awaiting further experience and documentation, as well as official statements by representative professional societies. Aborted SCD in the presence of L-ACAOS constitutes an adequate basis for intervention (generally surgical); in the presence of R-ACAOS, however, aborted SCD or other symptoms (such as dyspnea, syncope, or chest pain on exertion) necessitate further diagnostic workup. At our center, IVUS imaging of the pertinent coronary anatomy is routinely used to evaluate the severity of R-ACAOS. Unfortunately, the recommendations for treating ACAOS that have been issued by official organizations include few details and little supporting evidence. In general, it is currently agreed that ACAOS patients who have severe symptoms (dyspnea, chest pain, or syncope during exertion) or objective proof of ischemia on stress testing should have a revascularization procedure: surgery for L-ACAOS [11, 21] as well as R-ACAOS [21, 56–58]. For symptomatic R-ACAOS, our institution and other centers have recently implemented an experimental, institutional-review-board-approved protocol that calls for stent-angioplasty of the intramural segment, if a significantly stenosed segment is identified [57], as an attractive alternative to surgical treatment [4]. Treatment of patients who have minor symptoms or who lack evidence of ischemia on stress testing is subject to an ongoing discussion [18]. In addition, the question of genetic studies in familial cases of CAAs remains unsettled [18, 48, 56].

Conclusions

Recently, ACAOS has been recognized as one of the most frequent causes of SCD in athletes. Because L-ACAOS is the dominant pathology in these cases, the current emphasis is on excluding the presence of this condition in competitive athletes. In specific individuals, the severity of a given form of L-ACAOS or of some cases of R-ACAOS needs to be ascertained, by means of IVUS. Because SCD on the sports field should be avoided "at all costs," we recommend that relevant new information regarding the causes of SCD in athletes be disseminated to coaches and other staff members, as well as to athletes themselves. Victims of SCD should undergo aggressive resuscitation on the playing field, followed by referral to a specialized center for further diagnosis and treatment. As widespread screening for CAAs is introduced in clinical and population-based studies and as mechanisms of ischemia in ACAOS are clarified, more effective means of preventing the catastrophic consequences of CAAs can be expected to become available.

Acknowledgments The author thanks Virginia Fairchild of the Texas Heart Institute's Department of Scientific Publications for editorial assistance in preparing this chapter. He also thanks Melissa Mayo and Isabel Vasquez of the Texas Heart Institute's Visual Communications Services for help in preparing the figures.

References

1. Maron BJ, Roberts WC, McAllister HA, Rosing DR, Epstein SE. Sudden death in young athletes. Circulation. 1980;62(2):218–229.
2. Frescura C, Basso C, Thiene G, et al. Anomalous origin of coronary arteries and risk of sudden death: a study based on an autopsy population of congenital heart disease. Hum Pathol. 1998;29:689–695.
3. Corrado D, Basso C, Rizzoli G, Schiavon M, Thiene G. Does sports activity enhance the risk of sudden death in adolescents and young adults? J Am Coll Cardiol. 2003;42:1959–1963.
4. Maron BJ. Sudden death in young athletes. N Engl J Med. 2003;349:1064–1075.
5. Mirchandani S, Phoon CK. Management of anomalous coronary arteries from the contralateral sinus. Int J Cardiol. 2005;102:383–389.
6. Maron BJ, Thompson PD, Ackerman MJ, et al; American Heart Association Council on Nutrition, Physical Activity, and Metabolism. Recommendations and considerations related to preparticipation screening for cardiovascular abnormalities in competitive athletes: 2007 update: a scientific statement from the American Heart Association Council on Nutrition,

Physical Activity, and Metabolism: endorsed by the American College of Cardiology Foundation. Circulation. 2007;115:1643–1655.

7. Cheitlin MD, De Castro CM, McAllister HA. Sudden death as a complication of anomalous left coronary origin from the anterior sinus of Valsalva, a not-so-minor congenital anomaly. Circulation. 1974;50:780–787.
8. Maron BJ, Thompson PD, Puffer JC, et al. Cardiovascular preparticipation screening of competitive athletes. A statement for health professionals from the Sudden Death Committee (clinical cardiology) and Congenital Cardiac Defects Committee (cardiovascular disease in the young), American Heart Association. Circulation. 1996;94:850–856.
9. Taylor AJ, Byers JP, Cheitlin MD, Virmani R. Anomalous right or left coronary artery from the contralateral coronary sinus: "high-risk" abnormalities in the initial coronary artery course and heterogeneous clinical outcomes. Am Heart J. 1997;133:428–423.
10. Angelini P, Velasco JA, Flamm S. Coronary anomalies: incidence, pathophysiology, and clinical relevance. Circulation. 2002;105:2449–2454.
11. Angelini P, Walmsley RP, Libreros A, Ott DA. Symptomatic anomalous origination of the left coronary artery from the opposite sinus of valsalva. Clinical presentations, diagnosis, and surgical repair. Tex Heart Inst J. 2006;33:171–179.
12. Taylor AJ, Rogan KM, Virmani R. Sudden cardiac death associated with isolated congenital coronary artery anomalies. J Am Coll Cardiol. 1992;20:640–647.
13. Basso C, Maron BJ, Corrado D, Thiene G. Clinical profile of congenital coronary artery anomalies with origin from the wrong aortic sinus leading to sudden death in young competitive athletes. J Am Coll Cardiol. 2000;35:1493–1501.
14. Angelini P. Normal and anomalous coronary arteries: definitions and classification. Am Heart J. 1989;117:418–434.
15. Angelini P, Villason S, Chan AV, Diez JG. Normal and anomalous coronary arteries in humans. In: Angelini P, ed. Coronary Artery Anomalies. Philadelphia, PA: Lippincott, Williams & Wilkins; 1999:27–150.
16. Roberts WC. Congenital coronary arterial anomalies unassociated with major anomalies of the heart and great vessels. In: Roberts WC, ed. Adult Congenital Heart Diseases. Philadelphia, PA: Davis Co; 1987:583–663.
17. Angelini P, Flamm SD. Newer concepts for imaging anomalous aortic origin of the coronary arteries in adults. Catheter Cardiovasc Interv. 2007;69:942–954.
18. Cheitlin MD. Finding asymptomatic people with a coronary artery arising from the wrong sinus of valsalva: consequences arising from knowing the anomaly to be familial. J Am Coll Cardiol. 2008;51:2065–2067.
19. Eckart RE, Scoville SL, Campbell CL, et al. Sudden death in young adults: a 25-year review of autopsies in military recruits. Ann Intern Med. 2004;141:829–834.
20. Tomanek RJ. Formation of coronary vasculature during development. Angiogenesis. 2005;8:273–284.
21. Gersony WM. Management of anomalous coronary artery from the contralateral sinus. J Am Coll Cardiol. 2007;50:2083–2084.
22. Corrado D, Pelliccia A, Bjørnstad HH, et al; Study Group of Sport Cardiology of the Working Group of Cardiac Rehabilitation and Exercise Physiology and the Working Group of Myocardial and Pericardial Diseases of the European Society of Cardiology. Cardiovascular pre-participation screening of young competitive athletes for prevention of sudden death: proposal for a common European protocol. Consensus Statement of the Study Group of Sport Cardiology of the Working Group of Cardiac Rehabilitation and Exercise Physiology and the Working Group of Myocardial and Pericardial Diseases of the European Society of Cardiology. Eur Heart J. 2005;26:516–524.
23. Basso C, Frescura C, Corrado D, et al. Congenital heart disease and sudden death in the young. Hum Pathol. 1995;26:1065–1072.
24. Dimopoulos K, Di Mario C, Barlis P, et al. Haemodynamic significance of an anomalous right coronary with inter-arterial course assessed with intracoronary pressure measurements during dobutamine challenge. Int J Cardiol. 2008;126:e32–e35.

25. Waller BF, Hawley DA, Clark MA, Pless JE. Incidence of sudden athletic deaths between 1985 and 1990 in Marion County, Indiana. Clin Cardiol. 1992;15:851–858.
26. Maron BJ, Pelliccia A. The heart of trained athletes: cardiac remodeling and the risks of sports, including sudden death. Circulation. 2006;114:1633–1644.
27. Glover DW, Glover DW, Maron BJ. Evolution in the process of screening United States high school student-athletes for cardiovascular disease. Am J Cardiol. 2007;100:1709–1712.
28. Budoff MJ, Ahmed V, Gul KM, Mao SS, Gopal A. Coronary anomalies by cardiac computed tomographic angiography. Clin Cardiol. 2006;29:489–493.
29. Taylor AJ, Farb A, Ferguson M, Virmani R. Myocardial infarction associated with physical exertion in a young man. Circulation. 1997;96:3201–3204.
30. Devanagondi R, Brenner J, Vricella L, Ravekes W. A tale of two brothers: anomalous coronary arteries in two siblings. Pediatr Cardiol. 2008;29:816–819.
31. Iskandar EG, Thompson PD. Exercise-related sudden death due to an unusual coronary artery anomaly. Med Sci Sports Exerc. 2004;36:180–182.
32. Maron BJ, Poliac LC, Roberts WO. Risk for sudden cardiac death associated with marathon running. J Am Coll Cardiol. 1996;28:428–431.
33. Crawford MH. Screening athletes for heart disease. Heart. 2007;93:875–879.
34. Pelliccia A, Spataro A, Maron BJ. Prospective echocardiographic screening for coronary artery anomalies in 1,360 elite competitive athletes. Am J Cardiol. 1993;72:978–979.
35. Pelliccia A. Congenital coronary artery anomalies in young patients: new perspectives for timely identification. J Am Coll Cardiol. 2001;37:598–600.
36. Davis JA, Cecchin F, Jones TK, Portman MA. Major coronary artery anomalies in a pediatric population: incidence and clinical importance. J Am Coll Cardiol. 2001;37:593–597.
37. Maron BJ, Leon MB, Swain JA, Cannon RO 3rd, Pelliccia A. Prospective identification by two-dimensional echocardiography of anomalous origin of the left main coronary artery from the right sinus of Valsalva. Am J Cardiol. 1991;68:140–142.
38. Maron BJ, Gohman TE, Aeppli D. Prevalence of sudden cardiac death during competitive sports activities in Minnesota high school athletes. J Am Coll Cardiol. 1998;32:1881–1884.
39. Corrado D, Basso C, Pavei A, Michieli P, Schiavon M, Thiene G. Trends in sudden cardiovascular death in young competitive athletes after implementation of a preparticipation screening program. JAMA. 2006;296:1593–1601.
40. Lotfi K, White L, Rea T, et al. Cardiac arrest in schools. Circulation. 2007;116:1374–1379.
41. Harris KM, Sponsel A, Hutter AM, Maron BJ. Brief communication: cardiovascular screening practices of major North American professional sports teams. Ann Int Med. 2006;145:507–511.
42. Chaitman BR. An electrocardiogram should not be included in routine preparticipation screening of young athletes. Circulation. 2007;116:2610–2614.
43. Lawless CE, Best TM. Electrocardiograms in athletes: interpretation and diagnostic accuracy. Med Sci Sports Exerc. 2008;40:787–798.
44. Myerburg RJ, Vetter VL. Electrocardiograms should be included in preparticipation screening of athletes. Circulation. 2007;116:2616–2626.
45. Frommelt PC, Frommelt MA, Tweddell JS, Jaquiss RD. Prospective echocardiographic diagnosis and surgical repair of anomalous origin of a coronary artery from the opposite sinus with an interarterial course. J Am Coll Cardiol. 2003;42:148–154.
46. Lawless CE, Best TM. Electrocardiograms in athletes: interpretation and diagnostic accuracy. Med Sci Sports Exerc. 2008;40:787–798.
47. Liberman L, Pass RH, Kaufman S, Hordof AJ, Printz BF, Prakash A. Left coronary artery arising from the non-coronary sinus: a rare congenital coronary anomaly. Pediatr Cardiol. 2005;26:672–674.
48. Caracciolo EA, Davis KB, Sopko G, et al. Comparison of surgical and medical group survival in patients with left main coronary artery disease. Long-term CASS experience. Circulation. 1995;91:2325–2334.
49. SOS-KANTO study group. Cardiopulmonary resuscitation by bystanders with chest compression only (SOS-KANTO): an observational study. Lancet. 2007;369:920–926.

50. Bobrow BJ, Clark LL, Ewy GA, et al. Minimally interrupted cardiac resuscitation by emergency medical services for out-of-hospital cardiac arrest. JAMA. 2008;299:1158–1165.
51. Peberdy MA, Ornato JP. Progress in resuscitation: an evolution, not a revolution. JAMA. 2008;299:1188–1190.
52. Angelini P. Surgical standby: state of the art. In: Topol EJ, ed. Textbook of Interventional Cardiology. Philadelphia, PA: Saunders; 2008:541–548.
53. Maron BJ, Isner JM, McKenna WJ. 26th Bethesda conference: recommendations for determining eligibility for competition in athletes with cardiovascular abnormalities. Task Force 3: hypertrophic cardiomyopathy, myocarditis and other myopericardial diseases and mitral valve prolapse. J Am Coll Cardiol. 1994;24:880–885.
54. Thompson PD, Franklin BA, Balady GJ, et al; American Heart Association Council on Nutrition, Physical Activity, and Metabolism; American Heart Association Council on Clinical Cardiology; American College of Sports Medicine. Exercise and acute cardiovascular events placing the risks into perspective: a scientific statement from the American Heart Association Council on Nutrition, Physical Activity, and Metabolism and the Council on Clinical Cardiology. Circulation. 2007;115:2358–2368.
55. Maron BJ, Douglas PS, Graham TP, Nishimura RA, Thompson PD. Task Force 1: preparticipation screening and diagnosis of cardiovascular disease in athletes. J Am Coll Cardiol. 2005;45:1322–1326.
56. Brothers JA, Stephens P, Gaynor JW, Lorber R, Vricella LA, Paridon SM. Anomalous aortic origin of a coronary artery with an interarterial course: should family screening be routine? J Am Coll Cardiol. 2008;51:2062–2064.
57. Angelini P, Velasco JA, Ott D, Khoshnevis GR. Anomalous coronary artery arising from the opposite sinus: descriptive features and pathophysiological mechanisms, as documented by intravascular ultrasonography. J Invasive Cardiol. 2003;15:507–515.
58. Virmani R, Chun PK, Goldstein RE, Robinowitz M, McAllister HA. Acute takeoffs of the coronary arteries along the aortic wall and congenital coronary ostial valve-like ridges: association with sudden death. J Am Coll Cardiol. 1984;3:766–771.

Chapter 16
Participation in Sports for the Athlete with the Marfan Syndrome

Marla Mendelson

Introduction

The Marfan syndrome was first described in 1896 by Dr. Antoine Marfan, a French pediatrician [1, 2]. He described a young girl who manifested the classic musculoskeletal findings. This syndrome along with its propensity for aortic dilatation has been recognized across the world as one of the causes of sudden death in high-profile athletes receiving considerable media attention [3]. The Marfan syndrome with aortic dilatation is related to a mutation in the fibrillin I gene [1, 2]. The incidence in the general population is approximately 1 in 5,000 to 1 in 10,000, and it has an autosomal dominance pattern of inheritance [4, 5]. It is a syndrome comprising cardiovascular, visual, and skeletal manifestations, which will be discussed in this chapter. There are also several Marfan-like syndromes that carry this risk of sudden death from aortic dissection or rupture. The most common cause of sudden death in patients with the Marfan syndrome participating in athletics is aortic rupture; however, less often, complications of the mitral valve prolapse or degeneration may occur [6]. It is important to define the syndrome accurately, and various criteria have been formulated and are summarized in Table 16.1 [7, 8]. It is important for the severity of organ involvement to be established when formulating recommendations for participation in sports and physical activity [9]. Ultimately, the extent of aortic dilatation will determine their risk for participation. Other causes of progressive aortic dilatation are discussed (Table 16.2), such as the Ehlers–Danlos syndrome, Loeys–Dietz syndrome, Shprintzen–Goldberg syndrome, and patients born with bicuspid aortic valves [10–12].

Screening, as outlined in Table 16.3, the tall athlete, the basketball or volleyball player, for silent aortic disease is clinically advantageous [3]. This would include measurement of arm span and height with examination of the mouth, chest, and limbs. This should be routine in the preparticipation physical examination of athletes

M. Mendelson (✉)
Marfan Syndrome Program, Department of Cardiology, Northwestern Feinberg School of Medicine, Chicago, IL, USA
e-mail: m-mendelson@northwestern.edu

C.E. Lawless (ed.), *Sports Cardiology Essentials: Evaluation, Management and Case Studies*, DOI 10.1007/978-0-387-92775-6_16,

Table 16.1 Clinical recognition of the Marfan syndrome Ghent nosology

Diagnosis established by
Major criteria
Skeletal: pectus; arm span, wrist & thumb signs; scoliosis
Ectopic lens
Aortic root dilatation/dissection of ascending aorta
FBNI-mutation present
Family history: first-degree relative
Dural ectasia
Minor criteria
Skeletal: pectus excavation (moderate): joint hypermobility
High-arched palate
Facial features
Flat cornea; hypoplastic iris;
Mitral valve prolapse; pulmonary artery dilatation
Dilatation of descending thoracic or abdominal aorta
Spontaneous pneumothorax; apical blebs
Striae of the skin; incisional hernia

Adapted from [7, 8]

Table 16.2 Differential diagnosis of aortic dilatation

	Aortic dilatation	MVP	Differentiating features
Marfan syndrome	Yes	Yes	Body habitus Skeletal abnormalities
Bicuspid aortic valve	Yes	–	Aortic dilatation irrespective of valve pathology
Ehlers–Danlos (vascular type)	Yes	Yes	Multiple arteries involved skin and joint problems, craniosynostosis, club feet, PDA
Loeys–Dietz	Yes	–	Diffuse arterial aneurysms

Adapted from [11]

at risk. Any of these features would necessitate further, more specific evaluation for major and minor criteria of the Marfan syndrome. This may provide the initial opportunity to make the diagnosis before life-threatening complications arise. In addition to the Marfan syndrome, other heritable conditions may be identified. These syndromes are highlighted and compared (Table 16.2) to highlight the differential diagnosis of the cause of aortic dilatation [11, 13].

The Ehlers–Danlos syndrome occurs in approximately 1 to 5,000 births and is also of autosomal dominant inheritance [10]. Some of the clinical features overlap with those of the Marfan syndrome (Table 16.2) [11]. It is characterized by skin hyperextensibility, joint hypermobility, and easy bruising. There are different types of the Ehlers–Danlos syndromes including the kyphoscoliosis, vascular, and the

Table 16.3 Screening for the Marfan syndrome

History
Family history of aortic dissection or sudden death; relatives with the Marfan syndrome
Visual problems
Scoliosis
Physical
Body habitus: arm span compared to height
High arched palate
Pectus of chest
Murmur of mitral and/or aortic regurgitation
Mitral valve click
Arachnodactyly
Echocardiogram
Measure aortic root
Aortic valve Doppler assessment
Mitral valve Doppler assessment

hypermobility types. The kyphoscoliosis type has been associated with mitral and tricuspid valve prolapse [11]. The vascular type of the Ehlers–Danlos syndrome is associated with arterial rupture specifically in the bowel, intestine, and gravid uterus and is also associated with aortic dilatation [11]. The Loeys–Dietz syndrome is characterized by hypertelorism (widely set eyes), a bifid uvula, cleft palate, ascending aortic aneurysm, and dissection. These patients also present craniosynostosis (premature closure of cranial structures), Chiari malformations (cerebellum descends out of the skull compressing the spinal cord), club feet, and patent ductus arteriosus [11]. They may have aneurysms or dissections of the entire arterial tree; they may also have skin and joint abnormalities. They may have a more aggressive clinical course, and this may be the cause of the aortic dissection in young children. Other entities that could be confused with the Marfan syndrome would be congenital arachnodactyly, the Shprintzen–Goldberg syndrome associated with mental retardation, fragile X syndrome, and a syndrome which includes camptodactyly (permanent flexion of fingers), tall stature, and hearing loss [11].

Clinical recognition of the Marfan or other syndromes that result in silent, progressive aortic dilatation is of vital importance in the athlete being assessed prior to competitive sports or even the young, tall patient contemplating vigorous exercise [1, 8, 13–15]. The Ghent diagnostic nosology was established in 1996 to identify the syndrome summarized in Table 16.1 [7, 8, 11]. The major criteria of the Ghent nosology, including skeletal, ophthalmologic, aortic, genetic, and dural findings, establish major and minor criteria for the diagnosis of the Marfan syndrome, to identify patients to be followed closely for progressive aortic dilatation or mitral or aortic valve incompetence. It has been recommended that athletes who are taller than the average for the population be screened for the Marfan syndrome by patient and family history, physical examination, and specific diagnostic testing [9]. To establish the diagnosis, there must be two major criteria or one major and two minor areas of involvement. If the diagnosis is established, there should be an evaluation for aortic dilatation [4, 8].

Skeletal findings include long limbs, anterior chest (pectus) deformities due to rib overgrowth which may require surgery, arachnodactyly, elbow contractures, and scoliosis [11]. Four skeletal features must be present to meet the major criteria for diagnosis. This may include an arm span-to-height ratio greater than 1.05. Although a common clinical finding, joint hypermobility is considered "involvement" due to the syndrome or minor criteria, rather than major criteria [1, 11]. Arthritis may develop due to joint laxity [13, 14].

The facial features of the Marfan syndrome include downsloping, palpebral fissures, enophthalmos, a high arched palate, and tooth crowding [1, 11, 13]. These are considered "involvement" due to the Marfan syndrome. Lens dislocation, however, is considered a major criterion [11]. Other ophthalmologic findings include myopia, retinal detachment, cataracts, or glaucoma [13].

Cardiovascular criteria include a history of aortic root dilatation, dissection, or rupture [1, 11]. This usually occurs at the sinus of Valsalva. The majority of fatal events in the Marfan patient occur in early adulthood [11]. A study of normotensive athletes found that 0.96% of basketball and volleyball players had aortic dilatation, but not all of these patients met the criteria for the Marfan syndrome [4]. Aortic dilatation was diagnosed by echocardiography and defined as greater than 40 mm. The five subjects with severe dilatation were discouraged from participating in athletic activity and three complied. One patient collapsed from an aortic dissection after a game. Mitral valve dysfunction may occur in approximately 2/3 of patients with mitral valve prolapse, mitral regurgitation, and premature (before age 40) calcification of the mitral valve [16]. There also may be, in rare cases, primary myocardial dysfunction [13].

Other organ systems may be involved though do not constitute the major criteria. Skin manifestations include striae and inguinal hernias. Pulmonary manifestations may include apical blebs, recurrent spontaneous pneumothorax, pulmonary emphysema or dysfunction [11]. There may be restrictive lung disease from a severe pectus abnormality [11, 17]. The pulmonary artery may also be enlarged [11].

Dural ectasia (expansion of the dural sac around the spinal cord), a major criterion, may be found in up to 92% of patients and may also be seen in the Loeys–Dietz and Ehlers–Danlos syndromes [1, 11]. This could be diagnosed by CT scan or MRI. Often, the patients are asymptomatic; however, they may note low back pain, leg pain, or headaches.

Genetic findings and family history are major criteria for the diagnosis of the Marfan syndrome. The most compelling element of the family history in patients with the Marfan syndrome or the other heritable connective tissue disorders is a family history of aortic dissection or rupture. Family history of sudden death should be probed for an aortic etiology, especially if other clinical features are present. The fibrillin I gene on mutation on chromosome 15 can be identified in an index patient. At that time, the family is screened for the same mutation. If the gene mutation is present, further evaluation for anatomic evidence of the Marfan syndrome is indicated. New mutation may occur in about 27% of cases, and over 500 mutations have been described [1, 11, 13, 14]. Mutations in the gene result in proteolytic degradation of fibrillin I, resulting in abnormal microfibrils weakening the extracellular matrix. There may be flow-mediated dilatation of the large arteries [18]. It is speculated that this weakening may have affected the development of connective tissue. However, it appears that TGF-beta, a stimulator of inflammation and fibrosis, may cause connective tissue problems in the Marfan syndrome. Treatment strategies are now directed at medically suppressing TGF-beta, a potent stimulator of inflammation and fibrosis, to prevent loss of elasticity in the media [7]. Further molecular work has been done looking at the growth factor TGF beta [12, 19]. Excess TGF-beta may cause inherent weakness of connective tissue, and this has also precipitated new and exciting work in treatment options for these patients [7, 12].

The Evaluation

History

The patient may be experiencing chest pain referable to their mitral valve prolapse, back pain, or other joint laxity problems [1, 9, 13, 14, 20]. It is also important when taking history to establish the type of exercise that the athlete is already performing. Many of the young athletes work out with trainers who encourage weightlifting. It is important to determine the amount of weight that is being lifted and whether barbells are to be lifted overhead or lighter hand weights with lower weight and multiple repetitions which would be preferred. Aerobic exercise is usually well tolerated. It is very important to identify the type of sports in which the patient seeks to participate. Pertinent issues are summarized in Table 16.4 [21]. Family history of sudden premature death is important to establish as a major criterion of the Marfan syndrome [1, 6, 13, 14].

Table 16.4 Recommendations for sports participation in patients with the Marfan syndrome Ehlers Danlos and bicuspid aortic valve with aortic dilatation

Clinical presentations	Sports recommendations
Marfan syndrome	
1. No aortic dilatation	IA, IIA[a]
No moderate/severe mitral regurgitation	IA, IIA[a]
No family history of sudden death related to Marfan Syndrome	IA, IIA[a]
2. Aortic dimension 40 mm or greater	IA[a]
Prior surgical aortic root reconstruction	IA[a]
Moderate/severe mitral regurgitation	IA[a]
Family history of dissection or sudden death	
Bicuspid aortic valve	
Ascending aortic dilatation	No sports with collision
Ehlers Danlos: Vascular form (see text)	None

[a]Classification of sports. IA examples: billiards, bowling, cricket, curling, golf, riflery, and IIA examples: archery, auto racing, diving, equestrian, motorcycling
Adapted from [5,28,34]

Examination

The examination should include assessment for the major and minor diagnostic criteria (Table 16.1) [7, 8, 13]. The mouth should be checked for a high-arched palate and teeth crowding. The chest should be examined for the pectus abnormality. The pectus may either be a protuberance of the entire sternum causing the ribs to angle backwards (carinatum) or the sternum may appear to be sunken due to rib overgrowth (excavatum). The other type of pectus abnormalities may be in the transverse orientation in which the distal half of the sternum may grow inward causing a peaked appearance at the mid-sternum. The adult patient may have had surgery to correct the pectus in childhood to promote normal thoracic development. The heart examination in the patient with Marfan or suspected Marfan syndrome may reveal a downward displacement of the PMI. There may be murmurs consistent with mitral or aortic insufficiency. A mid-systolic click of mitral valve prolapse may be heard. Also, if there are abnormalities of the aortic valve, an ejection type click may be heard. Evaluation should include a complete vascular assessment for bruits over the aorta as well as the subclavian, renal, and the femoral arteries. Examination of the back should look for evidence of scoliosis. Limb deformities and lengthening may be seen; the distance between the heel and tibia may be greater than the femoral distance which can also be seen in the patients with Marfan syndrome. The arm span and height should be measured [1, 13, 14].

Diagnostic Testing

An electrocardiogram is often not useful for screening these patients [9, 22]. The cause of sudden death in these patients is rarely an arrhythmia. If significant mitral or aortic valve disease is present, there may be left ventricular hypertrophy, but this may be difficult in a younger patient to distinguish from a normal variant.

The echocardiogram is probably the best test to help establish the diagnosis of cardiovascular involvement with the Marfan syndrome [1, 9, 13, 15]. It also identifies the other causes of aortic dilatation. Ventricular dimensions and function can be identified. Valvar pathology such as mitral valve prolapse due to a severely myxomatous mitral valve with redundancy of the leaflets often causes clinically important mitral regurgitation. There also may be myxomatous changes of the aortic valve, resulting in aortic insufficiency. The bicuspid aortic valve that is associated with progressive aortic dilatation can also be identified by echocardiogram, and there may be aortic stenosis and/or aortic insufficiency. It has been noted that the aorta may increase in size irrespective of a valve pathology in patients with the bicuspid aortic valve. The aortic root should be measured at the level of sinuses of Valsalva and 4 cm above the aortic valve in the ascending aorta. If there is a suspicion of a fusiform dilatation beyond the borders of the image obtained by the echocardiogram, magnetic resonance imaging (MRI) or computed axial tomography (CT) should be considered to further elucidate any aortic enlargement [13]. MR or CT may be more accurate to assess enlargement of the sinus of Valsalva and outline ascending aorta.

This test may be performed serially if the site of greatest aortic dilatation is beyond the echocardiographic windows or if a severe pectus abnormality is present [1]. If there is correlation between the two tests, then the echocardiogram is easier to use serially and it also can give information regarding valve pathology.

Treatment

Medical

Patients identified as having aortic dilatation have traditionally been treated with beta-blockade to help slow the progression of aortic dilatation by decreasing the hemodynamic stress on the aorta walls [1, 7, 10]. These medications tend to slow the heart and therefore may interfere with peak exercise performance both in athletic activities and during the stress test. It is important to continue these medications to preserve and protect the aorta. New studies have found new treatment strategies that identify the TGF-beta signaling problem, novel angiotensin receptor blockers such as losartan have been identified to target this specific problem and thereby potentially prevent abnormal connective tissue development, when started early [12, 19, 23]. ACE inhibitors have also been used to reduce ejection impulse, but it is the angiotensin receptor blockers that appear to inhibit the TGF-beta signaling [12]. It is not clear whether this may reverse dilatation of the aorta or prevent further dilatation by stabilizing the connective tissue. Information regarding use of the new medications and eventual athletic participation has not been studied yet [7]. It has been suggested that the incidence of aortic dissection decreases after prophylactic beta blockade and early surgical intervention [5].

Surgical

Patients with progressive aortic dilatation are referred for surgery when the aorta has increased over 5 cm [1]. There are two types of surgery in common practice: the Bentall procedure, which requires a composite root replacement with a prosthetic mechanical valve, or the new valve-sparing surgery, where only the root is replaced [24, 25]. Participation in athletics after the surgery has not been well studied. The Bentall surgery does require postoperative lifelong coumadin therapy. A retrospective study compared the Bentall surgery and the valve-sparing surgery in patients who had aortic root operations after they were diagnosed with the Marfan syndrome [25, 26]. The late survival was actually lower in the Bentall group; however, those patients were older, had had more prior aortic dissections and emergent surgery and had larger aortic valve annulus at the time of operation [25]. They also had increased aortic insufficiency and had had concomitant coronary bypass grafting and mitral valve procedures. The valve-sparing procedure is being widely used in the younger patients, and further study regarding athletic participation after that surgery needs to be done.

Recommendation for Athletic Participation

Types of Exercise

In 2007, an AHA statement regarding exercise in patients with cardiovascular disease discussed the effects of resistance training [27]. Isometric exercise, the basis of resistance training, physiologically causes elevated systolic and diastolic blood pressure, elevated heart rate, vasoconstriction, and elevated peripheral vascular resistance. These hemodynamic changes would be contraindicated in patients with the Marfan syndrome if aortic dilatation is present. The Valsalva maneuver often performed during weightlifting is a forced expiration against a closed glottis increasing intrathoracic pressure and decreased venous return. Resistance training, also described as static or isometric exercise is therefore contraindicated in the Marfan syndrome, increasing the risk of aortic dissection by increasing peripheral resistance [1, 27]. Aerobic exercise is associated with an elevation in systolic blood pressure with only a modest increase in mean blood pressure and peripheral vascular resistance decreases [1].

General recommendations from the guidelines cautioned against bursts of exertion as in basketball, jogging, bicycling, soccer, and tennis [21]. Jogging, bicycling, and lap swimming are preferred. Environmental conditions must be considered such as climate extremes. Patients are advised to avoid exhaustion or excessive progressive training [21]. Table 16.4 gives specific examples of indicated and contraindicated activities [21, 28]. The activities assessed as intermediate risk may be permissible if there is little or no aortic root dilatation.

The 36th Bethesda conference studied the participation of young athletes with cardiovascular disease in sports [5, 28]. Sports were classified by their static and dynamic components, and recommendations were made regarding the patients with underlying disease. In Marfan patients, the authors recognize the risk of rupture associated with the aorta when the aorta is >50 mm [1, 6, 15]. It was also recommended that it is important to monitor the patients periodically for progressive dilatation of the aortic root. Mitral valve prolapse with mitral regurgitation and possible left ventricular systolic dysfunction as a cause of arrhythmias were identified as a possible cause of sudden death. In a study of young athletes who died suddenly, 3% died from a ruptured aortic aneurysm [29, 30]. Weightlifting was directly associated with aortic dissection in athletes with cystic medial necrosis and was therefore discouraged. There was decreased incidence of dissection with earlier surgery or beta-blocker use [1, 7, 10]. Whether medical treatment of the Marfan patients or surgery to correct their aortic dilatation renders them a candidate for an athletic participation is yet to be determined [5, 31, 32].

The Bethesda recommendations for sports participation in patients with aortic disease are summarized in Table 16.3 [5, 34]. These guidelines addressed patients who had no aortic dilatation but had moderate to severe mitral regurgitation and a family history of dissection or sudden death. The recommendations, which include participation only in 1A and 2A activities, are summarized in Table 16.5 [28]. The 1A recommended activities required low aerobic demands and a low static component and include billiards, bowling, cricket, curling, golf, and riflery. The 2A classification is for activities with moderate static demands but low dynamic or aerobic components, including archery, auto racing, driving, equestrian events, and motorcycling [5, 28]. For patients who have a >40- mm aortic transverse dimension or who have had prior reconstruction, and for patients with chronic dissection or who have moderate or severe mitral regurgitation or a family history of dissection or sudden death only 1A activities were recommended [1, 3, 28]. For the Ehlers–Danlos vascular type patients, it was recommended that they do not participate in competitive athletic activity because of the high risk of aortic rupture and rupture of branches of the aorta [5, 10, 11]. For all patients with suspected aortic disease, sports that require bodily collision were not advised. It is recommended that if the stigmata of the

Table 16.5 Examples of recommendations for physical activity in athletes with the Marfan syndrome

Permitted activities	
Modest hiking	
Tennis (doubles)	
Treadmill	
Stationary bicycle	
Bowling	
Golf	
Skating	
Snorkeling	
Brisk walking	
Intermediate risk	
Tennis (singles)	Basketball
Touch football	Raquetball
Biking	Running (sprinting)
Hiking	Skiing
Jogging	Soccer
Swimming laps	Baseball
Horseback riding	
Contraindicated	
Body building	
Ice hockey	
Rock climbing	
Windsurfing	
Motorcycling	
Surfing	
Weightlifting	
Scuba diving	

Adapted from [21]

Marfan syndrome are present; echocardiography and/or CT/MR for serial assessment of the aortic root is indicated [1].

Medical therapy may affect physical performance in the group of athletes with the Marfan syndrome [1, 29]. Beta-blockers are commonly prescribed to inhibit aortic dilatation, and they may inhibit heart rate response. The use of these drugs or even surgical intervention have not been assessed in terms of permitting competitive sports [29, 31–33].

There are specific progressive recommendations with regard to the patient with a bicuspid aortic valve with aortic enlargement who is also at risk for aortic dissection. When the aorta measures <40 mm and there is no aortic stenosis or regurgitation, the patient may participate in competitive sports. However, if the aorta is between 40 and 45 mm, they may participate in low/moderate dynamic sports (1A, 2A). They should avoid sports associated with collision or trauma. Low-intensity competitive sports are permitted only if the aorta is <45 mm [34].

In summary, the Bethesda recommendations for athletes with the Marfan syndrome who do not have an aortic root >40 mm; moderate to severe mitral regurgitation, or a family history of aortic dissection or sudden death may participate in IA and IIA activities (Table 16.4) [5, 21]. Athletes with aortic root dimensions >40 mm, prior surgical reconstruction, chronic dissection, moderate to severe mitral regurgitation or family history may only participate in IA activities. These patients should not participate in sports with risk of collision. It is recommended that patients diagnosed with the Ehlers–Danlos syndrome not participate in any competitive activity [5, 10, 21].

Case 1

An 18-year-old college freshman decides to go out for the volleyball team. She came from a small high school where she had played on the varsity team since her sophomore year. The college stipulated that she be seen by the team physician. She denied any cardiac symptoms at rest or with exertion. Her past medical history was notable for scoliosis which required her to wear a brace until age 16. The patient denied tobacco, drug, or alcohol use. She lives with her mother and stepfather. She ran 5 days weekly and worked out with a trainer 3 days per week. Family history was notable in that her father died suddenly at age 27, but further details were unavailable. She had no siblings. Review of systems was negative. Her examination was remarkable for a height of 70 in., an arm span of 75 in., and a weight of 150 pounds. She had a high-arched palate on examination of her mouth; her neck was normal, and there was no jugular venous distention. Her lungs were clear. Her chest exam was notable for a mild pectus abnormality. She had a normal S1, S2, a regular rate and rhythm. She had a systolic click with a holosystolic murmur. Her abdomen was benign. There were no bruits. Her fingers and toes were long and slim. There was a midline surgical scar on her back. The electrocardiogram was entirely normal. An echocardiogram was performed and revealed an aortic root enlargement of 4.3 cm and mitral valve prolapse.

Discussion

It is likely that the patient's father had the Marfan syndrome and died suddenly which may confer significant risk to this patient. The volleyball athlete is rather tall and gracile. Therefore, there should be a high index of suspicion for elements of the Marfan syndrome. The father's history and the echocardiography findings constitute a major criterion and establish the diagnosis of the Marfan syndrome. Her aorta is mildly enlarged. According to the Bethesda recommendation, the student should only participate in low dynamic (IA) and low static activities (IB) [21, 28]. It is not clear that beta-blockade or surgery alters this risk [31, 32].

Case 2

This is a 21-year-old male who presents for evaluation prior to participating in an exercise program. His only past medical history was two prior hospitalizations for spontaneous pneumothorax. His family history was unknown. He reported joint extensibility and easy bruising. His exam was entirely normal. His arm span was normal. His review of systems only noted easy bruisibility of his skin. An echocardiogram revealed an aortic root of 4.6 cm. Further evaluation revealed features of the vascular type Ehlers–Danlos Syndrome. He was restricted from competition sports because of the risk of arterial fragility.

Discussion

The patient's history of spontaneous pneumothorax and the dilated aortic root may suggest the Ehlers–Danlos or the Loeys–Dietz syndromes. The aortic root should be well studied in such patients, and if dilated, they may be at high risk of aortic rupture especially if presentation is due to the Ehlers–Danlos syndrome. Sports and exercise with risk of collision should be avoided.

Conclusion

Patients with aortic dilatation due to a variety of etiologies may be at risk by participating in vigorous sports. They are at significant risk with any activity that may involve bodily collision. Careful assessment of certain athletes such as volleyball and basketball players may diagnose the Marfan syndrome. However, other entities such as the bicuspid aortic valve which may be associated with aortic dilatation poses similar risk and may be less often clinically suspected.

References

1. Braverman, A. Exercise and the Marfan syndrome. Clinical Suppl: Cardiol. 1998:30:S387–S395.
2. Pyeritz, RE, Rimoin, DL, Conner, M, et al. Marfan syndrome and other disorders of fibrillin. In: Principles Practice of Medical Genetics. 3rd ed. New York: Churchill Livingston, 1997:1027–1066.
3. Saeed, IM, Braverman, AC. Approach to athlete with thoracic aortic disease. Curr Sports Med Rep. 2007:6:101–107.
4. Kinoshita N, Milmura, J, Obayashi, C, et al. Aortic root dilatation among young competitive athletes: Echocardiographic screening of 1929 athletes between 15 and 34 years of age. Am Heart J. 2000:139:723–728.
5. Maron, BJ, Ackerman, MJ, Nishimura, RA, et al. Task force 4: HCM and other cardiomyopathies, mitral valve prolapse, myocarditis, and Marfan syndrome. J Am Coll Cardiol. 2005:45:1340–1345.
6. Giese, EA, O'Connor, FG, Brennan, FH, et al. The athletic preparticipation evaluation: Cardiovascular assessment. Am Fam Physician. 2007:75:1008–1014.
7. Keane, MG, Pyeritz, RE. Medical management of Marfan syndrome. Circulation. 2008:117:2802–2813.
8. De Paepe, A, Devereux, RB, Dietz, HC, et al. Revised diagnostic criteria for the Marfan syndrome. Am J Med Genet. 1996:62:417–426.
9. Seto, CK. Preparticipation cardiovascular screening. Clin Sports Med. 2003:22:23–35.
10. Germain, DP. Ehlers-Danlos syndrome type IV. ORJD. 2007:2:32–41.
11. Callewaert, B, Malfait, F, Loeys, B, et al. Ehlers-Danlos syndromes and Marfan syndrome. Best Pract Res Clin Rheumatol. 2008:22:165–189.
12. Lacro, RV, Dietz, HC, Wruck, LM, et al. Rationale and design of a randomized clinical trial of B-blocker therapy (Atenolol) versus angiotensin II receptor blocker therapy (losartan) in individuals with Marfan syndrome. Am Heart J. 2007:154:624–631.
13. Ammash, NM, Sundt, TM, Connolly, HM. Marfan syndrome-diagnosis and management. Curr Probl Cardiol. 2008:33:7–39.
14. Dean, JC. Marfan syndrome: Clinical diagnosis and management. Eur J Hum Genet. 2007:15:724–733.
15. Maron, BJ, Douglas, PS, Graham, TP, et al. Task force 1: Preparticipation screening and diagnosis of cardiovascular disease in athletes. J Am Coll Cardiol. 2005:45:1322–1326.
16. Figueiredo, S, Martins, E, Lima, MR, et al. Cardiovascular manifestations in Marfan syndrome. Rev Port Cardiol. 2001:20:1203–1218.
17. Giske, L, Stanghelle, JK, Reid-Hendrikssen, S, et al. Pulmonary function, working capacity and strength in young adults with Marfan syndrome. J Rehabil Med. 2003:35:221–228.
18. Crilley, JG, Bendahan, D, Boehm, E, et al. Investigation of muscle bioenergeitics in the Marfan syndrome indicates reduced metabolic efficiency. J Cardiovasc Magn Reson. 2007:9:709–717.
19. Matt, P, Habashi, J, Carrel, T, et al. Recent advances in understanding Marfan syndrome: Should we not treat surgical patients with losartan? J Thorac Cardiovasc Surg. 2008:135:389–394.
20. Waseem, M, Ganti, S. Chest pain in an adolescent with Marfan syndrome. J Emerg Med. 2007:20:30–33.
21. Maron, BJ, Chaitman, BR, Ackerman, MJ, et al. Recommendations for physical activity and recreational sports participation for young patients with genetic cardiovascular disease. Circulation. 2004:109:2807–2816.
22. Lawless, CE, Best, TM. Electrocardiograms in athletes: Interpretation and diagnostic accuracy. Am Coll Sports Med. 2007:40:787–798.
23. Judge, DP, Dietz, HC. Therapy of Marfan syndrome. Annu Rev Med. 2008:59:43–59.
24. Patel, ND, Weiss, ES, Alejo, DE, et al. Aortic root operations for Marfan syndrome: A comparison of the Bentall and valve-sparing procedures. Ann Thorac Surg. 2008:85:2003–2011.

25. Kallenbach, K, Karck, M, Pak, D, et al. Decade of aortic valve sparing reimplantation. Are we pushing the limits too far? Circulation. 2005:112:I-253–I-259.
26. Sheick-Yousif, B, Sheinfield, A, Tager, S, et al. Aortic root surgery in Marfan syndrome. Isr Med Assoc J. 2008:10:189–193.
27. Williams, MA, Haskell, WL, Ades, PA, et al. Resistance exercise in individuals with and without cardiovascular disease: 2007 Update. Circulation. 2007:116:572–584.
28. Mitchell, JH, Haskell, W, Snell, P, et al. Task force 8: Classification of sports. J Am Coll Cardiol. 2005:45:1364–1367.
29. Maron, BJ, Zipes, DP. Introduction: Eligibility recommendations for competitive athletes with cardiovascular abnormalities-General considerations. J Am Coll Cardiol. 2005:45:0735–1097.
30. Maron, BJ. Sudden death in young athletes. N Engl J Med. 2003:349:1064–1075.
31. Januzzi, JL, Isselbacher, EM, Fattor, R, et al. Characterizing the young patient with aortic dissection: Results from the International Registry of Aortic Dissection (IRAD). J Am Coll Cardiol. 2004:43:665–669.
32. Shores, J, Berger, KR, Murphy, EA, et al. Progression of aortic dilatation and the benefit of long-term beta-adrenergic blockade in Marfans syndrome. N Engl J Med. 1994:330:1335–1341.
33. Yetman, AT, Bornemerier, RA, McCindle, BW. Long-term outcome in patients with Marfan syndrome: Is aortic dissection the only cause of sudden death? J Am Coll Cardiol. 2003:41:329–332.
34. Bonow, RO, Cheitlin, MD, Crawford, MH, et al. Task force 3: Valvular heart disease. J Am Coll Cardiol. 2005:45:1334–1340.

Chapter 17
Congenital Heart Disease: Exercise and Sports Participation

Marla Mendelson

Introduction

Athletes born with congenital heart disease may have previously undetected cardiac lesions that first come to medical attention during sports participation evaluation. Or, they may have had extensive corrective procedures and/or surgery in early childhood to reach young adulthood with fairly normal exercise capacity and the desire to compete. Recommendations for this group of patients need to be formulated based on the underlying cardiac problem, the propensity for sudden cardiac events, and the demands of planned activity. Each patient is unique with a different type of repair and different sequelae from the intervention or surgery. Therefore, each exercise prescription and recommendations for sports participation require a specific evaluation. Each lesion may have associated valvular or hemodynamic consequences that need to be anticipated. After surgical intervention, residual or sequelae may persist and pose further risk with time. Young adults who have not been diagnosed previously with a less complex congenital heart problem may, as adults, develop problems that could pose risks during sports participation. It is important to understand the basic anatomy and physiology of these patients in their repaired or unrepaired state. Each individual lesion, repaired and unrepaired, are discussed and specific recommendations detailed. Recommendations have been published by both the European Society of Cardiology and the 36th Bethesda Conference regarding sports participation in athletes with congenital heart disease [1, 2]. Full participation in all athletic endeavors may be permissible after full evaluation with periodic ongoing assessment, or there may be strict limitations.

It is important to encourage safe exercise because often patients with cardiac disease since childhood tend to be sedentary [3]. They may have been unnecessarily limited in their activity. They should be encouraged to participate in appropriate

M. Mendelson (✉)
Northwestern Adult Congenital Heart Center, Northwestern Feinberg School of Medicine, Chicago, IL, USA
e-mail: m-mendelson@northwestern.edu

C.E. Lawless (ed.), *Sports Cardiology Essentials: Evaluation, Management and Case Studies*, DOI 10.1007/978-0-387-92775-6_17,

physical activity to help forestall any future cardiac problem and for enhanced quality of life. After repair, in the absence of complications or hemodynamic problems, it has been noted that these patients may be generally more active than others with more complex diseases but are still below the national guidelines for exercise (30 min/day of moderate physical activity) [4].

The major concern when evaluating the patients with heart disease for exercise and athletic participation is their risk of sudden death [5]. In this population, arrhythmias and systemic ventricular failure are the most common causes, but not necessarily in all patients, before or after repair. The risk of sudden death in this population of patients may be actually due to the sequelae of their repair or due to the natural history of their congenital heart disease. Preparticipation evaluation must identify factors that may predispose the patient to sudden death [2, 6]. The most common causes of sudden death in athletes were due to coronary artery anomalies, aortic stenosis, or ruptured aortic aneurysms [7, 8].

Common Lesions in Adults with Congenital Heart Disease

Shunt Lesions

Atrial Septal Defect

The atrial septal defect (ASD) may be centrally located in the atrial septum, the secundum defect, involving the endocardial cushion, the primum defect, or in the superior aspect of the septum, the sinus venous defect. The ASD results in a shunting between the left atrium and right atrium. Because left atrial pressures are higher, shunting is left-to-right. Severe shunting causes the right atrium and eventually the right ventricle to enlarge. As a result, increased pulmonary blood flow over time causes pulmonary vascular changes and pulmonary vascular resistance increases resulting in Eisenmenger's physiology. The right-sided intracardiac pressures become higher, so shunting reverses and cyanosis ensues. This is a very rare entity in the adult population born with an ASD. An unrepaired secundum ASD with a relatively small shunt may not be detected until adulthood. If an ASD is found in a young adult, it is recommended that it be closed. Currently, it may be closed with a catheter-based device or by surgical closure. This would prevent enlargement of the right atrium and right ventricle over time.

The primum ASD is often associated with a cleft mitral valve which is repaired at the same time in childhood, but in the adult, there may be residual mitral regurgitation. After repair, patients may also be susceptible to atrial arrhythmias. The repair may have occurred during childhood, and the patient still may have a small increased risk of atrial arrhythmias. If corrected in childhood, there may be normalization of the right atrial and right ventricular dimension, and there may be little to no residual pulmonary hypertension.

Patent Foramen Ovale

The patent foramen ovale (PFO) is found in up to 20% of the adult population. Usually, this is detected as an incidental finding on an echocardiogram. It may be related to neurologic events caused by paradoxical emboli. At present, there is controversy in the medical community about closing these defects with a catheter-based device after neurologic events. In most patients, this is uncomplicated by other CHD. Due to the risk of paradoxical emboli, when this has been noted, the patient should avoid scuba diving. With decompression, there is a risk of paradoxical air emboli entering the systemic circulation [1]. Professional divers should be screened for PFO with an echocardiogram and bubble study. If necessary, a transesophageal echo could be performed for definitive diagnosis. In the present time, the risk of scuba diving is not an indication for closure of an uncomplicated PFO.

Ventricular Septal Defect

A ventricular septal defect (VSD) may appear in the subpulmonic, membranous, or muscular portion of the septum. The subpulmonic defect is often detected in childhood and closed surgically. The muscular septal defect may comprise multiple ventricular defects, and after surgery, small shunts may persist. VSDs may be complicated by the Eisenmenger's syndrome (described above) with increased pulmonary blood flow and increasing pulmonary pressure causing the shunt to reverse to right-to-left; Central cyanosis ensues. The VSD may also be associated with aortic valve regurgitation as the aortic valve leaflet moves abnormally to attempt to close the defect. There may be tricuspid valve pouching, and there is an increased risk of endocarditis with this defect. These patients are often diagnosed in childhood, and if it is an uncomplicated VSD with low pulmonary artery pressures, they may be not repaired and may not need to be repaired in the future. However, if there has been endocarditis, aortic regurgitation due to the abnormal aortic valve leaflet motion or increasing pulmonary pressures, it is recommended that these defects be closed. After repair, the electrocardiogram is usually abnormal with a right bundle branch block pattern present, but the repair is usually performed through the right atrium and tricuspid valve, and therefore, there should be no significant scar as a nidus for arrhythmia. The VSD may also be part of other complex congenital heart disease presentations.

Patent Ductus Arteriosus

The ductus arteriosus is an important structure in fetal circulation that usually closes at birth. It may remain patent allowing shunting oxygenated blood between the aorta and pulmonary artery. This should be either closed with a catheter-based occluding coil or surgically ligated and incised. If this is repaired in childhood, there are usually no significant residual problems such as pulmonary hypertension. Even when diagnosed later in life, there may not be significant shunting and pulmonary hypertension associated with this lesion. It may be associated with other congenital cardiac lesions [9]. A larger, unrepaired patent ductus may result in cardiomegaly and pulmonary hypertension.

Anomalous Venous Return

Total anomalous venous return (TAPVR) is when all four pulmonary veins enter into the right atrium, shunting oxygenated blood into the right heart or pulmonary circulation. This causes enlargement of the right atrium and ventricle [10]. This is usually detected and corrected in childhood [10]. After repair, there may be no residual hemodynamic sequelae or exercise restriction [11]. Partial anomalous venous return of one to three pulmonary veins may not be detected until adulthood. It may be associated with as ASD [10].

Eisenmenger's Syndrome and Pulmonary Hypertension

Any unrepaired shunt lesion may result in the Eisenmenger's Syndrome or physiology. In these patients, volume overload of the pulmonary circulation results in irreversible pulmonary vascular changes. As pulmonary artery pressure increases, the right-sided pressures increase, causing shunts to reverse with ensuing cyanosis. These patients will have the highest incidence of symptoms and physical limitations. They may participate in low dynamic, noncompetitive sports. Patients with pulmonary hypertension for other reasons have similar limitations.

Valvular Lesions

Bicuspid Aortic Valve

The bicuspid aortic valve is probably the most common congenital heart lesion occurring in approximately 1% of the adult population and may remain undiagnosed into adulthood [8, 9]. This can be associated with early calcification of the valve and development of aortic stenosis and/or aortic insufficiency. In the presence of a bicuspid aortic valve, there may be no significant valve abnormality, and yet, progressive aortic dilatation may occur (see the Marfan chapter) [12, 13]. Valvular heart disease is discussed elsewhere in this book, but certainly, issues regarding the young athlete should be considered. Particularly, an aortic dilatation carries a risk of aortic dissection and rupture as the aorta widens [13]. Bicuspid aortic valve is also associated with other congenital abnormalities such as coarctation of the aorta.

Aortic Stenosis

The level of participation in patients with aortic stenosis is dictated by severity of the stenosis [11, 14]. This has been defined as mild aortic stenosis (≤30 mm peak to peak systolic gradient at catheterization and a mean echocardiographic Doppler gradient of ≤25 mmHg or a peak instantaneous echo Doppler gradient of ≤40 mmHg). Mild stenosis from a bicuspid aortic valve is usually well tolerated. Moderate stenosis (peak systolic gradient and catheterization of 30–50 mmHg; mean echo Doppler gradient of 25–40 mmHg and a peak instantaneous Doppler gradient of 40–70 mmHg) may be associated with symptoms with exercise, and therefore, stress testing is quite helpful if there are no symptoms reported by the patient. Severe aortic stenosis (a peak-to-peak systolic gradient by catheterization of >50 mmHg a mean echocardiographic Doppler gradient of >40 mmHg and a peak instantaneous echo Doppler gradient of >70 mmHg) is often associated with severe left ventricular hypertrophy, exertional syncope, chest pain, or dyspnea [11, 14]. There may be characteristic left ventricular strain pattern on the electrocardiogram, and there is risk of sudden death particularly with physical exertion. If patients have aortic stenosis and remain asymptomatic, limited careful stress testing may help illicit symptoms that would precipitate intervention for the severity of stenosis [11].

Aortic stenosis was the cause of sudden death in approximately 1% of athletes studied [9, 15, 16]. Surgical intervention such as Ross procedure or valvuloplasty may have occurred. These patients may be able to participate and compete after full evaluation [9]. In a study of 81 athletes with bicuspid aortic valve, 30 were assessed as high risk and disqualified from competition. All showed subsequent clinical decline over the observation period [16]. The patient may have a bioprosthesis or a mechanical valve. They may require long-term anticoagulation, which poses a risk in sports that may result in collision [11, 14].

Aortic Insufficiency

Aortic insufficiency is often seen with a bicuspid aortic valve and may be well tolerated for years. There may be progressive asymptomatic increase in the size of the left ventricle which would need to be followed serially [14]. Left ventricular dilatation may be associated with a decrease in function, and the aortic valve should be repaired or replaced. Aortic regurgitation is important to assess left ventricular function periodically. Theoretically, with exercise, regurgitant volume should decrease in patients with aortic insufficiency. Therefore, stress testing with echocardiography may be helpful. Patients with mild-to-moderate aortic regurgitation may be completely asymptomatic and be able to participate in athletics. When severe aortic regurgitation is present and the left ventricle is enlarged, valve replacement should be considered. Dilatation of the aorta may occur and would be important to follow due to the risk of aortic enlargement rupture and dissection for the athlete or in the general population [11, 14]. Sports with collision risk should be avoided.

Patients who may have had a mechanical or bioprosthetic aortic valve placed may have residual normal valve function with normal left ventricular function and be asymptomatic. These patients would need to be further evaluated with exercise testing prior to participating in sports. The other consideration is that patients who have had a valve replacement, particularly a mechanical valve replacement, may be on anticoagulation, and therefore, there is a risk in participating in sports where there is a risk of bodily collision [11, 14].

Coarctation of the Aorta

Coarctation or narrowing of the descending thoracic aorta occurs distal to the origin of left subclavian artery and may remain undiagnosed into adulthood. In the uncorrected coarctation, there may be decreased blood flow to the lower body due to blood flow through bronchial collateral arteries. If not sufficient, the patient may experience leg fatigue. If diagnosed in childhood, the coarctation is corrected with either a grafting procedure, bypass from the subclavian artery to the aorta coarctation, or intravascular stenting. After repair, the aorta adjacent to the patch may become aneurysmal, or restenosis may have occurred which is important to identify prior to sport participation. Physical diagnosis in these patients may establish the diagnosis with decreased blood pressure in the lower extremity compared to arm pressures. This difference may approximate the actual gradient across a residual coarctation. There is often a bicuspid aortic valve present [9]. Chest X-rays reveal classic rib notching due to the enlarged collateral vessels. It may be an associated bicuspid aortic valve with stenosis and and/or insufficiency. If a bicuspid aortic valve is present, progressive aortic dilatation must also be considered. Systemic hypertension may be present before and after coarctation [9]. After repair, these patients may exhibit near-normal oxygen uptake with cardiopulmonary testing [17]. Many of these patients are NYHA Class I and have near-normal exercise performance [18]. As with any other aortic pathology, the risk of collision during sports must be considered [11, 14].

Pulmonic Stenosis

Pulmonary stenosis is often found as part of other complex congenital heart problems and as an isolated lesion that may be detected in childhood and treated with balloon valvotomy. If the stenosis is either above or below the valve itself, it may require surgical correction. In adulthood, mild-to-moderate pulmonary stenosis (peak gradient less than 60 mmHg) is often well tolerated but may become more problematic as it increases, or if there is a dynamic increase in the gradient with exercise [11]. Severe stenosis (peak gradient greater than 60 mmHg) should be treated with balloon valvotomy, and post-procedure recommendations depend on residual gradient [11]. Valvotomy may be indicated in the symptomatic adult prior to participation in sports [9]. Usually after childhood repair of isolated pulmonary valve stenosis, there are few residual problems [9]. Pulmonary valve insufficiency is often a result of surgical intervention for isolated pulmonary stenosis or a more complex presentation. Progressive pulmonary insufficiency is severe; there may be dilatation and often dysfunction of the right ventricle. Pulmonary valve replacement may be required to preserve right ventricular function. Severe pulmonary insufficiency and right ventricular enlargement pose significant risk for arrhythmias and, sometimes, sudden death [9].

Ebstein's Anomaly

Ebstein's anomaly is the arterializations of the right ventricle, and therefore, there is a small right ventricle, which may be nonfunctional as the septal leaflet or the tricuspid valve is downwardly displaced causing the effective right atrium to increase. This results in the tricuspid regurgitation, and an associated ASD may result in right-to-left shunting and cyanosis. This is often recognized when children present cyanosis. However, variability in severity is often found in the older population [11]. If there is abnormal functional capacity, surgery is recommended to realign or to attempt to realign the tricuspid valve and to decrease significant tricuspid regurgitation. These patients may also have associated bypass tract and atrial arrhythmias [11].

Complex Congenital Heart Lesions

The complex congenital heart patients will invariably have had repair before seeking to participate in rigorous physical activity or athletics. It is important to identify the type of surgery that they have had and to evaluate the patients for the expected sequelae of these problems. Each problem presents a unique anatomical variant, and often after repair, the anatomy is not restored although physiology may be reestablished. After repair, many of these patients have developed arrhythmias due to scar tissue. They may not have had an anatomic repair, and they may have had a physiologic repair. They may have had a repair requiring artificial material which has a finite life span, and they may require future surgeries. Many times, because of extensive scarring, these patients may ultimately require a pacemaker and that is certainly another consideration (see chapter regarding). Systemic ventricular function may progressively decline [19]. Even right ventricular function may become impaired over time [19].

Tetralogy of Fallot

Tetralogy of Fallot is the most common cyanotic congenital heart disease that is seen in the adult due to the advances in surgery performed early in life. Tetralogy of Fallot includes right ventricular outflow tract obstruction often at the pulmonary valve, right ventricular hypertrophy, a VSD with an overriding aorta. Pentology of Fallot may also include an ASD. The repair requires closure of the VSD as to redirect the aorta over the left ventricle and enlargement of the pulmonary outflow tract either with or without valve replacement. Many of the patients may not receive valve replacement or may have had an enlargement of a right ventricular outflow tract in progressive pulmonary insufficiency [19]. Sequelae of this repair may be arrhythmias and heart block, eventually requiring pacemakers. The repairs have been occurring earlier in childhood, and therefore, the patients may have experienced normal development of the heart after their repair with few residual problems and very good functional capacity [19]. The majority of these patients will be NYHA Class I and have near-normal exercise performance [18].

Transposition of the Great Vessels

In classic transposition of the great arteries, the aorta arises from the right ventricle, and the left ventricle is in continuity with the pulmonary artery. The surgical repair of this problem has changed over time. In the past, an atrial switch procedure (Mustard Senning) was performed reversing incoming blood flow. After removing the interatrial septum, a baffle was then placed to direct the venous blood flow from the superior and inferior vena cavae across the mitral valve into the left ventricle and out the pulmonary arteries to receive oxygenation. Oxygenated blood through the pulmonary veins is directed by way of another baffle across what has become the common atrium to the tricuspid valve of the right ventricle and out the aorta. After this procedure, because of the extensive surgery in the atria, patients were at risk for atrial arrhythmias, junctional rhythms, and heart block. Many patients require pacemakers. The major long-term concern is whether the right ventricle, which is the systemic ventricle, can sustain systemic ventricular function. It often dilates to improve its systolic function and may fail relatively early in life. More recently, patients have been undergoing an arterial switch operation to transect the great vessels switch position and reattach to their appropriate ventricles, and the coronary arteries are reimplanted (Jatene procedure). This surgery too may have sequelae later in life including coronary artery problems and aortic valve pathology but their ventricular function should be normal or near-normal.

In congenitally corrected transposition of the great arteries, the morphologic right ventricle is on the left side and in continuity with the aorta. Although there is appropriate flow of deoxygenated and oxygenated blood within the heart, it is the right ventricle that bears the systemic circulation and therefore may dilate over time. The natural history of congenitally corrected or L-transposition may entail arrhythmias, the development of progressive heart block, progressive pulmonic valve stenosis, and a VSD [11]. These patients may not present until adulthood when they develop heart block. The diagnosis is made by echocardiography, which reveals that the systemic ventricle is morphologically a right ventricle. The diagnosis may be made in childhood if associated with other congenital heart defects.

Single Ventricle Variants

Patients born with a single functioning ventricle or with a relatively normal ventricle and a diminutive right or left ventricle may have had surgery earlier in life to create an (extra cardiac) right ventricle as in the Glenn/Fontan procedures. Patients may have been born with a single functioning ventricle due to a variety of defects such as tricuspid atresia with an underdeveloped right ventricle. They may have a double-outlet right ventricle or double-inlet left ventricle variation. They would have had a series of operations to direct the systemic circulation to the aorta. The single ventricle, whether more physiologically a right or left ventricle, becomes the systemic ventricle. The single ventricle then becomes dedicated to the systemic circulation. The Glenn shunt directs superior vena cava blood flow into the right pulmonary artery. The Fontan procedure directs the inferior vena cava flow to the pulmonary artery either by way of the shunt or directly. Therefore, these patients do not have a functional right ventricle with pulsatile flow into the pulmonary arteries. Their ventricular function may be normal or impaired, and each patient is unique and needs to be evaluated. After Fontan surgery, 13–44% patients may require pacemaker implantation [19].

Tricuspid Atresia. Children born with a tricuspid atresia have a small or absent tricuspid valve, and therefore, there is rarely development of a normal right ventricle. Therefore, functionally they only have a left, systemic ventricle and undergo a Fontan procedure.

The morphologic right ventricle acting as a systemic ventricle may fail over the time. It is important to monitor ventricular function throughout life and institute appropriate therapy. These post-Fontan patients may demonstrate decreased oxygen uptake with cardiopulmonary testing [17].

Congenital Coronary Anomalies

Coronary artery anomalies are quite rare in the general population; however, it has been reported in up to 20% of sudden deaths during or immediately after sports [9, 20]. This diagnosis may not be made prior to the sudden death episode in young patients. The anomalous origin of the left main coronary artery from the pulmonary artery is often associated with sudden death in childhood or adulthood. It may have resulted in left ventricular dysfunction without an episode of sudden death. The anomalous origin of the left coronary artery also has been associated with sudden death when it passes between the aorta and the pulmonary artery. This may occur particularly with exertion. If this is known, the patients need to be restricted from exercise or undergo intervention [9]. This may be diagnosed by stress testing, multislice CT, or cardiac MRI/MRA.

These patients were in a study of sudden death occurring during athletic activity. 20% were due to anomalous coronary arteries in the athletes, and the difficult issue is that this may not have been previously diagnosed (see chapter regarding this topic) [9]. Sudden death is commonly associated with anomalies in left main artery originating from the sinus of Valsalva [3]. Other anomalies may affect older athletes.

Evaluation for Preparticipation Screening

As determined from the discussion above, each of these athletes/patients is unique, and each one should have an extensive evaluation and possibly even serial evaluations both prior to participating in physical activity or athletics. It is recommended that the preparticipation evaluation be conducted by both the primary care physician, in consultation with a cardiologist familiar in evaluating such athletes/patients. The athlete may enjoy full participation if certain criteria are met through the evaluation process.

History and Physical Examination

Highlights of the history and physical examination that are important to identify the patient at risk for participation during sports are summarized in Table 17.1. The history should include the history prior of the initial lesion at birth and the history of the interventions that have occurred since that time [9]. Operative notes are particularly useful to help describe the patient's current anatomy [9]. Records detailing prior intervention and surgery are important. There should be careful

Table 17.1 Pre-participation evaluation

History
Cardiac symptoms at rest and with activity
Prior intervention/surgery
Subjective functional assessment
Family history
Medications [1]
Examination
Arm – leg pressures; arterial pulses
Heart sounds
Murmurs, arrhythmias
Note scars from prior surgeries
Hepatomegaly
Edema
Electrocardiogram
Chamber enlargement/hypertrophy
Arrhythmias/bundle branch block
Ischemia
QRS duration
Ambulatory ECG monitoring
Arrhythmia detection
Periodic monitoring after repair
Echocardiography
Anatomy
Valve morphology and function
Ventricular function
Pulmonary vascular resistance estimate
Intracardiac shunting
Exercise testing
Functional capacity
Ventricular reserve
Arrhythmia provocation

Adapted from [1, 2, 11]

delineation of cardiac symptoms that could be a harbinger for problems during exercise [21]. The patient's subjective functional assessment may correlate with cardiopulmonary testing of maximal oxygen uptake [22]. It is also important to delineate the physical demands of the anticipated activity. Other medical problems that could impact on their participation during sports should be identified. Family history of others born with heart disease should be identified. Specifically, if there have been lesions associated with sudden death such as coronary artery anomalies, valvular heart disease, or aortic pathology [21]. Medications, vitamins, and dietary supplements should be identified [23].

The physical examination should include a general examination with focus upon all of the arterial pulses and on any differences between arm and leg pressures to help determine unpreviously undetected aortic coarctation [1, 2, 9, 11]. Complete cardiac examination for heart sounds, murmurs, or abnormal arrhythmias should be detected. Scars that may highlight prior surgeries that have not been discussed may also be noted at that time. The patient should be examined for hepatomegaly and certain other problems.

Electrocardiogram

Before or after repair, the adult with CHD might have an abnormal electrocardiogram (ECG). The screening ECG may help identify the athlete with previously undiagnosed CHD. The electrocardiogram may be useful in this patient population to determine evidence of heart block that often occurs after surgery. The electrocardiogram may detect bypass tracts as seen in the Wolff Parkinson White syndrome, or it may detect a prior infarction due to surgical complications or the presence of congenital coronary artery anomalies. For example, after VSD closure, a right bundle branch block may be present [24]. In a series of athletes with abnormal screening, ECG aortic stenosis, dilated cardiomyopathy, and coronary anomalies were detected [24]. ECG findings included left ventricular hypertrophy, bundle branch block, and prior infarct [23]. Ambulatory electrocardiographic monitoring (Holter, 30 day event monitor) should be performed regularly in patients at risk for sudden death. This mode of testing is useful to identify the cause of palpitations such as junctional arrhythmias, heart block, or supraventricular arrhythmias.

Echocardiogram

The echocardiogram is essential in diagnosing these patients. The echocardiogram can provide information regarding residual shunt, right and left ventricular function, and cardiac chamber dimensions. It also shows valvular function. The echocardiogram also permits visualization of the proximal aortic root. This test should be done serially and a schedule established for periodic testing to monitor valve function or ventricular function as needed. Pulmonary artery pressure may be estimated by Doppler echocardiography and the flow velocity of the tricuspid regurgitant jet [9]. A transesophageal echocardiogram may also be helpful for further identification of ASD or valvular abnormalities.

Stress Testing

Stress testing is important to assess functional capacity and for provocation of arrhythmia in this patient population and should be done periodically [3]. Sinus node dysfunction after surgery may limit the heart rate response to exercise [25]. This may take the form of cardiopulmonary testing to measure O_2 uptake and aerobic capacity, a treadmill with electrocardiographic monitoring alone or combined with imaging [17, 19, 25]. Imaging with echocardiography permits assessment of ventricular reserve and valve hemodynamics at rest and with exercise. Pulmonary artery pressure changes with exercise can also be estimated. A study of cardiopulmonary testing in patients with a variety of CHD revealed that patients with Eisenmenger's physiology, after Fontan repair, and CC-TGA had the lower uptake. Patients with aortic coarctation repair had near-normal values of oxygen uptake [17]. One explanation for lower exercise capacity in these patients is sinus node dysfunction resulting in limited heart rate response with exercise [25]. This testing should be done in asymptomatic patients who have had a complex repair to detect arrhythmias.

MRI/MRA and CT

MRI and CT scanning have an increasing role in the assessment of patients with congenital heart disease. Patients who have had a pacemaker or ICD may be referred for a CT scan and those without them may have an MRI to help find the anatomy to look at great vessel abnormality that may occur over time and to assess anatomic repairs. The CT angiogram or MRI/MRA (magnetic resonance angiography) may detect coronary artery anomalies [2]. The latter may be preferred so as to avoid large doses of radiation being administered to young individuals.

Cardiac Catheterization

Cardiac catheterization may be recommended for the best assessment of pulmonary artery pressures if a concern is raised by echocardiography and may be indicated. Cardiac catheterization may also be performed in anticipation of device closure for shunt lesion or for valvuloplasty with residual stenosis.

Recommendations

Recommendations for participation in exercise and athletic activities need to be uniquely tailored for the patients presenting diagnoses and sequelae of prior intervention. In general, patients with congenital heart disease may have sinus node

Table 17.2 General recommendations for patients with shunt lesions

Lesion	Hemodynamics/complications	Sports recommendation
ASD, unrepaired	Normal	All sports
	Mild pulmonary hypertension	IA[a]
	Cyanosis	No sports
	Mitral regurgitation	No sports
ASD, repaired	Arrhythmias	Individualized prescription
	Elevated pulmonary pressure or myocardial dysfunction	Individualized prescription
AV canal repair	Residual mitral regurgitation	IA, IB, IIA[a]
	None of the above (3–6 months after repair)	All sports
PFO	Residual shunt	No scuba diving
VSD, unrepaired	Normal	All sports
	Severe pulmonary hypertension	No sports
VSD, repaired	Arrhythmias/heart block	Individualized prescription
	Elevated pulmonary artery pressure	Individualized prescription
	Ventricular dysfunction	Further evaluation
	Severe pulmonary hypertension	No sports
	None of the above 3–6 months after repair	All sports
PDA, unrepaired	Normal LV	All sports
	LV enlarged from large shunt	Close first then evaluate
	Severe pulmonary hypertension	No sports
PDA, repaired	Residual pulmonary hypertension	(see below)
	Normal LV/pulmonary pressure (3 months after closure)	All sports
Total/partial anomalous venous return		
Unrepaired, partial	Normal	All sports
Repaired	Normal	All sports
Elevated pulmonary pressure	<30 mmHg	All sports
	>30 mmHg	Individual prescription
Eisenmenger's	Elevated pulmonary pressure, cyanosis	IA[a]/no competitive sports

Adapted from [1, 11, 14]

ASD atrial septal defect, *PFO* patent foramen ovale, *VSD* ventricular septal defect, *PDA* patent ductus arteriosus

[a] See Table 17.5

dysfunction and demonstrate a limited heart rate response to exercise [25]. Specific lesions are detailed in Tables 17.2–17.4 and divided into shunt lesions (Table 17.2), valvular lesions (Table 17.3), and complex congenital heart lesions (Table 17.4). These recommendations have been compiled from both the European Society of Cardiology [1] and the Bethesda consensus [11], but certainly each exercise and participation prescription needs to be individualized to the patient's needs and problems [16].

It is important to take into account the type of exercise that is required to complete the athletic activity and to participate fully. Exercise can be divided into

Table 17.3 General recommendations for patients with congenital valve disease

Lesion	Hemodynamics/complications	Sports recommendations
Bicuspid aortic valve		
Mild stenosis	Normal ECG/Stress test	All sports
Moderate stenosis	No symptoms or arrhythmias	
	No LVH on ECG	IA, IB, IIA[a]
	Normal stress test	
	SVT or VEA	IA, IB[a]
Severe stenosis	(see text to define)	No sports
After intervention/surgery	Residual AS-see above	Based on residual AS
Aortic insufficiency	Depends on LV and aortic root size	Individualized prescription
Aortic dilation	<40 mm	All sports
	40–45 mm	IA, IB, IIA, IIB (avoid collision)
	≥45 mm	IA only
Coarctation of the aorta		
Mild	No collaterals	All sports (avoid collision)
	No aortic root dilatation	All sports (avoid collision)
	Gradient ≤20 mmHg	All sports (avoid collision)
	Gradient ≥20 mmHg	
Moderately/severe	Exercise BP ≥230 mmHg	IA[a]
Pulmonary stenosis (PS)	Peak systolic gradient ≤40 mmHg	All sports
	Peak systolic gradient ≥40 mmHg	Consider valvuloplasty first: IA, IB, IIA[a]
After surgery/ valvuloplasty	Mild PS or 2–4 weeks after valvuloplasty	All sports
Pulmonary insufficiency	Severe RV enlargement	IA, IB[a]
After intervention	<1 year after intervention	IA, IB, IIA, IIB[a]
(3 months)	Aortic dilation	IA, IB[a]
Ebstein's anomaly	No cyanosis, normal RV	All sports
	No arrhythmias	
	Tricuspid regurgitation with moderate arrhythmia	IA, IB[a]; no competitive sports
Severe		No sports
After repair	No/mild tricuspid regurgitation	IA[a]
	No arrhythmias	

Adapted from [1, 9, 11, 14, 25]

LVH left ventricular hypertrophy, *ECG* electrocardiogram, *SVT* supraventricular tachycardia, *VEA* ventricular arrhythmias, *RV* right ventricle

[a] See Table 17.5

those activities that require dynamic or static effort. Dynamic activity results in increased oxygen uptake, increased heart rate, increased systolic pressure, and decreased diastolic pressure [27, 28]. Isometric or static exercises results in an increased heart rate, increased systemic blood pressure, and an increase in diastolic blood pressure which could be problematic in certain types of cardiac lesions [28]. Over time, these changes may result in left ventricular hypertrophy [9].

Table 17.4 General recommendations for patients with repaired complex congenital heart lesions

Lesion	Hemodynamics	Recommendation
Tetralogy of Fallot (repaired)	Normal right heart pressure	All sports
	No/mild RV volume overload	(avoid collision)
	No residual shunt	
	No arrhythmias	
	Pulmonary regurgitation or RV pressure >50 mmHg	IA[a]
	Arrhythmias	Individual prescription
Transposition of great arteries		
After atrial switch	No/mild chamber enlargement	IA, IIA[a]
	No atrial arrhythmias	
	No syncope	
	Normal stress test	
After arterial switch	Normal function with stress test	All sports
	No arrhythmias	
	Mild hemodynamic abnormality	IA, IB, IC[a]
	Ventricular dysfunction	IIA[a]
	Normal stress test	
Congenitally corrected	No symptoms	IA, IIA[a]
	No associated abnormalities	IB[a]
	No systolic ventricular enlargement	(no competitive)
	Normal stress test	
Postoperative Fontan	Normal ventricular function	IA, IB[a] (no competitive)

Adapted from [1, 11]
RV right ventricle
[a] See Table 17.5

Resistance training enhances strength and endurance but is contraindicated in the setting of pulmonary hypertension, decompensated congestive heart failure, aortic dissection, and uncontrolled arrhythmias [27].

Table 17.5 gives examples or particular activities associated with low or moderate dynamic and static activity to help understand the physical demands of a particular sport [28]. These recommendations are compiled from both the European Cardiac Society and 30th Bethesda Conference and should be considered as general guidelines [1, 11, 26, 27]. Also, it is important to look at the patient's risk of collision especially when there are grafts in place, as in a patient with coarctation or if the patient is on systemic anticoagulation and the risk of bleeding [2, 9]. It is important to identify the risk of sudden death in the athletes and the propensity for sudden death given their underlying cardiac problem, and this would be an important element to look at during the preparticipation evaluation [7–9]. The third major risk

Table 17.5 Intensity of sports: common examples

IA: Low static- low dynamic activity	
Billiards	Curling
Bowling	Golf
Cricket	Riflery
IB: Low static- moderate dynamic activity	
Baseball/softball[a]	Volleyball
Table tennis	Fencing
IC: Low static- high dynamic activity	
Badminton	Racquetball/squash[a]
Cross-country skiing	Running
Field hockey[a]	Soccer[a]
Orienteering	Tennis
Race walking	
IIA: Moderate static- low dynamic activity	
Archery	Equestrian[a]
Auto-racing[a]	Motorcycling[a]
Diving	

Adapted from [2, 6]
[a]Collision risk associated with this activity

that has been seen in the athletic population is the risk of aortic dissection. This would be risk for the patient with aortic dilatation from a bicuspid aortic valve, and certainly, participation in static exercise may further increase their risk [6]. Specific contraindications such as severe pulmonary hypertension, decompensated congestive heart failure, aortic dissection, and uncontrolled arrhythmias are important issues in this patient population [11].

Specific recommendations are detailed by lesions in Tables 17.2–17.4. In general, patients who are unrestricted from sports participation will have had an anatomic correction. They are subjectively NYHA Class I and have a normal physical examination, electrocardiogram, and stress testing. There have been no arrhythmias on Holter monitoring or stress testing. If minor abnormalities are present, the exercise prescription will need to be individualized. Patients generally prohibited from sports participation may only have had palliative procedures and have significant unoperated lesions or univentricular hearts. Patients will be restricted if the symptoms moderate activity (NYHA Class 2), palpitations, or syncope. Electrocardiographic evidence of ischemia, QRS prolongation, left ventricular hypertrophy, or arrhythmia will result in restricted activity. Elevated valvular gradients or pulmonary artery pressure by echocardiography would also necessitate restriction in athletic activities [1, 11].

Shunt lesions either unrepaired or repaired may be well tolerated in the young adult and adult population. Their level of participation really depends on the extended residual pulmonary artery pressure [9]. Specific recommendations are important regarding frequency of assessment as well as conditions for participations (Table 17.2).

The recommendations regarding participation in sports in patients with valvular heart disease depend upon the severity of the residual valve disease, whether it is unrepaired or it had been previously addressed (Table17.3). Residual left ventricular hypertrophy and symptoms may identify the patient at risk [9]. The particular population with valvular heart disease risk of sudden death would be associated with arrhythmias, sudden death, and left ventricular hypertrophy, and therefore, the evaluation would look for these elements, and the dictations may be required to be followed periodically to look for any development of arrhythmias, progression of aortic dilatation, or development of left ventricular hypertrophy.

Patients who have complex congenital heart lesions have had palliation or repair in childhood. These particular risks are unique to the type of surgery, sequelae of surgery, and residual lesions. These patients are extremely unique, and most of these patients in the young adult and adult population who seek participation in athletic events will have undergone a type of repair. They may need a series of repairs, and the preparticipation evaluation should identify the common lesions and valvular lesions, which are summarized in Table17.3.

Cases

Case 1: Bicuspid Aortic Valve

A 20-year-old soccer player was found to have a bicuspid aortic valve as an incidental finding. The echocardiogram revealed mild aortic regurgitation and normal ventricular function. The proximal ascending aorta measured 46 mm. The MRI revealed maximal aortic dimension of 47 mm.

Recommendation:
No competitive sports due to risk of aortic dissection or rupture.

Discussion:
A bicuspid aortic valve is the most common congenital lesion identified in the young adult/adult population, occurring in 1–2% of the population. Aortic dilatation may occur in the absence of aortic stenosis or regurgitation. Aortic dilatation poses a significant risk, and the aorta may increase in size over time.

Case 2

An 18-year-old male presented for preparticipation evaluation for a Division I college soccer team. He was born with Tetralogy of Fallot and had complete repair at age 2 years. He denied symptoms and had excellent functional capacity. An echocardiogram revealed minimal right ventricular enlargement, normal left ventricular function, and moderate pulmonary valve regurgitation.

A stress test with echocardiography revealed normal right and left ventricular reserve without worsening of pulmonic regurgitation. There were no provokable arrhythmias during the test. Holter monitoring was recommended and was negative for arrhythmia. He was approved for 1 year of participation provided no symptoms or changes in his functional capacity occurred in the interim. Despite pulmonary artery regurgitation, he demonstrated normal right ventricular reserve. The lack of arrhythmias during daily activity and with exercise needs to be established prior to sports participation.

References

1. Hirth, A, Reybrouck, T, Bjarnason-Wehrens, B, et al. Recommendations for participation in competitive and leisure sports in patients with congenital heart disease: a consensus document. Eur J Cardiovasc Prev Rehabil. 2006:13:293–299.
2. Maron, BJ, Douglas, PS, Thompson, PD. Task Force 1. Preparticipation screening and diagnosis of cardiovascular disease in athletes. J Am Coll Cardiol. 2005:45:1322–1326.
3. Thaulow, E, Fredriksen, PM. Exercise and training in adults with congenital heart disease. Int J Cardiol. 2004:97:35–38.
4. Dua, JS, Cooper, AR, Fox, KR, et al. Physical activity levels in adults with congenital heart disease. Eur J Cardiovasc Prev Rehabil. 2007:14:287–293.
5. Pigozzi, F, Rizzo, M. Sudden death in competitive athletes. Clin Sports Med.2008: 27:153–181.
6. Thompson, PD, Franklin, BA, Balady, GJ, et al. Exercise and acute cardiovascular events: Placing the risks into perspective. Circulation. 2007:115:2358–2368.
7. Scharhag, J, Meyer, T, Kindermann, I, et al. Bicuspid aortic valve. Clin Res Cardiol. 2006:95:228–234.
8. Maron, B. Cardiovascular disease in athletes. In Zipes, D, Libby, P, Bonow, R, Braunwald E (eds) Baunwald's heart disease: a textbook of cardiovascular medicine. 7th edition. Elsevier Saunders, Philadelphia. 2004:1985–1991.
9. Dent, JM. Congenital heart disease and exercise. Clin Sports Med. 2003:22:81–99.
10. Kaplan, S, Perloff, J. Survival patterns after cardiac surgery or Interventional catheterization. In Perloff JK, Child, J (eds) Congenital heart disease in adults. WB Saunders, Philapdelphia. 1998:54–58.
11. Graham, TP, Driscoll, DJ, Gersony, WM, et al. Task force 2: Congenital heart disease. J Am Coll Cardiol. 2005:45:1326–1333.
12. Stefani, L, Galanti, G, Toncelli, L, et al. Bicuspid aortic valve in competitive athletes. Br J Sports Med. 2008:42:31–35.
13. Galanti, G, Stefani, L, Vano, MC, et al. Effects of sports activity in athletes with bicuspid aortic valve and regurgitation. Br J Sports Med. 2010:44:275–279.
14. Bonow, RO, Cheitlin, MD, Crawford, MH, et al. Task force 3: Valvular heart disease. J Am Coll Cardiol. 2005:45:1334–1340.
15. Maron, BJ. Sudden death in young athletes. N Engl J Med. 2003:349:1064–1075.
16. Spataro, A, Pelliccia, A, Rizzo, M, et al. The natural course of bicuspid aortic valve in athletes. Int J Sports Med. 2008:29:81–85.
17. Giardini, A, Specchia, S, Berton, E, et al. Strong and independent prognostic value of peak circulatory power in adults with congenital heart disease. Am Heart J. 2007:154:441–447.

18. Dimopoulos, K, Okonko, DO, Diller, GP, et al. Abnormal ventilatory response to exercise in adults with congenital heart disease relates to cyanosis and predicts survival. Circulation. 2006:113:2796–2802.
19. Dimopoulos, K, Diller, GP, Piepoli, MF, et al. Exercise intolerance in adults with congenital heart disease. Cardiol Clin. 2006:24:641–660.
20. Vogt, S, Koenig, D, Prettin, S, et al. Unusual cause of exercise-induced ventricle fibrillation in a well-trained adult endurance athlete: a case report. J Med Case Reports. 2008:2:1–5.
21. Giese, EA, O'Connor, FG, Brennan, FH, PJ, et al. The athletic preparticipation evaluation: Cardiovascular assessment. Am Fam Physician. 2007:75:1008–1014.
22. Dimopoulos, K, Diller, GP, Okonko, D, et al. Exercise intolerance in adult congenital heart disease. Circulation. 2005:112:828–835.
23. Seto, CK. Preparticipation cardiovascular screening. Clin Sports Med. 2003:22:23–35.
24. Lawless, CE, Best, TM. Electrocardiograms in athletes: Interpretation and diagnostic accuracy. Med Sci Sports Exerc. 2008:40:787–798.
25. Ohuchi, H, Wantanabe, K, Kishiki, K, et al. Heart rate dynamics during and after exercise in postoperative congenital heart disease patients. Their relation to cardiac autonomic nervous activity and intrinsic sinus node dysfunction. Am Heart J. 2007:154:165–171.
26. Maron, BJ, Chaitman, BR, Ackerman, MJ, et al. Recommendations for physical activity and recreational sports participation for young patients with genetic cardiovascular disease. Circulation. 2004:109:2807–2816.
27. Williams, MA, Haskell, WL, Ades, PA, et al. Resistance exercise in individuals with and without cardiovascular disease: 2007 Update. Circulation. 2007:116:572–584.
28. Mitchell, JH, Haskell, W, Snell, P, et al. Task force 8: Classification of sports. J Am Coll Cardiolol. 2005:45:1364–1367.

Chapter 18
Athlete with a Device: Implantable Cardioverter Defibrillators and Pacemakers

Rachel Lampert and J. Philip Saul

Case 1. WK is a former collegiate varsity basketball player who at age 19 had a frank syncopal spell while running during practice. Cardiologic evaluation demonstrated unequivocal hypertrophic cardiomyopathy (HCM) and an implantable cardioverter defibrillator (ICD) was implanted. There was no family history of sudden cardiac death (SCD). Appeal was made to three Division I universities that he continue to play but all refused based on the Bethesda guidelines [1]. He finally played 2 years of varsity basketball at the University of Texas, El Paso, never receiving a shock. The ICD was interrogated after each practice game to insure lead integrity and proper device function. He now coaches basketball at a college in California [2].

Case 2. KB, a former collegiate varsity basketball player who suffered a cardiac arrest, was diagnosed with the long QT syndrome and received an ICD. After a year and half away from competition, she returned, and played 44 games. She then received three appropriate shocks during a game, and retired from play in 2006, describing that "it felt like a bomb exploding in my chest…it is no longer safe for me to play Division I basketball" [3].

Case 3. AF, an 18-year-old female, presented at 2 years of age with 2:1 atrioventricular (AV) heart block that progressed to complete heart block by 5 years of age. She did well with heart rates above 60 beats/min until the age of 7 when Holter monitoring demonstrated heart rates down to 27 beats/min and pauses of up to 3 s. She underwent transvenous dual-chamber pacemaker implantation from the left shoulder at the age of 7.5 years. At about 9 years of age, she began playing softball and eventually developed skills as a slow-pitch then fast-pitch right handed pitcher. A low level of traumatic risk to the device was discussed, as well as the fact that she had an adequate escape rhythm. After that discussion, her parents had a specially designed chest vest constructed with a circular offshoot that covers the device. She has played competitively at the high school and regional levels since

R. Lampert (✉)
Section of Cardiology, Yale University School of Medicine, New Haven, CT, USA
e-mail: rachel.lampert@yale.edu

C.E. Lawless (ed.), *Sports Cardiology Essentials: Evaluation, Management and Case Studies*, DOI 10.1007/978-0-387-92775-6_18,

then without pacemaker injury and has a scholarship to college where she plans to play softball competitively.

An increasing number of young athletes with serious electrical or structural cardiac abnormalities, most commonly HCM, long QT, Brugada syndrome, or arrhythmogenic right ventricular dysplasia, receive ICDs on clinically indicated grounds. Others, such as those with congenital complete heart block, or sinus or AV node dysfunction following surgery for structural congenital heart disease, may require permanent pacemakers [4]. Many wish to continue participation in organized sports. Whether they should be allowed to do so is currently a controversial subject [2, 5], and the situation can present a medical and ethical challenge for the treating physician. The conflict is quickly resolved if there is left ventricular dysfunction limiting exercise capacity or exercise-induced serious arrhythmias which would preclude competition. However, while patients with an ICD or pacemaker but no left ventricular compromise or other functional impairment may wish to continue high school or collegiate sports, current guidelines for ICD patients recommend against any competitive sports more vigorous than "Class IA" activities, such as bowling or golf [1], restricting competition in sports such as track, basketball, lacrosse, or field hockey, as well as sports with a likelihood of severe impact to the ICD, such as football and hockey. For patients with a pacemaker, the recommendation is avoidance of sports with danger of bodily collision, however, sports in which that danger is less may be practiced [1].

The postulated risks of sports, on which these restrictions are based, include increased frequency of ventricular arrhythmias, potential failure of a shock to convert a life-threatening arrhythmia, damage to the device or lead system, or risk of harm due to momentary loss of control from an arrhythmia or from the ICD shock itself [1]. The risk of exercise in patients with an ICD stems from their underlying arrhythmogenic myocardial substrate and not from the ICD itself. However, if the ICD effectively terminates arrhythmias during sporting activities, without adverse sequelae, participation in athletics becomes an issue of quality of life. Some data indicate that ICD shocks can decrease quality of life [6], yet restriction from sports may have a similar impact. For example, while collegiate athletes, in general, report higher quality of life than non-athlete students, on psychological as well as physical measures, quality of life for athletes sidelined even with a minor injury goes down, not only in comparison to students actively playing, but also in comparison with more sedentary individuals [7].

Postulated Risks of Sports

Triggering of Arrhythmia

It is highly likely that sports competition will in fact increase the likelihood of ventricular arrhythmias and subsequent ICD shocks. In the Physician's Health Study, exercise substantially increased the relative risk of SCD [8], and in a series of young victims of SCD, the relative risk for athletes was 2.5 [9], most of whom die during exercise [9, 10]. Exercise is known to exacerbate ventricular arrhythmias in HCM, arrhythmogenic right ventricular dysplasia, and the long QT syndrome [11]. Moderate exertion can trigger sustained ventricular arrhythmias in patients with an ICD [12].

Unknown Efficacy of the ICD During Sports

Whether the ICD can terminate ventricular arrhythmias occurring during exercise is unknown. Exercise increases potassium [13], which increases defibrillation thresholds (DFT) [14], decreases pH [15], and increases catecholamines [16], any of which could potentially render arrhythmias more difficult to terminate. For example, infusion of epinephrine at doses mimicking exercise minimally increased DFT and decreased first-shock efficacy in ICD patients undergoing DFT testing [17]. Other studies, however, have shown a beneficial [18] effect of epinephrine on DFT. The DFT is minimally higher, and first-shock efficacy less in the morning [19], the period of highest catecholamine levels [20]. The efficacy of anti-tachycardia pacing appears to be decreased with increased catecholamine levels during laboratory-induced mental stress in patients with an ICD; however, all shocks were effective [21]. Also, ischemia can increase the DFT [22] and is associated with an increased frequency of reinitiation of ventricular fibrillation [22]. However, it remains unknown whether there is a decreased success of the ICD in terminating ventricular arrhythmias during vigorous physical exertion.

Arrhythmic death in ICD patients is extremely rare [23–25], and this appears to be true during exertion. In 1,846 patients with an epicardial ICD, the reported incidence of tachyarrhythmic SCD was 0.8% [23], while it was 1% of 4,787 patients [24] and 1.8% of 4,889 patients [25] receiving a transvenous device. In all three series, electromechanical dissociation following multiple shocks was the most common mechanism of demise, followed by shock failure and incessantly recurrent ventricular arrhythmia. In most patients, advanced congestive heart failure or other underlying precipitants were present, and many had an increase in shocks in the preceding month [23], suggesting these were not acutely triggered events in otherwise stable patients such as those who would be participating in sports. Overall, the ICD effectively reduces SCD risk in multiple subgroups of patients including those with HCM [26, 27], arrhythmogenic right ventricular dysplasia [28], and the long QT syndrome [29].

There are two reported cases of shock failure during exercise. One patient died of intractable ventricular tachycardia during a treadmill test [23]. In this patient, an ethmozine-induced increase in DFT had been noted previously. A second patient during exercise following very heavy alcohol ingestion had stable ventricular tachycardia persist despite multiple ICD shocks [30]. Whether the ICD would be ineffective during exercise not complicated by Class IC anti-arrhythmic drugs or alcohol ingestion is unknown.

Several series do report successful conversions during exercise. Among a group of ICD recipients with HCM, 8 appropriate shocks were delivered during competitive sports and another 12 during vigorous noncompetitive activities. All were successful [27].

Nonarrhythmic Injury to the Athlete

A second potential risk of sports participation in ICD patients is the possibility of injury due to syncope from an arrhythmia or fall related to the shock itself. However, it seems unlikely that this risk would be greater during sports than during driving. Among participants in the AVID trial, most patients had resumed driving, and while shocks during driving occurred in 8%, the accident rate was actually lower than that of the general population [31].

Damage to the ICD System

The third potential risk of sports participation is damage to the ICD system due to direct trauma or repetitive arm motion.

Preliminary Safety and Efficacy Data: Survey Data

Three recent surveys of physicians caring for patients with an ICD or pacemaker have attempted to gather preliminary information about current sports participation in athletes with these devices [32–34].

Current Recommendations by Physicians

In 2006, all 1,687 physician members of the Heart Rhythm Society (HRS), a professional organization for electrophysiologists and others involved in the treatment of heart rhythm disturbances, were surveyed [33], with 614 responding. Recommendations by physicians to ICD patients regarding participation in sports varied widely (Fig. 18.1) and most respondents individualized recommendations. Few respondents (10%) counseled ICD patients to avoid all activities more vigorous than golf or bowling, but most did recommend against contact sports (76%). Some advised against competitive sports (45%) or sports with particular risk of injury (35%), including those involving heights, such as rock climbing or bungee jumping. Many physicians individualized recommendations based on underlying cardiac disease (71%). While there was consensus among many physicians that

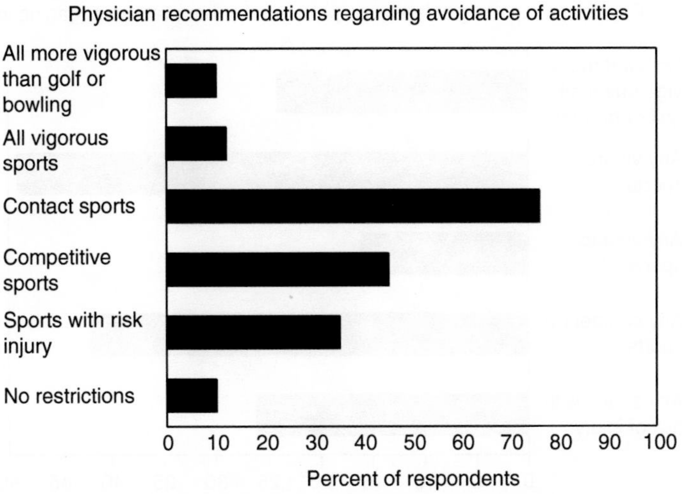

Fig. 18.1 Physician recommendations for restrictions (HRS survey). Reprinted from Lampert et al., "Safety of sports for patients with implantable cardioverter-defibrillators", J Cardiovasc Electrophysiol, 1/06, Blackwell Publishing. Permission has been granted from Blackwell Publishing

HCM, congestive heart failure, and ischemic disease should limit activity, opinions differed regarding how long QT syndrome and Brugada syndrome should affect sports participation. Some respondents lifted at least some restrictions after an arrhythmia-free period, most frequently 6 months or 1 year.

In a survey of members of the American Medical Society of Sports Medicine (AMSSM), 438 physicians responded, 91% of whom were team physicians and 17% of whom had cared for 81 athletes with an ICD. Their attitudes toward sports participation for patients with an ICD was similarly varied to the HRS cohort, with only 40% recommending against all vigorous sports, but a greater number recommending against contact sports [32].

Similarly, a recent survey of the Pediatric and Congenital Electrophysiology Society (PACES) found a wide variation in physician recommendations for sports participation for patients with pacemakers [34]. Among the 60 respondents, for a patient with an adequate escape rhythm, 18% of practitioners approved all sports, leaving 82% who did not allow at least one. Level of contact, level of competition, and adequacy of escape rhythm had the largest influence on recommendations.

Physician-Reported Sports Participation and Outcomes

In the HRS survey, sports participation by ICD patients appears to be common [33]. Overall, 70% of the HRS physicians reported that patients in their practice engaged in some form of sporting activity, with basketball, running, and skiing

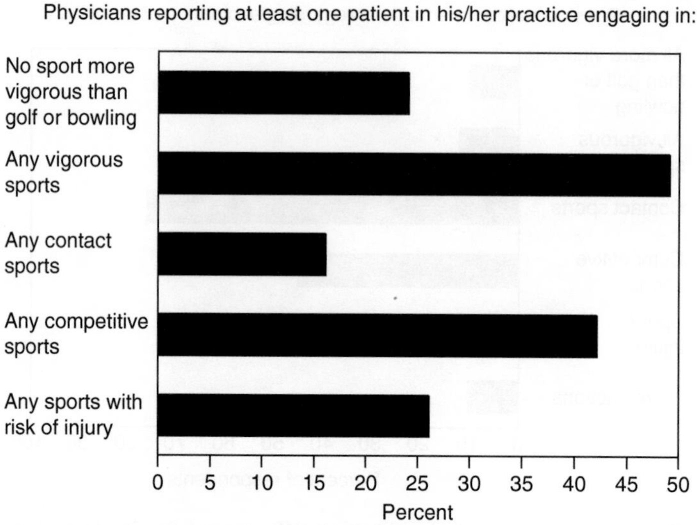

Fig. 18.2 Patients with ICDs: activities reported by physicians (HRS survey). Percentages refer to numbers of physicians reporting at least one patient in his/her practice engaging in each activity. Reprinted from Lampert et al., "Safety of sports for patients with implantable cardioverter-defibrillators", J Cardiovasc Electrophysiol, 1/06, Blackwell Publishing. Permission has been granted from Blackwell Publishing

being the most commonly reported (Fig. 18.2 and Table 18.1). Forty percentage of the respondents reported that patients had received ICD shocks during sports participation, with the most commonly reported sports being running and basketball (Table 18.1). While ICD shocks during sports were common, adverse outcomes of the arrhythmias and/or shocks received during sports were rare (Table 18.2). Overall, 1% of physicians reported known injury to a patient, 5% reported injury to an ICD system, and <1% reported the failure of shocks to terminate the arrhythmia. Of nine-specific ICD-related patient injuries described, six were minor. Major injuries included two head injuries due to falls, one during running, and one on a treadmill. A neck injury occurred during hunting. Two deaths were reported. One occurred due to the head injury on a treadmill, and no details were given of the other.

In the AMSSM survey, 30% of the 81 athletes described were reported to have received a shock at some point during their athletic career [32] (Fig. 18.3). Overall adverse event rate was 13.2%, but of the shocked athletes, 43.8% experienced some type of adverse event due to the shock, such as the failure of the shock to defibrillate (athlete survived), injury to the device, or injury to the athlete. Injury to the device included two lead fractures and one other nonspecified device injury, whereas injury to the athlete included abdominal laceration and two nonspecified injuries. Reasons for the differences in adverse events reported between these two surveys are not known.

Table 18.1 Patient participation in sports and shocks received (physician-reported)

Activity	Patient participation (any)	Patient participation (competitive)	Shocks received
Basketball	163 (27%)	92 (15%)	70 (11%)
Running/jogging/track	150 (24%)	61 (10%)[a]	107 (17%)
Skiing (snow/water)	96 (16%)	12 (2%)	42 (7%)
Tennis	83 (14%)	43 (7%)	44 (7%)
Baseball/softball	64 (10%)	45 (7%)	19 (3%)
Bicycling	63 (10%)	17 (3%)	36 (6%)
Swimming	57 (9%)	22 (4%)	38 (6%)
Soccer	47 (8%)	32 (5%)	15 (2%)
Hockey	30 (5%)	7 (1%)	12 (2%)
Football	22 (4%)	8 (1%)	5 (1%)
Weightlifting	17 (3%)	3 (<1%)	13 (2%)
Scuba	12 (2%)	0 (<1%)	3 (<1%)
Hunting	12 (2%)	0 (<1%)	9 (1%)
Volleyball	11 (2%)	6 (1%)	5 (1%)
Rock/mountain climbing	9 (1%)	0 (<1%)	5 (1%)
Lacrosse	7 (1%)	4 (<1%)	4 (<1%)
Surfing/windsurfing	7 (1%)	1 (<1%)	6 (1%)
Racquetball/squash	6 (1%)	6 (1%)	3 (<1%)
Ice/roller-skate/ skateboard	5 (1%)	1 (<1%)	2 (<1%)
Rugby	4 (<1%)	2 (<1%)	1 (<1%)
Wrestling	4 (<1%)	2 (<1%)	2 (<1%)
Rodeo/equestrian	4 (<1%)	4 (<1%)	1 (<1%)
Rowing	2 (<1%)	2 (<1%)	0
Sky-diving	2 (<1%)	0 (<1%)	0

Values refer to the number (%) of physicians citing at least one patient who participates in (first and second columns) or received a shock during (third column) each sport

Table reprinted from Lampert et al., "Safety of sports for patients with implantable cardioverter-defibrillators", J Cardiovasc Electrophysiol, 1/06, Blackwell Publishing. Permission has been granted from Blackwell Publishing

[a] Including marathon

The most common adverse events reported in all the surveys were lead fracture and lead dislodgement attributed to repetitive-motion activities, most commonly weightlifting and golf. The relative risk of lead fracture (or any adverse outcome) cannot be determined from these survey data, as physicians were not asked to report the total number of patients (unlikely to be accurate in a retrospective survey). However, most previous reports describe a low incidence of lead fracture of 0.4–4% [35, 36] (with one exception [37]). In the PACES survey, system damage to the pacemaker lead with a sports or leisure activity was uncommon [34]. Further, lead failure in children is quite common [38]; so the degree the damage was specifically related to the sports activity, rather than other factors such as growth, is not known.

Table 18.2 Adverse events reported due to arrhythmia or shock during sports participation

Adverse event	N
System damage	
Lead fracture/dislodgement	
Repetitive-motion activities (total)	28
Weightlifting	16
Golf	5
Tennis	2
Wood-chopping, swimming, waterskiing, hunting, "hanging from monkey bars"	1 each
Direct trauma (total)	10
Football	3
Basketball, hockey, biking, skiing, hit by golf ball, baseball wrestling	1 each
No details given	6
Generator damage (hit by softball)	1
Patient injury	
Minor injuries ("bruising, lacerations, soft tissue injury") (total)	6
Falls from bicycle	3
Falls due to syncope during golf, running, nonspecified	1 each
Major injuries (total)	3
Syncopal on treadmill with subdural hematoma	1
Syncopal while running with head injury	1
Fall during hunting with neck injury	1
Shock failure/multiple shocks (total)	4
Running	2
Football, basketball	1 each

Values refer to the numbers of events reported by physicians
Table reprinted from Lampert et al., "Safety of sports for patients with implantable cardioverter-defibrillators", J Cardiovasc Electrophysiol, 1/06, Blackwell Publishing. Permission has been granted from Blackwell Publishing

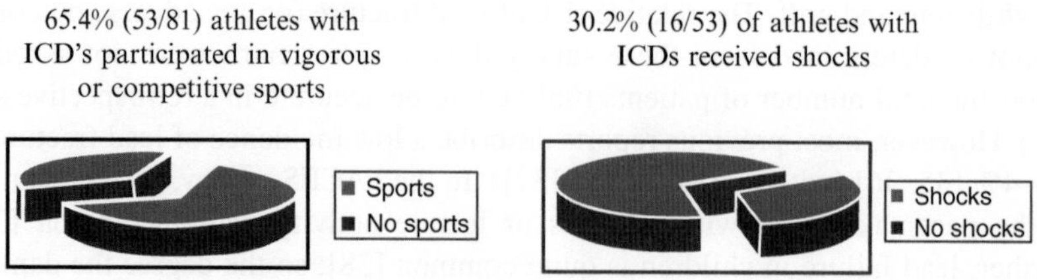

Fig. 18.3 Risk of shock during sports: AMSSM survey

Potential Safety-Related Precautions

Data from these surveys do not indicate that any sport is safe for any patient under any conditions. Patients participating in sports are a self- and perhaps physician-selected group. Many factors may decrease the potential risks of sports participation. One factor known to decrease exercise-related SCD is habitual exercise. In the Physician's Health Study, although SCD increased during exercise, habitual vigorous exercise, "enough to work up a sweat", reduced the risk of SCD during exercise sevenfold [8]. The "weekend athlete" phenomenon of intermittent high-intensity exercise should clearly be discouraged and patients wishing to exercise vigorously should be encouraged to do so regularly.

Another factor that decreases lethal arrhythmias [39] as well as ischemia [40] during exercise in coronary disease patients is compliance with target heart rate, defined as less than 85% of maximal heart rate on treadmill testing. Teaching patients to monitor and recognize a target heart rate will also decrease shocks due to sinus tachycardia, as will implantation of dual-chamber ICDs, with improved arrhythmia discrimination. In the PACES survey, many of the pediatric electrophysiologists did recommend specialized protective gear for patients with pacemakers participating in sports [34]. Whether the use of mechanical barriers such as a Kevlar vest decreases the risk of contact sports is unknown.

Current Bethesda guidelines [1] specifically restrict competitive sports. It has been suggested that recreational, versus competitive, activity may present less risk in some cardiac populations, perhaps providing "greater opportunity to exert reasonable control over the level of exercise, and ... recognize symptoms and terminate the activity" [41]. Whether the competitiveness of the activity significantly increases risk for patients with an ICD is unknown. In the HRS survey, patient participation in moderate-to-high intensity competitive sports was reported frequently, and significant adverse sequelae were rare. We did not attempt to define the level of competition in this retrospective survey. Whether the findings of this study would hold true for gifted athletes participating in athletics at the elite level requires further study.

Common sense suggestions for other at-risk cardiac populations have included avoidance of excessive activity or extreme weather conditions (skiing all day or in a snowstorm) or extreme sports such as hang-gliding [41]. These should apply to ICD patients as well. Further, given the high risk of syncope while swimming in dark water, such as a lake, river, or the ocean, some physicians recommend that ICD patients should probably always wear a life vest when swimming in such an environment whether they are being observed or not.

While shocks during sports were reported commonly, injury was rare and significant injury extremely rare. Current guidelines allow driving after 6 months free of arrhythmia [42], and similar restrictions on sporting activities might be appropriate.

The benefits of exercise are well-described, improving survival in healthy individuals [43] as well as patients with known coronary disease [44]. Inactive individuals are at increased risk of development of coronary artery disease [45], cardiac arrest

[46], and death [43]. While some studies have shown frequent brisk walking to be as beneficial as more vigorous exercise [46], most show a graded effect of exertion [43, 45]. Thus, vigorous exertion should perhaps be encouraged for ICD patients.

Limitations to Survey Data

There are a number of limitations to data from surveys, such as those described above. Relative additive risk of sports overall, or of a specific sport, for ICD shock or adverse outcome cannot be calculated. Also, as with any survey, respondents are self-selected, and recall of events can be selective: a patient shocked while surfing may be more memorable than one shocked while jogging. Factors predisposing to shock or shock frequency during sports, such as underlying heart disease or other factors, and factors perhaps predisposing to adverse outcome, such as rhythm resulting in shock, were not determined in any of these surveys.

Ongoing Research

Despite these many limitations, what these surveys do show is that patients with ICDs and pacemakers are participating in sports, regardless of guidelines and physician recommendations. Based on this information, a prospective study, the ICD Sports Safety Registry, has been instituted and is now in progress. The goal of this registry, currently open for enrollment (icdsports.registry@yale.edu), is to identify those individuals with an ICD who have made the decision to participate in sports, and follow them prospectively for 2 years. Adverse events will be quantified and risks determined, as well as factors that may influence risk, such as type of sport, or underlying diagnosis. Obtaining prospective data is crucial to determining risk and helping our patients with implanted devices make informed decisions about sports participation.

References

1. Maron BJ, Zipes DP: 36th Bethesda Conference: Eligibility recommendations for competitive athletes with cardiovascular abnormalities. J Am Coll Cardiol 2005; 45:1313–1375.
2. Lampert R, Cannom D: Sports participation for athletes with implantable cardioverter-defibrillators should be an individualized risk-benefit decision. Heart Rhythm 2008; 5:861–863.
3. Rardon JR: *Burt ends UW career*. 2006, Seattle Times, 1/6/06.
4. Bevilacqua L, Hordof A: Cardiac pacing in children. Curr Opin Cardiol 1998; 13:48–55.
5. Maron BJ, Zipes D: It is not prudent to allow all athletes with implantable cardioverter-defibrillators to participate in all sports. Heart Rhythm 2008; 5:864–866.
6. Schron EB, Exner DV, Yao Q, et al.: Quality of life in the antiarrhythmics versus implantable defibrillators. Circulation 2002; 105:589–594.
7. McAllister DR, Motamedi AR, Hame SL, et al.: Quality of life assessment in elite collegiate athletes. Am J Sports Med 2001; 29:806–810.

8. Albert CM, Mittleman MA, Chae CU, et al.: Triggering of sudden death from cardiac causes by vigorous exertion. N Engl J Med 2000; 343:1355–1361.
9. Corrado D, Basso C, Rizzoli G, et al.: Does sports activity enhance the risk of sudden death in adolescents and young adults? J Am Coll Cardiol 2003; 42:1959–1963.
10. Maron BJ, Shirani J, Poliac L, et al.: Sudden death in young competitive athletes: Clinical, demographic, and pathological profiles. JAMA 1996; 276:199–204.
11. Estes INAM, Link MS, Cannom D, et al.: Report of the NASPE policy conference on arrhythmias and the athlete. J Cardiovasc Electrophysiol 2001; 12:1208–1219.
12. Lampert R, Joska T, Burg MM, et al.: Emotional and physical precipitants of ventricular arrhythmia. Circulation 2002; 106:1800–1805.
13. Medbo JI, Sejersted OM: Plasma potassium changes with high intensity exercise. J Physiol 1990; 421:105–122.
14. Sims JJ, Miller AW, Ujhelyi MR: Regional hyperkalemia increases ventricular defibrillation energy requirements: Role of electrical heterogeneity in defibrillation. [see comment]. J Cardiovasc Electrophysiol 2000; 11:634–641.
15. Osnes JB, Hermansen L: Acid-base balance after maximal exercise of short duration. J Appl Physiol 1972; 32:59–63.
16. Kjaer M: Epinephrine and some other hormonal responses to exercise in man: With special reference to physical training. Int J Sports Med 1989; 10:2–15.
17. Sousa J, Kou W, Calkins H, et al.: Effect of epinephrine on the efficacy of the internal cardioverter-defibrillator. Am J Cardiol 1992; 69:509–512.
18. Suddath WO, Deychak Y, Varghese PJ: Electrophysiologic basis by which epinephrine facilitates defibrillation after prolonged episodes of ventricular fibrillation. Ann Emerg Med 2001; 38:201–206.
19. Venditti FJ, John RM, Hull ML, et al.: Circadian variation in defibrillation energy requirements. Circulation 1996; 94:1607–1612.
20. Turton MB, Deegan T: Circadian variations of plasma catecholamine, cortisol, and immunoreactive insulin concentrations in supine subjects. Clin Chim Acta 1974; 55:389–397.
21. Lampert R, Jain D, Burg MM, et al.: Destabilizing effects of mental stress on ventricular arrhythmias in patients with implantable cardioverter-defibrillators. Circulation 2000; 101:158–164.
22. Qin H, Walcott GP, Killingsworth CR, et al.: Impact of myocardial ischemia and reperfusion on ventricular defibrillation patterns, energy requirements, and detection of recovery. Circulation 2002; 105:2537–2542.
23. Pires LA, Lehmann MH, Steinman RT, et al.: Sudden death in implantable cardioverter-defibrillator recipients: Clinical context, arrhythmic events and device responses. J Am Coll Cardiol 1998; 33:24–32.
24. Pires LA, Hull ML, Nino CL, et al.: Sudden death in recipients of transvenous implantable cardioverter defibrillator systems: Terminal events, predictors, and potential mechanisms. J Cardiovasc Electrophysiol 1999; 10:1049–1056.
25. Mitchell LB, Pineda EA, Titus JL, et al.: Sudden death in patients with implantable cardioverter-defibrillators: The importance of post-shock electromechanical dissociation. J Am Coll Cardiol 2002; 39:1323–1328.
26. Maron BJ, Shen WK, Link MS, et al.: Efficacy of implantable cardioverter-defibrillators for the prevention of sudden death in patients with hypertrophic cardiomyopathy. N Eng J Med 2000; 342:365–373.
27. Begley DA, Mohiddin SA, Tripodi D, et al.: Efficacy of implantable cardioverter-defibrillator therapy for primary and secondary prevention of sudden cardiac death in hypertrophic cardiomyopathy. PACE 2003; 26:1887–1896.
28. Corrado D, Leoni L, Link MS, et al.: Implantable cardioverter-defibrillator therapy for prevention of sudden death in patients with arrhythmogenic right ventricular dysplasia. Circulation 2003; 108:3084–3091.
29. Zareba W, Moss AJ, Daubert JP, et al.: Implantable cardioverter-defibrillator in high-risk long QT syndrome patients. J Cardiovasc Electrophysiol 2003; 14:337–341.

30. Papaioannou GI, Klugar J: Ineffective ICD therapy due to excessive alcohol and exercise. PACE 2002; 25:1144–1145.
31. Akiyama T, Powell JL, Mitchell LB, et al.: Resumption of driving after life-threatening ventricular tachyarrhythmia. N Eng J Med 2001; 345:391–397.
32. Lawless CE: Safety and efficacy of implantable cardioverter-defibrillators and automatic external defibrillators in athletes. Clin J Sport Med 15(5):386–391.
33. Lampert R, Cannom D, Olshansky B: Safety of sports participation in patients with implantable cardioverter-defibrillators: A survey of Heart Rhythm Society Members. J Cardiovasc Electrophysiol 2006; 17:11–15.
34. Gajewski KK, Reed JH, Pilcher TA, et al.: Activity recommendations in paced pediatric patients: Wide variations among practitioners. Heart Rhythm 2008; 5:S95.
35. Kron J, Herre J, Renfroe EG, et al.: Lead- and device-related complications in the Antiarrhythmics versus Implantable Defibrillators Trial. Am Heart J 2001; 141:92–98.
36. Zipes DP, Roberts D, Pacemaker-Cardioverter-Defibrillator Investigators: Results of the International Study of the Implantable Pacemaker Cardioverter-Defibrillator. Circulation 1995; 92:59–65.
37. Luria D, Glikson M, Brady PA, et al.: Predictors and mode of detection of transvenous lead malfunction in implantable defibrillators. Am J Cardiol 2001; 87:901–904.
38. Fortescue EB, Berul CI, Cecchin F, et al.: Patient, procedural, and hardware factors associated with pacemaker lead failures in pediatrics and congenital heart disease. Heart Rhythm 2004; 1:150–159.
39. Hossack KF, Hartwig R: Cardiac arrest associated with supervised cardiac rehabilitation. J Cardiac Rehab 1982; 2:402–408.
40. Hauer K, Niebauer J, Weiss C, et al.: Myocardial ischemia during physical exercise in patients with stable coronary disease: Predictability and prevention. Int J Cardiol 2000; 75:179–186.
41. Maron BJ, Chaitman BR, Ackerman MJ, et al.: Recommendations for physical activity and recreational sports participation for young patients with genetic cardiovascular diseases. Circulation 2004; 109:2807–2816.
42. Epstein AE, Miles WM, Benditt DG, et al.: Personal and public safety issues related to arrhythmias that may affect consciousness: AHA/NASPE Medical/scientific statement. Circulation 1996; 94:1147–1166.
43. Paffenbarger RS, Hyde RT, Wing AL, et al.: Physical activity, all-cause mortality, and longevity of college alumni. N Eng J Med 1986; 314:605–613.
44. Wannamethee SG, Shaper AG, Walker M: Physical activity and mortality in older men with diagnosed coronary heart disease. Circulation 2000; 102:1358–1363.
45. Tanasescu M, Leitzmann MF, Rimm EB, et al.: Exercise type and intensity in relation to coronary heart disease in men. JAMA 2002; 288:1994–2000.
46. Lemaitre RN, Siscovick DS, Raghunathan TE, et al.: Leisure-time physical activities and the risk of primary cardiac arrest. Arch Intern Med 1999; 159:686–690.

Chapter 19
Long QT Syndrome and Other Channelopathies

Iwona Cygankiewicz and Wojciech Zareba

Introduction

Postmortem studies of exercise-related sudden death victims showed that in some cases no evidence for structural heart disease could be found. These cases had been for years classified as sudden deaths of unknown etiology, until the last decade brought a major breakthrough in elucidating the nature of at least some of these unexplained events as related to inherited or acquired cardiac ion channel disorders, so called "channelopathies" or "primary electric diseases" [1–3].

The most frequently recognized cardiac channelopathies include long QT syndrome (LQTS), short QT syndrome (SQTS), Brugada syndrome (BS), and catecholaminergic polymorphic ventricular tachycardia (CPVT). High frequency of life-threatening arrhythmias and structurally normal hearts constitute the common feature of these diseases [4–7]. Channelopathies can affect both sarcolemmal and internal sarcoplasmatic channels, with sodium, potassium, and calcium channels as the most frequently affected. Changes in the sodium and potassium channels by altering mainly the repolarization process may result in characteristic electrocardiographic patterns observed in surface ECG, as well as facilitate the occurrence of life-threatening arrhythmias and consequently increase the risk of sudden death [3, 8–10]. Recreational or especially competitive sport by various mechanisms may in some cases trigger the occurrence of life-threatening arrhythmias; therefore, athletes with channelopathies may be at an increased risk of dying suddenly while exercising.

This chapter reviews the current knowledge on the cardiac channelopathies with emphasis put on the practical aspects of the diagnosis and management.

W. Zareba (✉)
Heart Research Follow-up Program, University of Rochester Medical Center, Rochester, NY, USA
e-mail: wojciech_zareba@urmc.rochester.edu

C.E. Lawless (ed.), *Sports Cardiology Essentials: Evaluation, Management and Case Studies*, DOI 10.1007/978-0-387-92775-6_19,

Long QT Syndrome

Long QT syndrome (LQTS) is an inherited arrhythmia disorder characterized by a prolongation of QT interval in the electrocardiogram and a propensity to *torsades de pointes* ventricular tachycardia and sudden cardiac death [4, 11–13]. LQTS has been recognized for years as the Romano–Ward syndrome (familial occurrence with autosomal dominant inheritance, QT prolongation, and ventricular tachyarrhythmias) or the Jervell and Lange Nielsen syndrome (autosomal recessive inheritance, QT prolongation, ventricular tachyarrhythmias, and congenital deafness) [14–16]. Advances in genetics and basic electrophysiology within last decades brought a breakthrough in the understanding of etiology and mechanisms underlying LQTS. Mutations responsible for LQTS may be identified in approximately 60–70% of cases while in the remaining 30–40% LQTS is caused by yet unidentified mutations. Several genetic forms of LQTS have been identified; however, the most frequent: LQT1, LQT2, and LQT3 contribute to about 99% of all genotyped cases [17–21].

The clinical manifestations of affected LQTS patients may vary from completely asymptomatic individuals to fully symptomatic forms, even among patients harboring the same mutation. This phenomenon is defined as variable penetrance, and it represents a landmark feature of LQTS that may have a profound effect on clinical presentation, risk assessment, and management [21, 22]. Furthermore, the clinical course of LQTS has shown to be influenced by many factors, including gender, prior syncope, family history, QT-interval duration, genotype, type and location of the ion-channel mutation, and the risk of LQTS patients is age-dependent [13, 21–31].

Case Report #1

A 39-year-old female with a family history of sudden death was found unconscious from a water aspiration while swimming laps in the pool. She was pulled out of the pool and CPR was initiated; she was found to be in ventricular fibrillation, successfully defibrillated, and converted to a sinus rhythm. ECG recorded after defibrillation revealed a prolonged QT interval (QT/QTc = 536/491 ms) with broad-based T waves (Fig. 19.1). She had only one prior syncope 6 years prior to this event, at which time beta-blocker therapy was started. An ICD was implanted after her cardiac arrest, and genetic testing confirmed LQT1 gene mutation. Since implantation of her ICD she has had only one documented arrhythmia, which was ventricular fibrillation 1 month after implantation. The patient remains on beta-blockers and free of arrhythmias during subsequent follow-up.

LQT1 is the most frequent form of LQTS, found in 40–45% of patients with known gene mutations. LQT1 is caused by mutations of the KCNQ1 (KvLQT1) gene encoding α-subunit of potassium I_{Ks} channel. Patients with LQT1 are more likely to experience cardiac events during exercise [32, 33]. As documented by Schwartz et al. [33] in a study of 670 symptomatic LQTS patients, those with LQT1 experienced 62% of their lethal events during exercise, while only 3% of events occurred during rest/sleep. Therefore, in LQT1, exercise-related adrenergic activation seems to be the

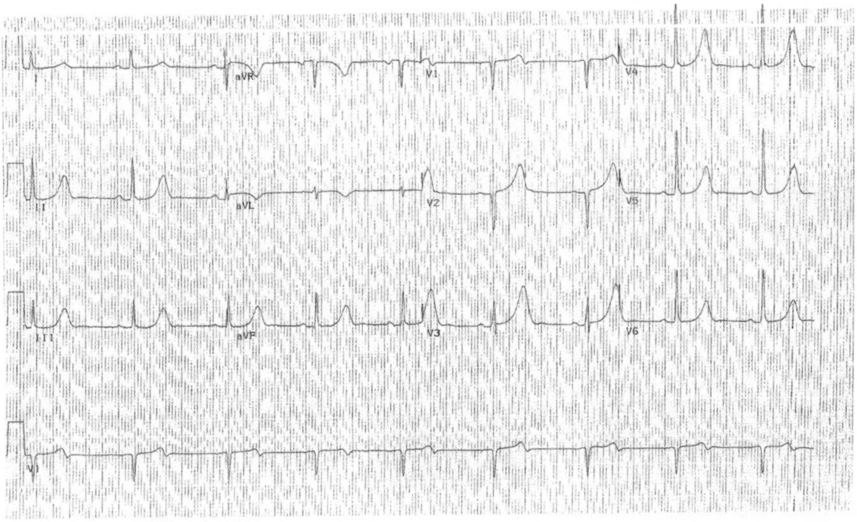

Fig. 19.1 Electrocardiogram of a 39-year-old woman diagnosed with long QT syndrome type 1. Note a prolonged QT interval and the presence of broad-based T waves typical for LQT1 patients

most important trigger for life-threatening arrhythmias. Exercise-related events in LQT1 patients occur early in life, especially in males, 94% of patients who experienced these events, presented them by the age of 20. From the pathophysiological point of view in patients with LQTS1, malfunctioning in I_{Ks} channel results in inadequate shortening of the QT interval during exercise-related increased heart rate. Inappropriate QT adaptation, together with an increased catecholaminergic release, favors early afterdepolarizations, and then facilitates ventricular tachycardia.

Swimming was recognized as a specific trigger for lethal events in LQTS patients yet in pregenetic era [11, 34–36] and a few case reports have been described so far [36–40]. In a study by Schwartz et al. [33], swimming-triggered cardiac events were observed in 33% of LQT1 patients, and on the other hand 99% of patients who experienced cardiac arrest while swimming were identified as LQT1. The exact mechanism, why swimming is such a specific trigger, is not fully understood; however, it is presumed that cardiac events might be triggered by a combination of sympathetic stimulation and fear, but also immersion in cold water provoking diving reflex might contribute to these events [33, 34, 36, 41].

Case Report #2

A 33-year-old woman with a history of two syncopal episodes after phone ringing at the age of 17 and 18 was diagnosed recently as having LQTS syndrome. The ECG revealed a prolonged QT interval with the presence of low-amplitude T waves (Fig. 19.2). A week after diagnosis she died in her sleep. Based on genetic testing received, she was diagnosed with LQT2.

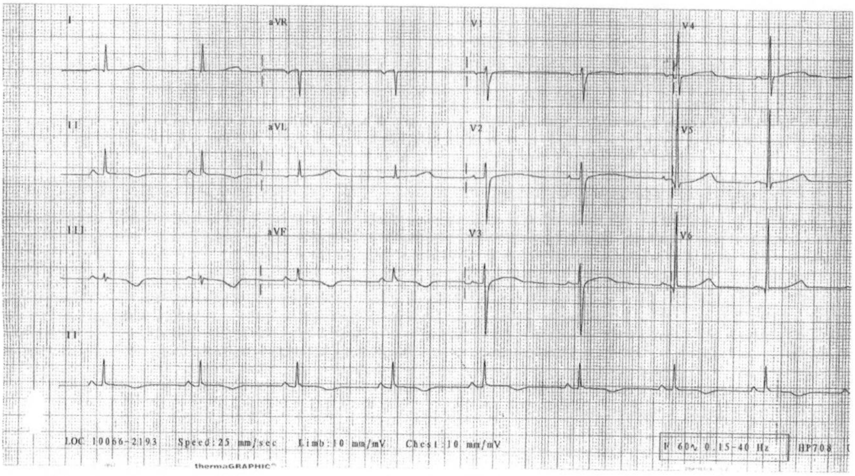

Fig. 19.2 Electrocardiogram of a 33-year-old female diagnosed with long QT syndrome type 2. Note a prolonged QT interval and the presence of low-amplitude T waves typical for LQT2 patients

LQT2 is the second most frequent form of the LQTS occurring also in about 40–45% of cases. This form of LQTS is caused by mutations of the KCNH2 (HERG) gene encoding subunit of potassium I_{Kr} channel [4]. Patients with LQT2 are less likely to experience life-threatening events during exercise (13%) and are more likely to experience them in relation with emotions (49%) or at rest/sleep without arousal (29%). Sleep-related events tend to appear later in a lifetime as those exercise-related [33, 35]. Analysis of specific triggers showed that auditory-related stimuli are characteristic for this subgroup. The most typical past history of such a patient, as the one presented above, would reveal a history of syncopal episodes shortly after morning wake up with an alarm clock or with a wake up call. Even though no case reports have been reported so far, auditory stimuli, like pistol shot, may be potential triggering events for athletes participating in competitions.

Case Report #3

A 28-year-old male with several syncopal episodes since childhood considered initially as having vasovagal etiology. Treatment with beta-blockers was initiated at that time. At the age of 17, he passed out during vigorous physical exercise (running up and down stairs at wrestling practice). CPR was started and he regained consciousness briefly before losing consciousness again. He was taken to a hospital, where the ECG revealed a prolonged QT interval (QTc = 604 ms) with peaked T waves after a long-lasting ST segments (Fig. 19.3). Dose of beta-blocker was increased and ICD was implanted. Following the guidelines, the patient was discouraged from further sport activities. Within a next year, the patient experienced a

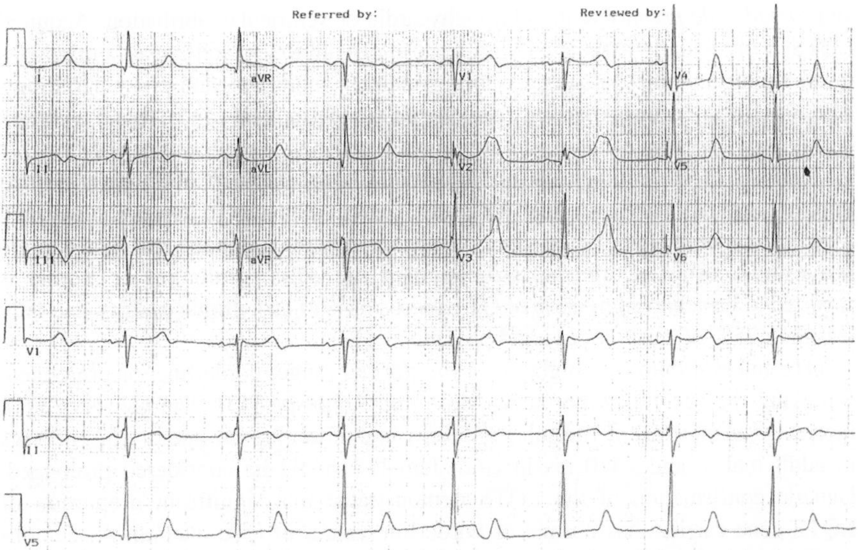

Fig. 19.3 Electrocardiogram of a 28-year-old patient with long QT syndrome type 3. Note a prolonged QT interval and the presence of peak T waves after a long ST segment typical for LQT3 patients

few VT episodes and flecainide was added to beta-blocker therapy. In addition, several inappropriate ICD shocks occurred over the next 3 years, triggered by the episodes of atrial fibrillation and once to T wave oversensing during tachycardia. After ICD was exchanged and programming parameters adjusted, no further symptoms/shocks have been observed.

Only 5–8% of known cases are recognized as LQT3 type caused by the mutations of SCN5A gene. In LQT3, persistent inward sodium current contributes to prolonged repolarization [4]. Typical ECG shows peaked, frequently asymmetrical T waves after a long ST segment. LQT3 patients are predisposed to experience their syncopal episodes and/or SCD with no relation to exercise. However, even in this subgroup, exercise-related syncopal episodes were reported in 13% of cases [33].

As demonstrated above, LQTS patients constitute a very heterogeneous group from clinical, electrocardiographic, and genetic point of view. The LQTS is usually suspected after the patient experienced palpitations, syncope, an aborted cardiac arrest, or sudden death/cardiac arrest in a relative [4, 11–13]. The differential diagnosis includes a spectrum of arrhythmogenic disorders including hypertrophic cardiomyopathy, arrhythmogenic right ventricular cardiomyopathy/dysplasia (ARVC/D), LQTS, drug-induced QT prolongation, and Brugada syndrome [3]. The circumstances of the syncopal episodes may be suggestive of type of arrhythmogenic disorder or type of the LQTS, as discussed above. Obtaining information regarding family history is important for revealing a pattern of syncopal or sudden death episodes in first-degree and more remote relatives. Information regarding medications taken needs to be acquired since some drugs may contribute to significant QT prolongation and *torsades de pointes* ventricular tachycardia or ventricular fibrillation. Acquired LQTS is particularly associated with the use of antibiotics, antifungal, antiarrhythmics, antihistaminines, antidepressants, proteinase inhibitors, and prokinetic drugs. The entire list of drugs potentially prolonging the QT interval can be found on www.qtdrugs.org. Physical examination infrequently adds to the diagnosis of LQTS.

Analysis of all available ECGs is essential since repolarization duration and morphology may vary over time. Every ECG should have QTc duration measured, which is sometimes neglected since physicians rely on automatic readings that are not always correct. Correct classification of the QT as prolonged or normal is reported to be achieved by 96% of QT experts, 62% of arrhythmia experts, and only less than 25% of cardiologists and physicians [42].

QTc interval duration might be in the normal range, borderline, or prolonged, following the criteria proposed by Moss and Robinson [43]. The values of QTc (corrected using Bazett' formula) >460 ms in children by the age of 15, >450 ms in adult males, and >470 ms in adult females should be considered prolonged. Genetic confirmation of the LQTS demonstrated that significant proportion of LQTS gene carriers has normal or borderline values of QTc interval. As demonstrated in the above presented case reports, careful analysis of T-wave morphology in a 12-lead ECGs may be important for the diagnosis of LQTS patients especially with borderline QTc duration (420–470 ms). Patients with LQT1 present with broad base T waves, those with LQT2 have low-amplitude T waves, while in LQT3 peaked, late-onset T waves segment are characteristic [44–46].

The above-mentioned changes in QTc duration and T-wave morphology should be analyzed in light of the clinical history of the evaluated individual. The meaning of a QTc duration of 460 ms will be different if there is a history of frequent syncopal episodes in the past or if there is sudden death at young age in the family. In patients with QTc prolongation >500 ms, usually there is not much doubt regarding the diagnosis. Individuals with QTc <500 ms are frequently referred for exercise ECG testing and 24-h Holter monitoring. The presence of QTc > 500 ms at heart rates <100 beats per minute during exercise testing or Holter recordings may be indicative of LQTS, whereas values below 500 ms are within physiologic range.

Genetic testing improves the diagnosis of LQTS. There are data indicating that the clinical course is different by genotype, and the effectiveness of therapy with beta-blockers also differs in LQT1 than LQT2 and LQT3 patients [21, 22, 47]. Knowing the genetic mutation in a proband provides an opportunity to conduct genotyping of family members who frequently cannot be diagnosed just based on ECG findings. Genetic testing of individuals suspected for LQTS with QTc < 500 ms is particularly useful since an overlap between affected and unaffected individuals in this category of patients is very substantial. Standard genotyping usually focuses on the most frequent LQTS genes: LQT1, LQT2, LQT3, LQT5, and LQT6, whereas the remaining genes (LQT4, LQT7–10) are tested less frequently since mutations of these genes are very infrequent.

In addition to diagnosing patients, clinicians need to evaluate potential risk for cardiac events to determine optimal therapy for the patients. Low-risk subjects might need to be just observed and treated with beta-blockers; in case of high-risk subjects, ICD therapy might be implemented. Risk stratification of the LQTS patients is based on several factors including QTc duration, history of cardiac events (timing and frequency of syncopal events, cardiac arrest), gender, age, genotype, and family history [4, 21, 23, 27, 28, 48]. It is well documented that patients with QTc > 500 ms are at higher risk of cardiac events than those with shorter QTc. Recent (within prior 2 years) episodes of syncopal episodes indicate significantly increased risk of future cardiac events [25]. Gender modulates the risk of cardiac events depending on age; in children, male gender is associated with higher risk of cardiac events than female gender [28] while in adults females are at higher risk. Genotype is of more importance for predicting cardiac events defined as syncope [21], whereas in case of more severe endpoints (aborted cardiac arrest or death) clinical presentation is more important than genetic background of the LQTS [25].

Case Report #4

A 28-year-old female, who had syncopes of unknown origin for several years, occurring on exertion before being diagnosed with LQTS on the basis of ECG findings (QTc = 520 ms). First, the subject was started on beta-blockers and became symptomatic with bradycardia. A pacemaker was implanted a year later and beta-blocker therapy was continued. Despite this therapy, she lost consciousness and received CPR, although she never needed defibrillation. An ICD was implanted and later upgraded to allow AV pacing. Subsequently, the subject stopped beta-blocker treatment as she became symptomatic with sinus bradycardia, and fatigue due to increasing doses of beta-blockers. A few years later, she was exercising strenuously doing power walking and received one appropriate ICD shock for VF followed by two inappropriate shocks due to sensing problems. Next year, the subject was skiing down hill and received two appropriate VT shocks from her ICD (Fig. 19.4).

Therapeutic options in patients with LQTS include pharmacotherapy, implantation of cardioverter defibrillator, surgical procedures, or combination of above-mentioned strategies [4]. Adrenergic stimulation is considered as the most important triggering factor for most of the cardiac events in LQTS patients, therefore, protection with beta-blockers for many years has been considered as the first line of therapy [33]. Data from the LQTS registry based on 869 patients treated with beta-blockers demonstrated a 68% reduction in cardiac events in probands and 42% reduction in cardiac events in affected family members [49]. Last decades brought evidence that the effectiveness of beta-blocker therapy depends on the genotype, with the highest efficacy observed in LQT1 patients. In patients with LQT2 and LQT3 relatively high rate of events (22 and 33%, respectively) was observed despite beta-blocker treatment [47]. In LQT3, known to be linked to the SCN5A gene mutation, sodium channel blockers may shorten QT duration and may be considered as an alternative therapeutic approach. In patients who remain symptomatic despite pharmacological treatment, implantable cardioverter defibrillator and/or adjunctive left cardiac sympathetic denervation should be considered. ICDs

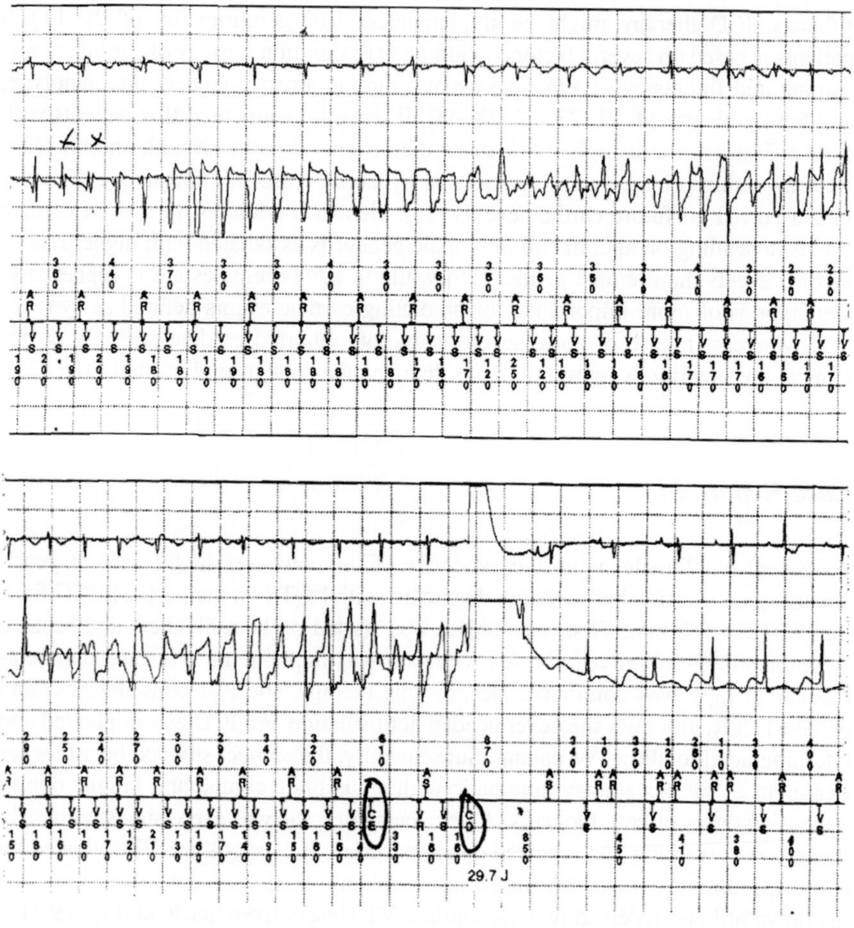

Fig. 19.4 Intracardiac electrogram with ventricular tachycardia related to exercise and terminated by ICD shock in a LQT1 patient

have been documented as an effective strategy for all patients with indications for secondary prevention and in high-risk patients for primary prevention [50–52]. Risk stratification of LQTS patients is based on clinical and family history, ECG findings, and genotype. Beta-blockers should be continued in nearly all patients with ICD. As shown in a case report, discontinuation of pharmacological treatment may result in increased frequency of arrhythmias and subsequent ICD shocks. The surgical procedure of left cardiac sympathetic denervation was introduced into LQTS therapy before beta-blockers became widely available; however, currently its application is limited to patients with ICD who develop electrical storms and ICD discharges despite being on beta-blocker therapy [53, 54]. Recently, a new therapeutic device, wearable cardioverter defibrillator (WCD), has been introduced and could be potentially applied to patients at high risk of arrhythmias who have contraindications or refused to be implanted with an ICD. Figure 19.5 shows a strip of

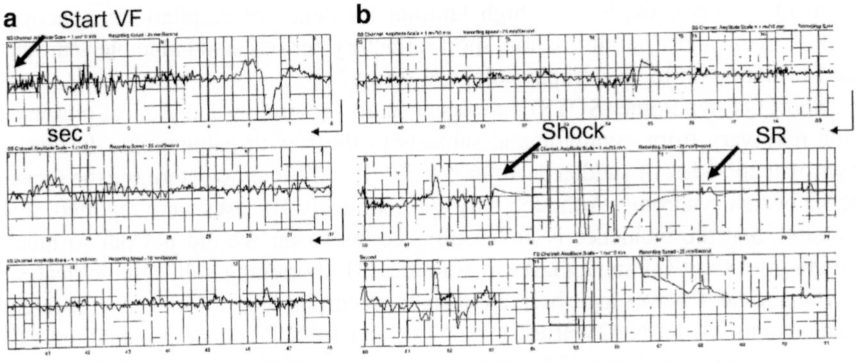

Fig. 19.5 Ventricular fibrillation terminated by a shock from wearable defibrillator. Two-channel electrocardiogram recorded by a device

ECG recording from the WCD showing the termination of ventricular fibrillation by DC shock of the WCD in an acrobat with LQTS syndrome who refused to be implanted with ICD but has been successfully treated several times with defibrillation from wearable defibrillator over the last few years.

It is important to emphasize that the above-mentioned therapeutic options should be accompanied by preventive measures aiming to decrease the risk of arrhythmic events including elimination of auditory stimuli, restriction of sport or specifically water activities, education of patients and their families regarding drugs that could prolong QT interval. Automated external defibrillators accompanying patients at home, at sport events, and other occasions provide an additional protection allowing for immediate reaction in case of life-threatening ventricular arrhythmias. Patients should also be educated regarding consequences of poor compliance when taking beta-blockers. Many cases of recurrent arrhythmias are associated with interruptions in beta-blocker therapy which should be avoided.

Short QT Syndrome

For many years, attention was paid exclusively to prolonged, and not too short, QT interval. First observation on the potential role of shortened QT interval in sudden death pathogenesis was based on a study by Algra et al. [55] who from the study of Holter recordings of 6,693 patients concluded that both prolonged (>440 ms) and short (<400 ms) QTc intervals were associated with similar, twofold increased risk of sudden death during a 2-year follow-up as compared to subjects with QTc within a normal range. However, it was in 2000 when Gussak et al. [56] for the first time described a family with idiopathic short QT interval and high incidence of atrial fibrillation. In 2003, Gaita et al. reported on two families with short QT interval and an increased risk of sudden death [57], and the term "short QT syndrome" was coined. It is nowadays defined as a genetic syndrome characterized by constant short QT interval (≤320 ms), high familial incidence of palpitations, syncope, sudden death and atrial fibrillation, short refractory periods, and inducible ventricular fibrillation during electrophysiological study.

Short QT syndrome (SQTS) may occur in all age groups and clinical presentation may vary from asymptomatic subjects to those with palpitations, dizziness, syncopal episodes, or sudden death [6, 57, 58]. It is difficult to determine the prevalence of this syndrome. Although only approximately 50 cases were reported, it is possible that the incidence is underestimated, as so far we did not put so much attention to short QT in ECG. Apart from the QT shortening, tall, symmetrical, or asymmetrical T waves are observed in right precordial leads. So far, five different gene mutations: KCNH2 (HERG), KCNQ1, and KCNJ2-encoding potassium cardiac ion channels and loss-of-function mutations in CACNB2b and CACN1C genes encoding subunits of cardiac L-type calcium channels have been linked to a SQTS [59–62]. Apart from genetic background, an acquired transient QT interval shortening may be related to an increase in heart rate, ionic changes (hypercalcemia and hyperkaliemia), acidosis, autonomic nervous system imbalance, or drug influence (digitalis), and these potential mechanisms should be taken into account while diagnosing patients with a short QT.

Up to now, ICD implantation is the only available method of treatment in these patients; however, high percentage of inappropriate ICD discharges due to T-wave oversensing was reported [63, 64]. Different drugs potentially influencing repolarization have been studied but only quinidine was shown to normalize the QT interval in patients with a SQTS and therefore could be considered as an adjunctive therapy [65]. No data on athletes with SQTS exist so far.

Brugada Syndrome

Case Report #5

A 35-year-old man with a past history of syncope 2 months prior to referral was found to be staggering around in the bathroom, where he lost consciousness and hit his head against a cabinet. The group home workers noted him to be unresponsive. No convulsions or bowel or bladder incontinence was noted during the episode. He recovered spontaneously before EMS was summoned and was brought to the hospital. The ECG recorded showed an ST-segment coved-type elevation in leads V1–V3 (Fig. 19.6). Physical examination, imaging tests (echocardiogram and cardiac MRI), and exercise stress tests were unremarkable. There was frequent QRS-ST variation with varying J-point depression throughout the Holter recording, with no episodes of VT. Due to the characteristic ECG findings and his clinical syncope, he underwent implantation of a single chamber ICD without arrhythmic events under general anesthesia. He has done well since then without any noted recurrent episodes of syncope or ICD documented arrhythmia.

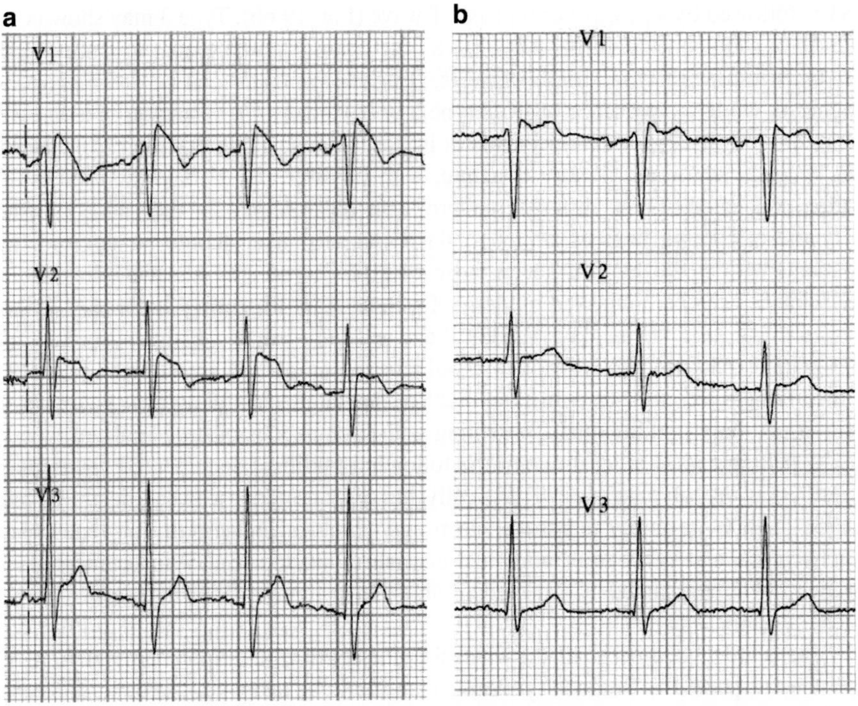

Fig. 19.6 Typical pattern of Brugada syndrome type 1 (**a**) with coved ST elevation in right precordial leads, and type 2 (**b**) with saddleback ST-segment elevation in V1–V3

The characteristic setting of Brugada syndrome, as shown in our case report, is a middle-aged man with a history of syncopal episodes or cardiac arrest at rest, no structural heart disease, and an abnormal ECG with a specific pattern of ST-segment elevation in right precordial leads [5, 66].

The prevalence of Brugada syndrome is relatively low, estimated at 5:10,000 inhabitants in Europe and the USA and up to 12–58/10,000 in Southeast Asia, but this syndrome was documented to be responsible for at least 20% of sudden death cases in patients with structurally normal hearts [67, 68]. There is a striking difference in the prevalence of Brugada syndrome by gender, estimated at 8:1 ratio, in men as compared to women. Even though the exact pathomechanism of these differences have not been elucidated so far, it seems that hormonal and gender-related changes in repolarization may play a role [69, 70]. Brugada syndrome has documented genetic background as an inherited autosomal dominant disease with various penetration linked to the SCN5A gene, encoding the α-subunit of the cardiac sodium channel. So far, nearly 80 mutations of SCN5A gene have been described [71].

Three typical ECG patterns have been described in patients with Brugada syndrome. In type 1, a coved ST-segment elevation greater or equal to 2 mm followed by a negative T wave is seen in more than one right precordial leads (V1–V3) (Fig. 19.6a). In type 2, saddleback configuration of ST-T segment is observed and

ST is followed by a positive or biphasic T wave (Fig. 19.6b). Type 3 may show both coved or saddleback configuration, but ST-elevation is less or equal to 1 mm [72].

Only in case of type 1 ECG changes, Brugada syndrome can be definitely recognized, while the presence of ECG type 2 or 3 should raise suspicion of a disease and further tests should be performed. It is worth emphasizing that the ECG pattern in Brugada syndrome is very dynamic, with possible day-to-day variation or is often concealed. Three different patterns can be observed in the same patient. Therefore, careful analysis of sequential ECH recording should be advised. In patients with concealed form or in those with ECG type 2 or 3, typical diagnostic ST changes can be unmasked by drugs, fever, or other triggering factors [72–75].

To diagnose a "Brugada syndrome," and not only isolated Brugada electrocardiographic pattern, ECG changes should be accompanied by clinical findings. According to a consensus published in 2005, the diagnosis of Brugada syndrome is confirmed only in individuals presenting with spontaneous or drug-induced type 1 ECG pattern and/or at least one of the following findings: documented ventricular fibrillation or polymorphic VT, a family history of sudden cardiac death, coved (type 1) ECG in family members, electrophysiological inducibility of ventricular tachycardia, and syncope or nocturnal agonal respiration [67]. As documented in patients with implanted ICDs, cardiac arrest in patients with Brugada syndrome occur usually at night [76].

There are two aspects in the analysis of electrocardiographic presentation of patients suspected of Brugada syndrome that should be taken into account: differential diagnosis of possible ECG variants mimicking Brugada syndrome pattern and patients with ECG pattern 2 or 3, in whom further evaluation should be performed to warrant the diagnosis. Abnormalities that may lead to ST-segment elevation in the right precordial leads include: right bundle branch block, left ventricular hypertrophy, acute myocardial infarction (especially right ventricle ischemia), acute myo- or pericarditis, hypothermia, dissecting aortic aneurysm, pulmonary embolism, neurologic disorders, and electrolyte changes (hypercalcemia and hyperkaliemia) [67]. In majority of cases, clinical picture will allow for differentiating. In athletes, frequently observed early repolarization pattern as well as possibility of ARVD may evoke potential differential diagnosis problems. Bianco et al. observed "Brugada-like" pattern of ECG in 8% of 155 studied male athletes and found that the amplitude of ST-elevation (greater in BS) and QRS duration (wider in BS) were the only two patterns differentiating athletes with an early repolarization syndrome from patients with BS [77]. Early repolarization pattern, observed in the majority of highly trained athletes, is benign in nature, while the diagnosis of Brugada syndrome results in restriction from competitive sports. In respect to differential diagnosis with ARVD, some major discrepancies include the history of exercise-related syncope, monomorphic VT, and persistent ECG changes in ARVD patients, as opposite to Brugada syndrome presenting with syncope at rest, polymorphic VT, and dynamic ECG pattern. To exclude the potential presence of ARDV, assessment of structural function of the heart by imaging techniques should be considered as the first step.

In patients suspected for Brugada syndrome but with ECG pattern type 2 or 3, additional tests have to be performed. Provocation of characteristic ECG abnormalities with sodium channel blockers (ajmaline, flecainide, procainamide, and pilsicainide) and the use of electrophysiological study to induce ventricular tachycardia or ventricular fibrillation are considered as procedures to be performed in patients diagnosed with Brugada syndrome. A high likelihood of Brugada syndrome can be assumed if the ECG pattern 1 can be induced by drugs in patients with type 2 or 3, and is associated with clinical symptoms [67].

Risk stratification of patients with Brugada syndrome is based on the past history, ECG pattern, and EPS findings. Patients with aborted sudden death are considered as the highest risk subset, followed by symptomatic patients with spontaneous type 1 ECG pattern. Among asymptomatic patients, those with spontaneous type 1 ECG and inducible VT are at the highest risk. Asymptomatic patients with only drug-induced ECG changes are considered as "low risk" [78, 79]. Regarding genetic testing, the presence of SCN5A mutation confirms the diagnosis, nevertheless it can be found in only 15–30% of patients with Brugada syndrome [71]. Therefore, currently diagnosis, risk stratification, and management of these patients should be based rather on clinical findings than on genetic assessment.

So far, only ICD therapy has been proven to be effective in patients with Brugada syndrome [80]. As recommended by the consensus on Brugada syndrome, implantation of cardioverter defibrillator is indicated as secondary prevention in patients with a documented history of cardiac arrest (class I) and as primary prevention in symptomatic patients with spontaneous type 1 ECG (class I) or drug-induced ECG changes (class IIa). It should also be recommended in asymptomatic patients with spontaneous type 1 ECG pattern and inducible VT/VF (class IIa), or drug-induced type 1 ECG, family history of sudden death, and positive EPS study (class IIb) [67]. In our case report, no drug challenge or EPS study was performed due to the presence of ECG-type 1 in a symptomatic patient.

From pathophysiological point of view, drugs decreasing outward positive currents, as well as those increasing inward positive currents theoretically, should be effective in the therapy of Brugada syndrome. So far, quinidine is the most widely studied drug, and proposed as the alternative for ICD treatment; however, no randomized data on effectiveness of this pharmacotherapy is available [80, 81]. Beta-adrenergic drugs have been proven to be effective in the treatment of electrical storms in patients with BS [82]. Taking into account the specific triggers of ECG changes and potentially life-threatening arrhythmias, some general considerations of management of patients with Brugada syndrome should be underlined. It is not likely for patients with Brugada syndrome to experience syncopal episodes during exercise. On the other hand, bradycardia, hyperthermia, and electrolyte disturbances in athletes might lead to unfavorable combination of triggering factors and induce not only ECG changes but also increase the risk of lethal arrhythmias. Antiarrhythmic drugs (sodium channel blockers from class IA and IC, calcium antagonists, and beta-blockers), psychotropic drugs, first generation antihistaminics, alpha-adrenergic agonists, and potassium channel opening drugs are among the most important drugs to be avoided [67]. Careful management of supraventricular arrhythmias and optimal ICD programming should also be warranted in BS patients as frequent inappropriate ICD discharges have been reported in these patients in relationship with improperly detected supraventricular arrhythmia [83]. Even though athletes are known to present with supraventricular arrhythmias more frequently than within the general population, no data exists on the above-mentioned inappropriate ICD therapy in these subjects.

Catecholaminic Polymorphic Ventricular Tachycardia

Catecholaminic Polymorphic Ventricular Tachycardia CPVT, is a rare, but highly lethal, inherited channelopathy characterized by exercise- or emotion-induced palpitations and/or blackouts in subjects with no structural heart disease [7, 84]. In majority of cases, patients become symptomatic in early childhood with the mean age of symptoms between 7 and 9 years old. Typical electrocardiographic presentation includes bidirectional ventricular tachycardia with alternating 180°-QRS axis on beat-to-beat basis, even though sometimes polymorphic VT may be observed [7]. Adrenergic-induced bidirectional VT may be self-terminating but sometimes may degenerate to ventricular fibrillation, therefore cardiac arrest can be frequently found as the first manifestation of CPVT. It is also worth emphasizing that a positive family history of sudden death before the age of 40 can be found in approximately 30% of cases [85].

Even though CPVT is rare, with the prevalence estimated at 1:10,000, the mortality rate is very high, 30–50% at the age of 30 years. Analysis of the database of 119 CPVT patients showed that 80% of these patients experienced cardiac events before the age of 40 [7]. On the other hand, Priori et al. reported approximately 2 years delay since the first symptoms in establishing CPVT diagnosis in patients with exercise-related syncopal episodes, which may significantly contribute to high mortality rate in untreated patients [85]. Unlike previously described channelopathies, CPVT is even more difficult to recognize if based only on a surface ECG. Even though tendency to bradycardia or prominent U wave have been reported in CPVT patients, usually a surface electrocardiogram is normal. Apart from exercise-induced ventricular arrhythmias, supraventricular arrhythmias, especially atrial fibrillation, has also been reported as frequent in CPVT patients [86].

As resting ECG is irrelevant for the diagnosis in patients suspected of CPVT, further cardiovascular evaluation should include imaging exams to rule out the presence of structural heart disease, Holter monitoring to assess the presence of arrhythmia during daily activities and under emotional stress, and above all exercise stress test to evaluate the relationship of ventricular arrhythmia with increasing workload. Ventricular arrhythmia usually appears at the heart rate of 110–130 bmp and tends to aggravate in number and complexity with an increasing heart rate. Typical pattern observed during an increased workload includes gradual progression from isolated premature beats to bigeminy, couplets, runs of nonsustained VT, and finally to a sustained bidirectional VT, not rarely degenerating into ventricular fibrillation. Sometimes, isoprotenelol infusion is used to reproduce VT pattern. On the other hand, it should be emphasized that CPVT is not inducible by programmed electrical stimulation [80–82].

CPVT was first described as a syndrome in 1970s. After decades it has been documented that CPVT is associated with mutations in two genes: RYR2 encoding the cardiac ryanodine receptor channel (autosomal dominant form) and CASQ2 encoding calsequestrin, a calcium binding protein of sarcoplasmatic reticulum (autosomal recessive form). RYR2 mutation is observed in 50–55% of CPVT cases. Genetic defects result in abnormal calcium release from sarcoplasmatic reticulum and subsequent calcium diastolic overload leading to delayed afterdepolarizations and triggered activity [84, 85].

Beta-blockers and ICD implantations are the only therapeutic options in patients with CPVT. Beta-blockers should be titrated under the control of exercise stress test and this test should be repeated to control the efficacy of treatment during every routine follow-up visit [87]. It is estimated that up to 30% of patients on beta-blockers will still present ventricular arrhythmia during exercise stress test. Apart from patients with a history of cardiac arrest with ICD indications for secondary prevention, also in patients in whom beta-blockers fail to suppress ventricular arrhythmia, ICD should be advised.

Recommendations for Sport Participation in Patients with Channelopathies

Recommendations for patients with channelopathies to perform competitive sports or participate in sport-related leisure activities are based on four main documents: Bethesda Conference [88] and the consensus of the European Society of Cardiology [89] referring to the eligibility of athletes with cardiovascular disorders to participate in competitive sports, recommendations for patients with genetic cardiovascular diseases performing recreational sports [90] by American Heart Association, and recommendations for patients with arrhythmias participating in both leisure time and competitive sports edited by European Association for Cardiovascular Prevention and Rehabilitation [91]

Patients with inherited cardiac channelopathies are at greater risk of developing life-threatening arrhythmia while participation in sport and subsequently are at greater risk for sudden death during or after exercise. Larger population of patients with genetic disorder wishes to participate in recreational, rather than competitive sports. Eligibility of these subjects to participate in leisure time and competitive sports depends on both type of exercise and clinical picture of a patient. Not surprisingly, eligibility criteria are more strict for subjects willing to participate in competitive activities. However, it should be emphasized that independently on the mode of exercise – recreational or competitive, some general rules should be followed. In general, patients with inherited genetic disorders should avoid sports characterized by an abrupt onset with acceleration over a short time that may be associated with sudden increase in catecholamine levels and should undertake rather sports with long-lasting stable exercise level. This is of special importance in patients with LQTS and CPVT when adrenergic overdrive is a well-recognized triggering factor (Table 19.1). Water sports like swimming, diving, surfing, and windsurfing are contradicted in

Table 19.1 Clinical, ECG and genetic characteristics of channelopathies

	LQT1	LQT2	LQT3	SQTS	Brugada	CPVT
Estimated prevalence	1:3,000–5,000	1:3,000–5,000	1:10,000–15,000	Difficult to estimate	5:10,000 (1:2,000 in endemic regions in Southeast Asia)	1:10,000
Age of the first symptoms	Adolescence, young adulthood	Adolescence, young adulthood	Adolescence, young adulthood	Average 35 years, but may appear at any age	Average 41 years	Childhood (average 7–9 years)
Gender	Similar	Similar	Similar	Similar	M:F 8:1	Similar
Exercise-related	Yes	Rarely	Rarely		Rather not	Yes (+++)
Specific triggers	Swimming	Auditory stimuli	Sleep		Fever and sleep	Any exercise
ECG findings	Prolonged QT, broad-based T waves	Prolonged QT low-amplitude T waves	Prolonged QT peaked, late-onset T waves	Shortened QT	Coved ST elevation (type 1) or saddleback ST elevation (type 2) in right precordial leads	Normal surface ECG
Exercise test	Abnormal QT adaptation to increasing HR	Abnormal QT adaptation to increasing HR	Adaptation to increasing HR frequently normal		Possible unmasking of ECG changes	Aggravation of ventricular arrhythmia

Holter monitoring	Prolonged QT, ventricular arrhythmia, Torsade de pointes	Prolonged QT, ventricular arrhythmia, Torsade de pointes	Prolonged QT, ventricular arrhythmia, Torsade de pointes	Shortened QT	Consistent or intermittent abnormal repolarization pattern	Ventricular arrhythmia related to exercise or emotions
Drug provocative tests	Epinephrine				Sodium channel blockers	Isoproterenol
Typical type of arrhythmia	Torsade de pointes	Torsade de pointes	Torsade de pointes	VT	Polymorphic VT	Bidirectional and/or polymorphic VT
Gene mutations	KCNQ1 (KvLQT1)	KCNH2 (HERG)	SCN5A	KCNH2 (HERG), KCNQ1, KCNJ2, CACNB2b, and CACN1C	SCN5A	RYR2 (autosomal dominant form) CASQ2 (calsequestrin)
Therapy	Beta-blockers	Beta-blockers + ICD	Beta-blockers + ICD, flecainide	ICD, quinidine	ICD, quinidine	ICD, beta-blockers

Table 19.2 Factors to avoid in patients with channelopathies based on the recommendations of the American Heart Association Committee on Exercise, Cardiac Rehabilitation, and Prevention (Maron et al. [89])

- Exertion characterized by rapid accelerations and decelerations
- Extreme environmental conditions for temperature, humidity, and altitude
- Excessive participation in sports activities
- Specific triggers like swimming, diving, and abrupt loud noises
- Sports at high risk of traumatic injury
- Amusement park rides
- Paired athletic activities when a second part might be at risk
- Extreme sports
- Substances like cocaine, anabolic steroids, and nutritional supplements

LQT1 patients, while all activities potentially related with sudden auditory stimuli are not recommended for LQT2 subjects. In general, dehydration, electrolyte imbalance, and extreme temperatures are to be avoided as potential factors facilitating arrhythmia occurrence. Table 19.2 summarizes factors that should be avoided in patients with channelopathy.

Independently of the level, professional or recreational, sports can be categorized according to the level of intensity. Basketball, body building, tennis, running, and skiing are considered as high-intensity level sports while billiards, bowling, cricket, curling, golf, and riflery as low intensity. In respect to competitive sport, according to Bethesda Conference, participation in all competitive sports, except from those in class IA (sports with low dynamic and low static component), should be restricted in a patient with a past history of cardiac arrest or a suspected LQTS precipitated syncopal episode regardless of the QTc value or genotype. Asymptomatic patients with a prolonged QT interval (QTc > 470 ms in men and >480 ms in women) should be restricted to class IA sports. Genotype-positive but asymptomatic patients with no prolonged QT interval may be allowed to participate in competitive sports. European Society of Cardiology edited similar recommendations for patients with overt LQTS and/or proven mutations, but they are more restrictive for silent gene carriers in whom the same restrictions as for overt patients are applied. Patients with SQTS should be restricted to perform class IA activities and patients with CPVT should be restricted from all competitive sports. Table 19.3 summarizes recommendations for competitive sport participation according to the American and the European guidelines [88, 90].

Regarding recreational sport activities, patients with channelopathies according to the AHA recommendations may participate in the majority of low and moderate intensity sports, paying attention to avoid triggers specific for a given disease. Furthermore, eligibility for participation in sport activities was assessed on a graded scale from 0 to 5 points. Activities categorized as 0–1 are generally not advised or discouraged; those with 4–5 are probably permitted, while the remaining 2–3 should be assessed individually (Table 19.4). Recommendations for eligibility to perform particular sports in patients with LQTS and Brugada syndrome are presented in Table 19.4. The AHA statement emphasize that decisions to allow

Table 19.3 Recommendations for participation in competitive sport activities [88, 91]

Clinical setting		According to Bethesda Conference [88]	According to European Association for Cardiovascular Prevention and Rehabilitation [91]
LQTS	Symptomatic	Restricted to class IA sports	No competitive sports allowed
	Asymptomatic, phenotypically overt	Restricted to class IA sports; more liberal approach toward LQT3 allowed	No competitive sports allowed
	Asymptomatic, phenotypically (–), genetic (+)	Allowed to participate in competitive sports	No competitive sports allowed
	Specific considerations	Avoid specific triggers like swimming (LQT1) and abrupt loud noise (LQT2)	
SQTS	Phenotypically overt	Restricted to class IA sports	Only low static/dynamic sports allowed
	Silent gene carrier	–	Only low static/dynamic sports allowed
Brugada syndrome	Overt	Restricted to class IA sports advisable	Only low demand sports allowed
	Silent gene carrier; Brugada-like pattern	–	Low to moderate sports allowed
	Specific considerations	Avoid hyperthermia	
CPVT	Symptomatic	Restricted to class IA sports	No competitive sports
	Asymptomatic with inducible VT	Restricted to class IA sports	No competitive sports
	Asymptomatic with no inducible VT	Less restrictive approach allowed	No competitive sports
	Specific considerations	Swimming not allowed	
Patients with channelopathies after ICD implantation		Restricted to class IA sports Avoid sports with risk of traumatic injury	

Sports included in Class IA according to Bethesda Conference: billiards, bowling, cricket, curling, golf, and riflery. Class I corresponds to low static component (<20% of maximal voluntary contraction) while Class A corresponds to activities with low dynamic component (<40% of maximal oxygen uptake

Table 19.4 Recommendations for leisure-time sport participation in patients with channelopathies according to American Heart Association Committee on Exercise, Cardiac Rehabilitation and Prevention (modified from Maron et al. [89])

Scale for eligibility				
	Level of exercise intensity	0–1 Not advised	2–3 Allowed on an individual basis	4–5 Probably permitted
LQTS	High	Basketball	Racketball/squash	
		Body building[a]	Skiing downhill[a]	
		Ice hockey [a]	Skiing cross country	
		Rock climbing [a]		
		Running		
		Soccer		
		Tennis (singles)		
		Windsurfing[b]		
	Moderate	Motorcycling	Jogging	Biking
		Surfing[b]	Sailing	Modest hiking
		Swimming[b]	Hiking	Tennis (doubles)
		Weightlifting [a]		Treadmill
	Low	Scuba diving[b]	Horseback riding[a]	Bowling
		Snorkelling[b]		Golf
				Skating
				Non-free weights
				Brisk walking
Brugada syndrome	High	Body building[a]	Basketball	Skiing cross country
		Ice hockey[a]	Racketball/squash	
		Rock climbing[a]	Running	
		Skiing downhill[a]	Soccer	
		Windsurfing[b]	Tennis (singles)	
	Moderate	Surfing	Motorcycling[a]	Baseball/softball
				Biking
				Modest hiking
				Jogging
				Sailing[b]
				Swimming[b]
				Tennis (doubles)
				Treadmill
				Hiking
		Free weight lifting[a]		
	Low	Scuba diving[b]	Horseback riding[b]	Bowling
				Golf
				Skating
				Snorkelling[b]
				Non-free weights
				Brisk walking

[a]Risk of traumatic injury

[b]Risk of impaired consciousness with water-related activities

sport activity should be based on an individual basis taking into account the risk to benefit ratio for a patient and the specific environmental factors [90].

There is an ongoing debate on how to approach patients with an implanted ICD who wish to participate in leisure or even competitive sports [92–94]. Uncertainty is related to the lack of data on the natural course of sport participants after ICD implantation. Patients with channelopathies constitute the higher challenge as they are not limited by functional capacity of their circulatory system, as they have no structural heart disease, but at the same time they are at high risk of arrhythmic events, a risk that may be even exaggerated during exposure to exertion and emotions. The most common reasons to discourage athletes from sport participation include increased probability of experience arrhythmia and subsequently appropriate or inappropriate ICD shocks in some cases, potential risk of device failure to restore a normal rhythm, damage to the device or ICD leads, or injuries related to syncopal episodes or ICD-delivered treatment during sport activities. In patients with channelopathies having repolarization abnormalities, incidents of inappropriate ICD therapy due to T wave oversensing have been reported.

Patients after ICD implantation should not be allowed to participate in competitive sports, apart from those with low cardiovascular demand and low risk for a patient or the other related to experience syncopal episode. Leisure time sports are allowed but patient should be treated with pharmacotherapy decreasing the risk of arrhythmic events, and a careful evaluation of the maximal sinus rate and preponderance to atrial fibrillation should be performed. In general, patients should avoid any sport-related situation which may cause ICD malfunctioning due to bodily impact or extreme movements of arms. According to ESC after any ICD intervention, a 6-week refraining from sports should be applied, and change in pharmacotherapy and ICD parameters reprogramming should be considered.

Acknowledgments We would like to acknowledge Dr. David Huang and Dr. Helmut Klein for sharing with us clinical cases illustrating patients with inherited channelopathies and Betty Mycking for her assistance in data collection.

References

1. Tester DJ, Ackerman MJ. The role of molecular autopsy in unexplained sudden cardiac death. Curr Opin Cardiol 2006;21:166–72
2. Tan HL, Hofman N, van Langen IM, van der Wal AC, Wilde AAM. Sudden unexplained death. Heritability and diagnostic yield of cardiological and genetic examination in surviving relatives. Circulation 2005;112:207–13
3. Lehnart SE, Ackerman MJ, Benson DW Jr, Brugada R, Clancy CE, Donahue JK, George AL Jr, Grant AO, Groft SC, January CT, Lathrop DA, Lederer WJ, Makielski JC, Mohler PJ, Moss A, Nerbonne JM, Olson TM, Przywara DA, Towbin JA, Wang LH, Marks AR. Inherited arrhythmias: a National Heart, Lung, and Blood Institute and Office of Rare Diseases workshop consensus report about the diagnosis, phenotyping, molecular mechanisms, and therapeutic approaches for primary cardiomyopathies of gene mutations affecting ion channel function. Circulation 2007;116:2325–45

4. Goldenberg I, Moss AJ. Long QT syndrome. J Am Coll Cardiol 2008;51:2291–300
5. Benito B, Brugada R, Brugada J, Brugada P. Brugada syndrome. Progress Cardiovasc Dis 2008;51:1–22
6. Schimpf R, Borggrefe M, Wolpert C. Clinical and molecular genetics of the short QT syndrome. Curr Opin Cardiol 2008;23:192–8
7. Napolitano C, Priori SG. Diagnosis and treatment of catecholaminergic polymorphic ventricular tachycardia. Heart Rhythm 2007;4:675–8
8. Marcus FI. Depolarization/repolarization, electrocardiographic abnormalities, and arrhythmias in cardiac channelopathies. J Electrocardiol 2005;38(Suppl. 4):60–3
9. Antzelevitch C. Heterogeneity and cardiac arrhythmias: an overview. Heart Rhythm 2007;4:964–72
10. Boussy T, Paparella G, de Asmundis C, Sarkozy A, Chierchia GB, Brugada J, Brugada R, Brugada P. Genetic basis of ventricular arrhythmias. Cardiol Clin 2008;26(3):335–53
11. Moss AJ, Schwartz PJ. Sudden death and the idiopathic long QT syndrome. AM J Med 1979;66:6
12. Moss AJ, Schwartz PJ, Crampton RS, Locati E, Carleen E. The long QT syndrome: a prospective international study. Circulation 1985;71:17–21
13. Moss AJ, Schwartz PJ, Crampton RS, et al. The long QT syndrome. Prospective longitudinal study of 328 families. Circulation 1991;84:1136–44
14. Jervell, FL-N. Congenital deal-mutism, functional heart disease with prolongation of the Q-T interval and sudden death. Am Heart J 1957;54:59–68
15. Romano C, Gemme G, Pongiglione R. Rare cardiac arrhythmias of the pediatric age. Ii. Syncopal attacks due to paroxysmal ventricular fibrillation (Presentation of 1st case in Italian pediatric literature). Clin Pediatr (Bologna) 1963;45:656–83
16. Ward OC. A new familial cardiac syndrome in children. J Ir Med Assoc 1964;54:103–6
17. Tester DJ, Will ML, Haglund CM, Ackerman MJ. Compendium of cardiac channel mutations in 541 consecutive unrelated patients referred for long QT syndrome genetic testing. Heart Rhythm 2005;2:507–17
18. Splawski I, Shen J, Timothy KW, et al. Spectrum of mutations in long-QT syndrome genes: KVLQT1, HERG, SCN5A, KCNE1, and KCNE2. Circulation 2000;102:1178–85
19. Napolitano C, Priori SG, Schwartz PJ, et al. Genetic testing in the long QT syndrome. Development and validation of an efficient approach to genotyping in clinical practice. JAMA 2005;294:2975–80
20. Moss AJ, Kass RS. Long QT syndrome: from channels to cardiac arrhythmias. J Clin Invest 2005;115:2018–24
21. Zareba W, Moss AJ, Schwartz PJ, et al. Influence of genotype on the clinical course of the long-QT syndrome. International Long-QT Syndrome Registry Research Group. N Engl J Med 1998;339:960–5
22. Priori SG, Napolitano C, Schwartz PJ. Low penetrance in the long-QT syndrome: clinical impact. Circulation 1999;99:529–33
23. Priori SG, Schwartz PJ, Napolitano C, et al. Risk stratification in the long-QT syndrome. N Engl J Med 2003;348:1866–74
24. Hobbs JB, Peterson DR, Moss AJ, et al. Risk of aborted cardiac arrest or sudden cardiac death during adolescence in the long-QT syndrome. JAMA 2006;296:1249–54
25. Sauer AJ, Moss AJ, McNitt S, et al. Long QT syndrome in adults. J Am Coll Cardiol 2007;49:329–37
26. Vincent GM, Timothy KW, Leppert M, et al. The spectrum of symptoms and QT intervals in carriers of the gene for the long-QT syndrome. N Engl J Med 1992;327:846–52
27. Locati EH, Zareba W, Moss AJ, et al. Age- and sex-related differences in clinical manifestations in patients with congenital long-QT syndrome: findings from the International LQTS Registry. Circulation 1998;97:2237–44
28. Zareba W, Moss AJ, Locati EH, et al. Modulating effects of age and gender on the clinical course of long QT syndrome by genotype. J Am Coll Cardiol 2003;42:103–9

29. Moss AJ, Shimizu W, Wilde AA, et al. Clinical aspects of type-1 long-QT syndrome by location, coding type, and biophysical function of mutations involving the KCNQ1 gene. Circulation 2007;115:2481–9
30. Goldenberg I, Moss AJ, Zareba W, et al. Clinical course and risk stratification of patients affected with the Jervell and Lange-Nielsen syndrome. J Cardiovasc Electrophysiol 2006;17:1169–71
31. Kaufman ES, McNitt S, Moss AJ, Zareba W, Robinson JL, Hall WJ, Ackerman MJ, Benhorin J, Locati ET, Napolitano C, Priori SG, Schwartz PJ, Towbin JA, Vincent GM, Zhang L. Risk of death in the long QT syndrome when a sibling has died. Heart Rhythm 2008;5(6):831–6
32. Schwartz PJ, Zaza A, Locati E, Moss AJ. Stress and sudden death. The case of the long QT syndrome. Circulation 1991;83(Suppl. II):II71–80
33. Schwartz PJ, Priori SG, Spazzolini C, et al. Genotype-phenotype correlation in the long-QT syndrome: gene-specific triggers for life-threatening arrhythmias. Circulation 2001;103:89–95
34. Ackerman MJ, Tester DJ, Porter CJ. Swimming, a gene-specific arrhythmogenic trigger for inherited long QT syndrome. Mayo Clin Proc 1999;74:1088–94
35. Moss AJ, Robinson JL, Gessman L, et al. Comparison of clinical and genetic variables of cardiac events associated with loud noise versus swimming among subjects with the long QT syndrome. Am J Cardiol 1999;84:876–9
36. Choi G, Kopplin LJ, Tester DJ, Will ML, Haglund CM, Ackerman MJ. Spectrum and frequency of cardiac channel defects in swimming-triggered arrhythmia syncopes. Circulation 2004;110:2119–24
37. Ott P, Marcus FI, Moss AJ. Ventricular fibrillation during swimming in a patient with long QT syndrome. Circulation 2002;106:521–2
38. Ackerman MJ, Porter BJ. Identification of a family with inherited Long QT syndrome after a pediatric near drowning. Pediatrics 1998;101:306–8
39. Batra AS, Silka MJ. Mechanism of sudden cardiac arrest while swimming in a child with the prolonged QT syndrome. J Pediatr 2002;141:283–4
40. Lunetta P, Levo A, Laitinen PJ, Fodstad H, Kontula A, Sajantila A. Molecular screening of selected long QT syndrome (LQTS) mutations in 165 consecutive bodies found in water. Int J Legal Med 2003;117;115–7
41. Katagiri-Kawade M, Ohe T, Arakaki Y, Kurita T, Shimizu W, Kamiya T, Orii T. Abnormal response to exercise, face immersion, and isoproterenol in children with the long QT syndrome. Pacing Clin Electrophysiol 1995;18(Pt 1):2128–34
42. Viskin S, Rosovski U, Sands AJ, Chen E, Kistler PM, Kalman JM, Rodriguez Chavez L, Iturralde Torres P, Cruz FFE, Centurion OA, Fujiki A, Maury P, Chen X, Krahn AD, Roithinger F, Zhang L, Vincent GM, Zeltser D. Inaccurate electrocardiographic interpretation of long QT: the majority of physicians cannot recognize a long QT when they see one. Heart Rhythm 2005;2:569–74
43. Moss AJ, Robinson JL. Long QT syndrome. Heart Dis Stroke 1992;1:309–14
44. Moss AJ, Zareba W, Benhorin J, et al. ECG T-wave patterns in genetically distinct forms of the hereditary long QT syndrome. Circulation 1995;92:2929–34
45. Zhang L, Timothy KW, Vincent GM, et al. Spectrum of ST-T-wave patterns and repolarization parameters in congenital long-QT syndrome: ECG findings identify genotypes. Circulation 2000;102:2849–55
46. Zareba W. Genotype-specific patterns in long QT syndrome. J Electrocardiol 2006;39:S101–6
47. Priori SG, Napolitano C, Schwartz PJ, et al. Association of long QT syndrome loci and cardiac events among patients treated with β-blockers. JAMA 2004;292:1341–4
48. Zareba W, Moss AJ, le Cessie S, Locati EH, Robinson JL, Hall WJ, Andrews ML. Risk of cardiac events in family members of patients with long QT syndrome. J Am Coll Cardiol 1995;26:1685–91
49. Moss AJ, Zareba W, Hall WJ, et al. Effectiveness and limitations of beta-blocker therapy in congenital long-QT syndrome. Circulation 2000;101:616–23

50. Groh WJ, Silka MJ, Oliver RP, Halperin BD, McAnulty JH, Kron J. Use of implantable cardioverter-defibrillators in the congenital long QT syndrome. Am J Cardiol 1996;78:703–6
51. Zareba W, Moss AJ, Daubert JP, et al. Implantable cardioverter defibrillator in high-risk long QT syndrome patients. J Cardiovasc Electrophysiol 2003;14:337–41
52. Daubert JP, Zareba W, Rosero SZ, Budzikowski A, Robinson JL, Moss AJ. Role of implantable cardioverter defibrillator therapy in patients with long QT syndrome. Am Heart J 2007;153(Suppl. 4):53–8
53. Moss AJ, McDonald J. Unilateral cervicothoracic sympathetic ganglionectomy for the treatment of long QT interval syndrome. N Engl J Med 1971;285:903–4
54. Schwartz PJ, Priori SG, Cerrone M, et al. Left cardiac sympathetic denervation in the management of high-risk patients affected by the long-QT syndrome. Circulation 2004;109:1826–33
55. Algra A, Tjissen JG, Roelandt Pool J, Lubsen J. QT interval variables from 24 hour electrocardiography and the two-year risk of sudden death. Br Heart J 1993;70:43–8
56. Gussak I, Brugada P, Brugada J, Wright RS, Kopecky SL, Chaitman BR, Bjerregaard P. Idiopathic short QT interval: a new clinical syndrome? Cardiology 2000;94:99–102
57. Gaita F, Giustetto C, Bianchi F, Wolpert C, Schimpf R, Riccardi R, et al. Short QT syndrome: a familial cause of sudden death. Circulation 2003;103:965–70
58. Giustetto C, Di Monte F, Wolpert C, Borggrefe M, Schimpf R, Sbragia P, Leone G, Maury P, Anttonen O, Haissaguerre M, Gaita F. Short QT syndrome: clinical findings and diagnostic-therapeutic implications. Eur Heart J 2006;27:2440–7
59. Brugada R, Hong K, Dumaine R, Cordeiro J, Gaita F, Borggrefe M, Menendez TM, Brugada J, Pollevick GD, Wolpert C, Burashnikov E, Matsuo K, Wu YS, Guerchicoff A, Bianchi F, Giustetto C, Schimpf R, Brugada P, Antzelevitch C. Sudden death associated with short QT syndrome linked to mutations in HERG. Circulation 2004;109:30–5
60. Bellocq C, van Ginneken AC, Bezzina CR, Alders M, Escante D, Mannens MM, Baro I, Wilde AA. Mutation in KCNQ1 gene adding to the short QT interval syndrome. Circulation 2004;109:2394–7
61. Priori SG, Pandit SV, Rivolta I, Berenfed O, Ronchetti E, Dhamoon A, Napolitano C, Anumonwo J, di Barleta MR, Gudapakkam S, Bosi G, Stramba-Badiale M, Jalife J. A novel form of short QT syndrome (SQT3) is caused by a mutation in the KCNJ2 gene. Circ Res 2005;96:800–7
62. Antzelevitch C, Pollevick GD, Cordeiro JM, et al. Loss-of-function mutations in the cardiac calcium channel underlie a new clinical entity characterized by ST-segment elevation, short QT intervals, and sudden cardiac death. Circulation 2007;115:442–9
63. Schimpf R, Bauersfeld U, Gaita F, Wolpert C. Short QT syndrome: successful prevention of sudden death in an adolescent by implantable cardioverter-defibrillator treatment for primary prophylaxis. Heart Rhythm 2005;2:416–7
64. Schimpf R, Wolpert C, Bianchi F, Giustetto C, Gaita F, Bauersfeld U, et al. Congenital short QT syndrome and implantable cardioverter defibrillator: inherent risk for inappropriate shock delivery. J Cardiovasc Electrophysiol 2003;14:1273–7
65. Gaita F, Guistetto C, Bianchi F, Schimpf R, Haissaguerre M, Calo L, et al. Short QT syndrome; pharmacological treatment. J Am Coll Cardiol 2004;43:1494–9
66. Brugada P, Brugada J. Right bundle branch block, persistent ST segment elevation and sudden cardiac death: a distinct clinical and electrocardiographic syndrome. A multicenter report. J Am Coll Cardiol 1992;20:1391–6
67. Antzelevitch C, Brugada P, Borggrefe M, Brugada J, Brugada R, Corrado D, Gussak I, LeMarec H, Nademanee K, Perez Riera AR, Shimizu W, Schulze-Bahr E, Tan H, Wilde A. Brugada syndrome: report of the second consensus conference. Heart Rhythm 2005;2(4):429–40
68. Hermida JS, Lemoisne JL, Aoun FB, Jarry G, Rey JL, Quiret JC. Prevalence of the Brugada syndrome in an apparently healthy population. Am J Cardiol 2000;86:91–4
69. Shimizu W, Matsuo K, Kokubo Y, Satomi K, Kurita T, Noda T, Nagaya N, Suyama K, Aihara N, Kamakura S, Inamoto N, Akahoshi M, Tomoike H. Sex hormone and gender difference – role of testosterone on male predominance in Brugada syndrome. J Cardiovasc Electrophysiol 2007;18:415–21

70. James AF, Choisy SC, Hancox JC. Recent advances in understanding sex differences in cardiac repolarization. Prog Biophys Mol Biol 2007;94(3):265–319
71. Antzelevitch C. Genetic basis of Brugada syndrome. Heart Rhythm. 2007;4:756–7
72. Brugada R, Brugada P, Brugada J. Electrocardiogram interpretation and class I blocker challenge in Brugada syndrome. J Electrocardiol 2006;39(Suppl. 4):S115–8
73. Brugada R, Brugada J, Antzelevitch C, Kirsch GE, Potenza D, Towbin JA, Brugada P. Sodium channel blockers identify risk for sudden death in patients with ST-segment elevation and right bundle branch block but structurally normal hearts. Circulation 2000;101(5):510–5
74. Miyazaki T, Mitamura H, Miyoshi S, Soejima K, Aizawa Y, Ogawa S. Autonomic and antiarrhythmic drug modulation of ST segment elevation in patients with Brugada syndrome. J Am Coll Cardiol 1996;27(5):1061–70
75. Antzelevitch C, Brugada R. Fever and Brugada syndrome. Pacing Clin Electrophysiol 2002;25:1537–9
76. Mizumaki K, Fujiki A, Tsuneda T, Sakabe M, Nishida K, Sugao M, Inoue H. Vagal activity modulates spontaneous augmentation of ST elevation in the daily life of patients with Brugada syndrome. J Cardiovasc Electrophysiol 2004;15:667–73
77. Bianco M, Bria S, Gianfelici A, Sanna N, Palmieri V, Zeppilli P. Does early repolarization in the athlete have analogies with the Brugada syndrome? Eur Heart J 2001;22:504–10
78. Priori SG, Napolitano C, Gasparini M, Pappone C, Della Bella P, Giordano U, Bloise R, Giustetto C, De Nardis R, Grillo M, Ronchetti E, Faggiano G, Nastoli J. Natural history of Brugada syndrome: insights for risk stratification and management. Circulation 2002;105: 1342–7
79. Brugada J, Brugada R, Antzelevitch C, Towbin J, Nademanee K, Brugada P. Long-term follow-up of individuals with the electrocardiographic pattern of right bundle-branch block and ST-segment elevation in precordial leads V1 to V3. Circulation 2002;105:73–8
80. Brugada J, Brugada R, Brugada P. Pharmacological and device approach to therapy of inherited cardiac diseases associated with cardiac arrhythmias and sudden death. J Electrocardiol 2000;33(Suppl):41–7
81. Alings M, Dekker L, Sadée A, Wilde A. Quinidine induced electrocardiographic normalization in two patients with Brugada syndrome. Pacing Clin Electrophysiol 2001;24(9 Pt 1):1420–2
82. Tanaka H, Kinoshita O, Uchikawa S, Kasai H, Nakamura M, Izawa A, Yokoseki O, Kitabayashi H, Takahashi W, Yazaki Y, Watanabe N, Imamura H, Kubo K. Successful prevention of recurrent ventricular fibrillation by intravenous isoproterenol in a patient with Brugada syndrome. Pacing Clin Electrophysiol 2001;24(8 Pt 1):1293–4
83. Sarkozy A, Boussy T, Kourgiannides G, Chierchia GB, Richter S, De Potter T, Geelen P, Wellens F, Spreeuwenberg MD, Brugada P. Long-term follow-up of primary prophylactic implantable cardioverter-defibrillator therapy in Brugada syndrome. Eur Heart J 2007;28:334–44
84. Mohamed U, Napolitano C, Priori SG. Molecular and electrophysiological bases of catecholaminergic polymorphic ventricular tachycardia. J Cardiovasc Electrophysiol 2007;18:791–7
85. Priori SG, Napolitano C, Memmi M, Colombi B, Drago F, Gasparini M, DeSimone L, Coltorti F, Bloise R, Keegan R, Cruz Filho FE, Vignati G, Benatar A, DeLogu A. Clinical and molecular characterization of patients with catecholaminergic polymorphic ventricular tachycardia. Circulation 2002;106(1):69–74
86. Leenhardt A, Lucet V, Denjoy I, Grau F, Ngoc DD, Coumel P. Catecholaminergic polymorphic ventricular tachycardia in children. A 7-year follow-up of 21 patients. Circulation 1995;91:1512–9
87. Sumitomo N, Harada K, Nagashima M, Yasuda T, Nakamura Y, Aragaki Y, Saito A, Kurosaki K, Jouo K, Koujiro M, Konishi S, Matsuoka S, Oono T, Hayakawa S, Miura M, Ushinohama H, Shibata T, Niimura I. Catecholaminergic polymorphic ventricular tachycardia: electrocardiographic characteristics and optimal therapeutic strategies to prevent sudden death. Heart 2003;89:66–70
88. Zipes DP, Ackerman MJ, Estes III M, Grant AO, Myerburg R, Van Hare G. 36th Bethesda Conference. Task Force 7: Arrhythmias. J Am Coll Cardiol 2005;45:1354–63

89. Pelliccia A, Fagard R, Bjørnstad HH, Anastassakis A, Arbustini E, Assanelli D, Biffi A, Borjesson M, Carrè F, Corrado D, Delise P, Dorwarth U, Hirth A, Heidbuchel H, Hoffmann E, Mellwig KP, Panhuyzen-Goedkoop N, Pisani A, Solberg EE, van-Buuren F, Vanhees L, Blomstrom-Lundqvist C, Deligiannis A, Dugmore D, Glikson M, Hoff PI, Hoffmann A, Hoffmann E, Horstkotte D, Nordrehaug JE, Oudhof J, McKenna WJ, Penco M, Priori S, Reybrouck T, Senden J, Spataro A, Thiene G; Study Group of Sports Cardiology of the Working Group of Cardiac Rehabilitation and Exercise Physiology; Working Group of Myocardial and Pericardial Diseases of the European Society of Cardiology. Recommendations for competitive sports participation in athletes with cardiovascular disease: a consensus document from the Study Group of Sports Cardiology of the Working Group of Cardiac Rehabilitation and Exercise Physiology and the Working Group of Myocardial and Pericardial Diseases of the European Society of Cardiology. Eur Heart J. 2005;26(14):1422–45
90. Maron BJ, Chaitman BR, Ackerman MJ, Bayes de Luna A, Corrado D, Crosson JE, Deal BJ, Driscoll DJ, Estes NA 3rd, Araujo CG, LIang DH, Mitten MJ, Myerburg RJ, Peliccia A, Thompson PD, Towbin JA, Van Camp SP. Working Groups of the American Heart Association Committee on Exercise, Cardiac Rehabilitation, and Prevention; Councils on Clinical and Cardiovascular Disease in the Young. Recommendations for physical activity and recreational sports participation for young patients with genetic cardiovascular diseases. Circulation 2004;109:2807–16
91. Heidbuchel H, Corrado D, Biffi A, Hoffmann E, Panhuyzen-Goedkoop N, Hoogsteen J, Delise P, Hoff PI, Peliccia A. Study Group on Sports Cardiology of the European Association for Cardiovascular Prevention and Rehabilitation. Recommendations for participation in leisure-time physical activity and competitive sports of patients with arrhythmias and potentially arrhythmogenic conditions. Eur J Cardiovasc Prev Rehabil 2006;13:676–86
92. Lampert R, Cannom D, Olshansky B. Safety of sports participation in patients with implantable cardioverter defibrillators: a survey of Heart Rhythm Society Members. J Cardiovasc Electrophysiol 2006;17:11–5
93. Maron BJ, Zipes DP. It is not prudent to allow all athletes with implantable cardioverter defibrillators to participate in all sports. Heart Rhythm 2008;5:864–6
94. Lampert R, Cannom D. Sports participation for athletes with implantable cardioverter-defibrillators should be an individualized risk-benefit decision. Heart Rhythm 2008;5:861–3

Chapter 20
Cardiac Effects of Ergogenic Aides and Supplements

Holly J. Benjamin and Joseph A. Congeni

Introduction

Great concern exists that athletes who regularly exercise are using dietary supplements and other purported ergogenic aids as a means for enhancing athletic performance and altering body composition. Twelve billion dollars is estimated to have been spent in 1999 in the USA alone on supplements [1]. It is not surprising that athletes have followed this trend. What the athletes often fail to recognize is the lack of evidence in controlled trials demonstrating the true effects on performance. Many popular products are largely unregulated and their purity is unknown. Widespread use of combination products has also contributed to a higher number of doping infractions and adverse medical consequences. In 2001, Green published the results from an NCAA survey from 13,914 students from 30 sports competing at 637 NCAA Division I, II, and III schools. This accounted for a 64.3% response rate. Notable findings included a wide variation in substance abuse according to sport. Amphetamine use was highest in DIII, cocaine use in DII, ephedrine use in both DII and DIII. Androgenic anabolic steroid (AAS) use was reported at 1.1% overall across DI–DIII but was higher in some sports like football and ranged from 0 to –5% for men vs. 0–1.5% for women. 32.1% of AAS users obtained their steroids from a physician that was not the school's team physician [2].

In 2002, the International Olympic Committee (IOC) [3] released a report that examined 634 supplements from 215 manufacturing companies in 13 different countries. The results showed that 94 products (15%) contained banned or restricted substances and an additional 66 supplements (10%) contained unlabeled substances in borderline doping levels. Lastly, 41% of the supplement manufacturers in the USA had produced at least one sport supplement that tested positive for a banned or restricted substance.

H.J. Benjamin (✉)
Associate Professor of Pediatrics and Surgery, Section of Academic Pediatrics, Section of Orthopedic Surgery and Rehabilitation Medicine, Director of Primary Care Sports Medicine, The University of Chicago, 5841 S. Maryland Ave. MC 6082
e-mail: hbenjamin@peds.bsd.uchicago.edu

C.E. Lawless (ed.), *Sports Cardiology Essentials: Evaluation, Management and Case Studies*, DOI 10.1007/978-0-387-92775-6_20,

Table 20.1 A sample list of prohibited substances and known cardiac side effects

Drugs and supplements of abuse	SCD	Arrhythmias	Thrombosis/ embolisms	CAD	MI	HF	CM	LVH	HTN
AAS	Yes	Yes	Yes	Yes	Yes	Yes	Yes	Yes	yes
hGH	Yes	Yes	Yes			Yes	Yes	Yes	
EPO			Yes			Yes			yes
Amphetamines	Yes	Yes	Yes		Yes	Yes	Yes		yes
Cocaine	Yes	Yes	Yes		Yes	Yes	Yes		Yes
Ephedrine	Yes	Yes	Yes		Yes		Yes		Yes
Caffeine	Yes	Yes							yes

AAS hGH EPO see text for abbreviations. CAD = coronary artery disease, MI = myocardial infarction, HF = heart failure, CM = Cardionmyepathy, LVH = left vaerticular hypertrophy, HTN = hypertension, SCD = sudder cardiac death

The true magnitude of the supplement industry and its lack of regulation cannot be measured at this time. It is clear that serious side-effects can occur as a result of the use and/or misuse of sport supplements and ergogenic aids. The cardiovascular side-effects of doping appear to clearly be the most deleterious to the athlete – whether elite, amateur, or recreational [4]. This chapter will highlight known cardiovascular effects such as sudden cardiac death, myocardial infarction, thrombosis, arrythmogenesis, heart failure, hyperlipidemia, and hypertension with regard to the most popular drugs and supplements of abuse including anabolic-androgenic steroids, dihydroepiandrostenedione (DHEA), human growth hormone (hGH), erythropoietin (EPO), amphetamines, cocaine, and caffeine (Table 20.1).

Anabolic Androgenic Steroids

AAS have been associated with significant systemic multiorgan system effects (Table 20.2); none more concerning than cardiovascular adverse effects. Cardiac effects range from altered lipid levels and hypertension to myocardial infarction, ischemic heart disease, cardiomyopathy, and sudden death. More recently, these drugs have been associated with atrial fibrillation and even implicated in the development of histologic hypertrophic structural changes to the heart [5].

In 1995, Melchert and Welder categorized AAS-induced cardiovascular effects into four hypothetical models: an atherogenic model for lipoprotein effects, a thrombogenic model for clotting factors and platelet effects, a vasospasm model and a direct myocardial injury model (Table 20.3) [5]. Many factors influence the severity of the doping effects on individual athletes including the type, quantity and duration of drug used, organ system sensitivity, the sport, and the presence of polysubstance abuse. AAS use and abuse is common in all athletes in most sports including elite, professional, amateur, and recreational independent of age, gender, or race. AAS use has been reported in youth athletes as young as age 10 in both males and females [6]. Thus health-care professionals in the field of sports medicine

Table 20.2 Common side effects of anabolic steroid use

Heart arrhythmias
Reduction in HDL, increased fatty deposits
Hypertension
Liver, prostate, and kidney cancer
Blood coagulation disorders
Psychiatric problems (depression, labile emotions, aggression)
Musculoskeletal injuries
Growth suppression in skeletally immature youth
HIV from shared needles
Epistaxis
Acne vulgaris
Extremity edema
Reduced or increased libido
Breast growth in males
Testicular atrophy, reduced sperm counts
Baldness
Body hair growth in females
Masculinization, clitoral enlargement and breast reduction in females

Table 20.3 Four proposed models for AAS-induced cardiovascular effects

Model	AAS effects
Atherogenic	Lipoprotein concentrations
Thrombogenic	Clotting factors and platelets
Vasospasm	Vascular nitric oxide system
Direct myocardial injury	Myocardial cell injury and death

must be familiar with and highly vigilant to warning signs of AAS use/abuse in all athletic populations. The American College of Sports Medicine has strongly condemned the use of anabolic androgenic steroids and other related drugs. In 2007, ACSM recommended mandatory drug testing in major league baseball and previously in 2003 called for increased vigilance to identify and eradicate steroid use in sports (http://www.acsm.org).

Atherogenic

Altered lipid levels in anabolic androgenic steroid users are reflected in increased low-density lipid protein, and decreased high-density lipid protein. This results in an increased risk to AAS users for myocardial infarction [7–9]. The oral C17 alkylated steroids seem to exert the greatest effects on the lipid profile [10–12]. Thrombus formation has been postulated by way of these adverse lipid changes, and is supported further by findings of AAS-induced, increased platelet aggregation, enhanced coagulation, enzyme activity, and coronary vasospasm [13].

Thrombogenic

AAS decrease fibrinolytic activity, suppress prostacyclin synthesis, increase release of proteins S and C, and increase platelet aggregation. AAS abuse may also increase the production and activation of thrombin and plasmin. All of these factors can increase the risk of vascular occlusion, particularly in the setting of strenuous exercise [4].

Vasospasm

Testosterone has been to increase the systemic vascular response to norepinephrine. Sadler et al. found that AAS use resulted in impaired vessel reactivity but not endothelial dysfunction [7].

Direct Myocardial Effects

Hypertension in AAS users has been reported and results in blood volume increases and fluid retention [8,13,14]. This effect as well as the finding of increased septal thickness and left ventricular mass recorded in AAS users [15, 16] can lead to significant detrimental cardiac remodeling.

Myocardial structural changes appear to contribute to AASs pro-arrhythmic effects. They affect the electrical stimulation threshold of the heart and can alter electrolyte concentrations. Numerous case reports discuss the induction of atrial fibrillation in AAS users [17]. Ventricular fibrillation is also frequently observed [4]. The inter-related and cross-reactive cardiovascular effects of anabolic androgenic steroids lead to a significant increased risk of sudden cardiac death in users.

Are the Cardiac Effects of Anabolic Steroid Use Reversible?

Cardiac hypertrophy associated with AAS use results in increased fibrosis and is therefore irreversible and pathological as compared to the physiologic hypertrophy observed in weightlifters and other highly trained resistance athletes. Urhausen studied three groups of German weightlifters: current AAS users, ex-AAS users (most recent use >12 months prior) and nonusers. He demonstrated that even several years after discontinuation of AAS abuse, strength athletes still show a slight increase in concentric left ventricular hypertrophy in comparison with AAS-free strength athletes. As systolic blood pressure was higher in current users compared to former users or nonusers, the observed myocardial changes may have represented a cause or an effect of the higher blood pressure [18].

Polysubstance Abuse

Polysubstance abuse can exponentially increase the athlete's risk of complications and side effects, some of which have serious long-term consequences. The interactions between drugs and supplements are highly complex and have great variability in individual responses. Clark and Schofield [19] reported a case of a 40-year-old man who developed new-onset congestive heart failure and severe acute hepatitis several months after he began using anabolic-androgenic steroids, ephedra and gamma-hydroxybutyrate supplements. Evidence of polysubstance abuse in any athlete is highly concerning, even potentially life-threatening, and must be addressed in a comprehensive manner, often requiring a multidisciplinary health-care approach. The following highly publicized case of a major league baseball star illustrates this poignantly. In 2004, Ken Carminiti, 41, died a sudden cardiac death attributed at the time to drug abuse with cocaine and opiates. Cocaine is known for causing an increased risk of an acute myocardial infarction or a life-threatening arrhythmia. However, a coroner's report revealed that underlying coronary artery disease and cardiac hypertrophy were contributing factors, and in 2002, Carminiti had admitted to using steroids in the 1996 when he won the National League's MVP award [20]. Thus, it is more likely that the cause of death was related to the use of both cocaine and steroids.

Dehydroepiandrosterone (DHEA)

DHEA is a 19-carbon steroid, often called a prohormone, it is officially classified as an androgen. It is produced in the adrenal gland and exists in two forms: an unconjugated form (DHEA) and DHEAS, a sulfate ester-conjugated form. DHEAS is an abundant, biologically active steroid hormone that circulates and serves as a major precursor of DHEA. DHEAS is strongly bound to albumin, DHEA less so. DHEA circulates in response to the secretion of adrenocorticotrophic hormone [21].

The mechanism of action for DHEA is liver absorption following oral administration with subsequent conversion to DHEAS. It is a precursor for both androgens and estrogens which is synthesized and converted into peripheral tissues to testosterone, dihydrotestosterone, estrogens, and sex hormones.

DHEA first achieved notoriety in the early 1990s when it was marketed in France as an "aging cure" [22]. Use in athletes has been aimed at increasing androstenediol and testosterone, although increases may be transient. Rise in estrogen levels is more predictable and may be an unwanted side effect in athletes. DHEA use rose in popularity when the 1985 FDA ban was lifted in 1994 to allow over-the-counter sales as a dietary supplement. Despite this, use of DHEA by athletes is banned by the IOC and the NCAA [21].

Evidence that DHEA has a true ergogenic effect in the athletic population is lacking. One theory (Corrigan) [21] that contributed to initial enthusiasm for

DHEA use by athletes was that both testosterone and epitestosterone would rise such that the TE ratio used during mandatory urine drug screening tests would remain below the cutoff of 6 [23]. However, limited studies have resulted in conflicting data and use of DHEA has currently fallen out of favor. The number of athletes currently using DHEA cannot be estimated currently and its long-term effects on the endocrine system are unknown.

Case 1. Twenty-three-year-old Asian male body builder presented to a sports medicine clinic for evaluation of concentration difficulty, minor mood swings, and for a routine physical. His past medical history was unremarkable. Sports history was notable for taking up weight-lifting 5 years ago and bodybuilding for 2 years. He had a history of elevated liver transaminases 1 year ago. He denied use of medications, but admits to taking protein supplements and has a history or intermittent creatine supplementation. Further history reveals a 20 lb weight gain in the last year. Social history includes a report of moderate school-related stress as a first year law student. FMH was unremarkable.

Physical examination revealed a muscular male 5 ft 6 in. tall in no distress. Mild striae in his armpits were noted; otherwise, his exam was unremarkable. He requested lab work to recheck his liver enzymes. Additional questioning into the mood swings, weight gain and history of abnormal liver enzymes resulted in the patient admitting he started using anabolic steroids 18 months ago to aid him in his bodybuilding and to improve his appearance and self-esteem for dating. At that point during the office visit he opened up a spreadsheet on his laptop and showed a detailed log of anabolic steroid use. He used both oral and injectable forms. Most of the supply came from Mexico via the internet. He logged type of steroid, dates of use, doses and had "stacked" steroids three times. When he started to experience side effects such as liver enzyme effects or the mood swings he would cycle off. He did admit to a period of testicular atrophy in the past. When counseled on the serious negative and potentially irreversible effects of anabolic steroids then patient stated that was why he kept the log and cycled on and off – i.e. to minimize effects. He emphatically stated that he intended to continue to use steroids to body build as he felt his dosing and cycling regimen was safe. He asked if he could come in to clinic two to three times a year for check ups and blood work to monitor him while on steroids.

Peptide Hormones and Analogues

Human Growth Hormone (hGH)

The first documented abuse of hGH occurred in the early 1980s, almost a decade after anabolic steroid use achieved international notoriety in the sports world [24]. hGH was felt to offer several advantages over anabolic steroids most notable of which was the inability to detect hGH on random urine drug screens. To date, there have been few randomized double-blind placebo-controlled studies that have examined the effect of hGH on muscle strength in athletes. One 1993 study evaluated 22 adult male athletes who were given recombinant human growth hormone (rhGH) at a dose similar to the supraphysiologic dose used to treat children with Turner Syndrome, or placebo daily at bedtime for 6 weeks. Each study subject trained 8–14 h/week [25]. Results were reported on 18 of the subjects and showed significant increase in biceps and quadriceps strength in both groups but no difference between the rGh and placebo groups. Urine was monitored for concurrent anabolic steroid use. Three subjects withdrew due to experiencing hand edema and one had carpal tunnel symptoms.

Mechanism of Action

GH physiology describes a pulsatile secretion that is highly variable among various individuals and has daily variations related to sleep, exercise, and nutritional status. Acute exercise stimulates pulsatile GH secretion by five- to tenfold. Longstanding malnutrition and obesity suppress normal GH secretion. The half-life of a spontaneous GH pulse is approximately 20 min. GH is not secreted intact in the urine and that coupled with wide variability in GH levels has made it difficult to develop an effective screening test for abuse [26].

Adverse Effects of GH Abuse

There are five categories of known adverse GH effects and are related to long-term uses (Table 20.4). These include fluid retention, insulin resistance, mandibular overgrowth, malignancies, and blood borne disease due to contaminated needle use [27].

Specific Cardiovascular Concerns

Dilated cardiomyopathy is a known complication of excess growth hormone levels due to interstitial fibrosis, myocardial hypertrophy, and lymphomononuclear

Table 20.4 Adverse GH effects

Categories	Systemic effects
Fluid retention	Arthralgias, carpal tunnel syndrome, and pseudotumor cerebri
Insulin resistance	Impaired glucose tolerance, type II diabetes mellitus, hypertension, increased cardiovascular disease, dyslipidemia
Acromegaloid features	Mandibular overgrowth
Malignancies	Predominantly GI tract
High risk behavior such as needle sharing	HIV, hepatitis

infiltration with necrosis [28]. Arrhythmias and sudden cardiac death have also been reported [4].

Future Concerns

There appears to be little change in body composition in healthy, lean, trained athletes. This is in direct contrast to the significant, often dramatic, changes seen in GH-deficient children. Of concern is the concomitant use of GH with gonadotropin-releasing hormone analogues in pre-adolescent and adolescent athletes that participate in height sensitive sports such as volleyball and basketball [29]. Combined use could results in delayed puberty and increased growth in children. Future research and education is needed to decrease the illicit use of hGH in athletes as well as to better understand the adverse effects on the human body.

Despite the lack of evidence, the high cost of hGH and the warnings about potential long-term dangers of hGH, it continues to be a popular drug of abuse in the athletic population [27]. Research in the area of testing for hGH abuse has evolved to the extent that a testing procedure for hGH was implemented at the 2004 Olympic Games in Athens, Greece. Testing procedures for hGH will continue to evolve in sports.

Erythropoietin (EPO)

Recombinant human erythropoietin misuse has been reported predominantly in endurance athletes, most notably competitive cyclists. EPO use results in a dose-dependent effect on the hematologic and cardiovascular systems resulting in increased blood viscosity and increased afterload to the heart. Thrombosis, embolisms, arterial hypertension, and cardiac dysfunction have been reported [28, 30, 31]. Anti-doping regulation is difficult with EPO abuse which has contributed to its use in the more elite athletic populations [30, 32].

Stimulants

Stimulant use results in central nervous systems effects by enhancing the secretion of epinephrine, norepinephrine, dopamine, and serotonin. Stimulants are often used by athletes who hope to see physiological responses that delay time to exhaustion and increase perceived energy levels and alertness. Little evidence exists that any sympathomimetic drugs actually affect athletic performance; however, they continue to have widespread popularity and frequent use. The most commonly used stimulants are amphetamines, cocaine, ephedrine alkaloids, and caffeine. These stimulant substances are prohibited in competition according to the WADA prohibited substance lists (http://www.wada-ama.org) [33]. Caffeine is prohibited in a dose-dependent range meant to reflect excessive intake rather than routine dietary use. The sale and/or use of cocaine is illegal in the USA yet is still sold in large quantities on the black market. Use of stimulant substance by athletes is of great concern due to the frequency and severity of the effects on the cardiovascular system.

Amphetamines

Amphetamines appear to mask the physiological perception of fatigue thus may increase time to exhaustion in athletes. Amphetamines are taken orally and can be inhaled. Amphetamine intoxication can result in rhythm disturbances, acute coronary events, strokes, systemic hypertension, cardiogenic shock, and death [34].

Cocaine

Cocaine is an alkaloid extracted from erythroxylon coca. It has a potent sympathomimetic and a vagolytic effect on the heart. Ventricular arrhythmias, A-V conduction disorders, QT and PR-interval prolongation syndromes are risks for sudden death in cocaine users than appears to be independent of any underlying cardiovascular disease due to direct myocardial effects and adrenergic responses [35]. Myocardial ischemia, myocardial infarction, and coronary artery thrombosis are consequences of cocaine use. Chronic cocaine use may result in other cardiac pathology including myocarditis, dilated cardiomyopathy, infective endocarditis, hypertension, thromboembolic events, strokes, and/or life-threatening aneurysms [36].

Ephedra and Ephedrine

Ephedra containing sympathomimetic products have enjoyed great popularity in the last decade or so in their guise of weight-loss aid and athletic performance enhancer. In its heyday, ephedra enjoyed the position of being classified as a nutritional supplement and therefore any regulation of its use was essentially absent. Despite widespread intentional use, it is likely that some athletes were unaware that they were ingesting ephedrine in unknown quantities. Derived from ephedra containing plants such as Ma Huang, ephedrine is often considered a "natural" product, leaving consumers unaware of their consumption.

In 2003, Shekelle et al. [37] published a meta-analysis in *JAMA* that reviewed the safety and efficacy of ephedra for weight loss and athletic performance. Fifty-two controlled trials and 65 case reports were included in the analysis. The results noted that ephedrine was more effective than placebo in promoting weight loss. Ephedrine combined with caffeine was similarly effective in promoting weight loss. In the athletic population, exercise capacity after a single dose of ephedra and caffeine combined was improved by 20–30%. No improvements were seen with either ephedra or caffeine used independently as a single dose [37]. Recently, Williams et al. studied three groups of resistance-trained athletes that ingested placebo, caffeine (300 mg) or caffeine (300 mg) plus ephedra (300 mg). Maximal strength was tested by bench press (1 RM), latissimus dorsi pull down, and a 30 s Wingate test. No significant effects on strength, endurance or peak anaerobic power were found. Increased alertness and enhanced mood was reported in the caffeine plus ephedra study group [38].

Cardiovascular and Systemic Side Effects

Ephedrine is structurally similar to amphetamine. Cardiovascular side effects predominate and often occur in the absence of any pre-existing heart disease. Ephedrine and ephedra (with or without caffeine) were shown to be associated with higher odds ratios over placebo for psychiatric symptoms, heart palpitations, tachycardia, upper gastrointestinal tract symptoms, autonomic hyperactivity, and headache. There were 17,842 adverse events reported in JAMA. About one-half of the serious adverse events occurred in persons under 30 years of age. Serious events included 5 myocardial infarctions, 5 deaths, 11 cerebrovascular events, 4 seizures, and 8 psychiatric cases attributed to ephedra/ephedrine ingestion. This meta-analysis concluded that there was insufficient evidence to support performance enhancing effects of ephedra/ephedrine in athletes [37, 39]. The report was notable for resulting in the US government's decision to remove all ephedra-containing supplements from sale in December, 2003.

Ephedra/Ephedrine as a Controlled or Restricted Drug in Sport

Anti-doping rules exist for the NCAA and the IOC regarding the use of ephedra containing supplements and are still enforced today. A positive doping test includes a urinary concentration greater than 10 mcg/ml [40]. These substances are prohibited during in-competition times yet use is strongly discouraged at all times.

Case two. Sean Riggins, a 16-year-old football player from Illinois, suffered a sudden cardiac arrest and could not be resuscitated. History revealed he had been "partying quite a bit" and during a football game he became nauseated and later passed out at home. He then was taken to his physician's office where he suffered sudden cardiac arrest from which he could not be resuscitated. Cardiac enzymes were significantly elevated, and the Logan County coroner ruled his death to be due to acute myocardial infarction due to vasoconstrictive properties. Questioning of fellow teammates indicated that several team members were using ephedra in the form of Yellow Jackets that they had purchased at a local truck stop. The product was labeled as a dietary supplement and high energizer, containing 25 mg ephedra, and 300 mg of caffeine. Sean's death prompted the State of Illinois legislature to pass a law banning sale of ephedra. Late in 2003, a similar federal law was passed.

Caffeine/Gaurana

Caffeine is perhaps the most widely consumed stimulant substance in the world. From 1998 to 2003, an increase of 465% was seen in the sale of energy drinks in the USA. Sales approximated $5 billion with teens and young adults accounting for $2.3 billion spent [41]. Caffeine is consumed in a variety of forms including beverages, medications, dietary supplements and foods. It may enhance physical performance, increase aerobic endurance, strength, and reaction time. These effects on sport performance are dose dependent and extremely variable [42]. Ergogenic effects have been reported with doses of 3–6 mg/kg and doses might reach 13 mg/kg body weight in some athletes. Caffeine is structurally similar to adenosine, binding in its place to cell membrane receptors, in turn blocking adenosine's actions. Caffeine can potentiate stimulant effects or can counteract others. It appears to be taken up by all body tissues. Other side effects of caffeine intake include increased heart rate, raised systolic and diastolic blood pressure, diuresis, increased attentiveness, increased speech rate and motor activity, tremors, sleep disturbances, and improved mood [43].

Some athletes are unaware of the amounts of caffeine they are ingesting on a routine basis and they ingest caffeine from multiple dietary sources without regard to amount of caffeine or recommended serving size. Examples of popular energy drinks and their caffeine content are contained in Table 20.5 [41].

In the athletic population it is difficult to independently evaluate the organ systems of interest, specifically central nervous system, musculoskeletal and fat in regards to effects of caffeine on the exercising body. Multiple additional factors

Table 20.5 Typical ingredients of popular energy drinks (based on average 8 oz serving)

Energy drink	Caffeine content (mg/8 oz serving)
Arizona Caution Extreme Energy Shot[a]	100 mg
Cocaine[a]	280 mg
Full Throttle(sold as 16 oz)[a]	72 mg
Red Bull[a]	80 mg
Rock Star Energy (sold as 16 oz)[a]	80 mg
Rock Star Juiced (sold as 24 oz)[a]	80 mg
Spike Shooter	300 mg

Source: J Am Pharm Assoc® American Pharmacists Association

[a] Each contains other dietary supplements such as ginseng, taurine, and guarana

affect both experimental design and individual responses such as previous history of caffeine use, nutritional status, the type, duration and intensity of exercise, and the caffeine dose [42].

Caffeine as a Controlled or Restricted Drug in Sport

Caffeine is a "controlled or restricted drug" in the college and elite athletic world. Drug testing is performed for caffeine use/abuse. The IOC considers urinary levels greater than 12 mcg/mL post-competitions illegal. The National Collegiate Athletic Association (NCAA) defines urinary levels greater than 15 mcg/mL as illegal in the USA (http://www.ncaa.org) [44]. Only about 0.5–5% of orally ingested caffeine reaches the urine as most is metabolized by the liver. Therefore, it is difficult to reach urinary caffeine levels exceeding 12 mcg/mL by routine dietary ingestion alone. For example, a 70 kg adult athlete would have to drink more than four mugs of regular coffee about 1 h before exercise (>6 mg/kg body weight) in order to produce a postexercise urine sample (1–1 ½ h later) that might approach illegal levels. Urinary levels of caffeine that exceed 12 mcg/mL likely indicate deliberate ingestion of caffeine, often in the form of tablets or suppositories and should be investigated [42].

Effects of Caffeine Intake in Children

There are concerns of the use of caffeine in children. A study by Ellison reported that children ages 6–10 years old reported caffeine intake approximately 8 of 10 days on average. Other studies have reported caffeine intakes in children approximating 16 mg/day in 7–8 year olds and 24 mg/day in 9–10 year olds vs. 37.4 mg/day in 5–18 year olds [45, 46]. Concerns regarding the effects of caffeine on the developing neurological system exist as well as on the cardiovascular system (hypertension and cardiovascular disease). Caffeine intake should be eliiminated from a child's diet. This will be consistent with the AAP policy on caffeine and energy drinks that is currently in press and the 2.5-4 mg restriction was edited out in favor of the recommendation of complete restriction from caffeine. Caffeine withdrawal has been seen in children consuming more than 300 mg/day or 10 mg/kg/day [47]. The primary dietary source of caffeine for children appears to be soft drinks [48].

Guarana

Caffeine is a component of guarana. Guarana is marketed to increase energy, enhance physical performance and promote weight loss. One gram of guarana is equal to approximately 40 mg caffeine. Guarana may increase the total caffeine in an energy drink [49]. The presence of caffeine in the form of guarana or kola nut may confuse the consumer through either intentional or unintentional misdirection on product labels. Improvements in education and consumer labeling of products containing stimulant substances is greatly needed and should be supported by all members of the sport community.

Conclusion

The quality, safety, content, and labeling of each supplement must be sought such that athletes and all consumers can be counseled and educated appropriately regarding the risks and benefits of product use. Due to the widespread use and abuse of anabolic-androgenic steroids and a wide variety of unregulated dietary supplements and stimulants, serious cardiovascular consequences are of great concern to the health-care professional and sport scientist. Almost all illicit drugs can cause cardiac symptoms including cardiomyopathies, myocarditis, coronary abnormalities, valvular diseases, and primary electrical disorders. Cardiac arrhythmias frequently result either directly or indirectly from illicit drug use and often occur in the absence of any underlying cardiac abnormalities. However, illicit drug use that precipitates cardiac arrhythmias may signal the presence of latent heart disease such as inherited cardiomyopathies or life-threatening arrhythmogenic heart disease. The presence of new onset cardiac disease or unexplained cardiac symptoms associated with sport participation and exercise prompts an immediate and thorough investigation into the cause and must include a thorough screen for drug/supplement use or abuse.

It is the responsibility of all health-care professionals in the field of sports medicine to educate themselves as to the warning signs and risks of illicit drug and supplement use in the athletic population. Support of efforts aimed at youth athletes through professional level competitors that provide education and encourage drug free sport participation hopefully will result in a national and international decline in doping practices and experimentation in the future. The most current international standard prohibited substance list and the World Anti-doping Code of Ethics is available at http://www.wada-ama.org (the home website of the World Anti-Doping Agency). Additional resources are available at http://www.ncaa.org and http://www.usoc.org.

References

1. Herbal treatments: the promises and pitfalls. *Consum Rep.* 1999;64:44–48.
2. Green GA, Uryasz FD, Petr TA, et al. NCAA study of substance use and abuse habits of college student-athletes. *Clin J Sport Med.* 2001;11:51–56.
3. IOC Press release. 4 April, 2002; http://www.olympic.or/uk/news/publications/press_ik.asp?release=266.

4. Deligiannis A, Bjöornstad H, Carre F, et al. ESC Study Group of Sports Cardiology. ESC Study Group of Sports Cardiology Position Paper on adverse cardiovascular effects of doping in athletes. *Eur J Cardiovasc Prev Rehabil.* 2006;13:687–694.
5. Melchert RB, Welder AA. Cardiovascular effects of androgenic-anabolic steroids. *Med Sci Sports Exerc.* 1995;27:1252–1262.
6. Kerr JM, Congeni JA. Anabolic-androgenic steroids: use and abuse in pediatric patients. *Pediatr Clin N Am.* 2007;54:771–785.
7. Sadler MA, Griffiths KA, McCredie RJ, et al. Androgenic anabolic steroids and arterial structure and function in male bodybuilders. *J Am Coll Cardiol.* 2001;37:224–230.
8. Hickson RC, Ball KL, Falduto MT. Adverse effects of anabolic steroids. *Med Toxicol Adverse Drug Exp.* 1989;4:254–271.
9. Glazer G. Arthogenic effects of anabolic steroids on serum lipid levels. *Arch Intern Med.* 1991;151:1925–1933.
10. Hartgens F, Kuipers H. Effects of androgenic-anabolic steroids in athletes. *Sports Med.* 2004;34:513–554.
11. National Institute on Drug Abuse Research Report – Steroid Abuse and Addiction. *National Institutes of Health Education Publication No. 00–3721.* Bethesda (MD): National Institutes of Health; 2000.
12. Hartgens F, Reitjens G, Keizer HA, et al. Effects of androgenic-anabolic steroids on apolipoprotiesn and lipoproteins (a). *Br J Sports Med.* 2004;38:253–259.
13. Sullivan ML, Martinez CM, Gennis P, et al. The cardiac toxicity of anabolic steroids. *Prog Cardiovasc Dis.* 1998;41:1–15.
14. Riebe D, Fernhall B, Thompson PD. The blood pressure response to exercise in anabolic steroid users. *Med Sci Sports Exerc.* 1992;24:633–637.
15. McKillop G, Todd IC, Ballantine D. Increased left ventricular mass in a bodybuilder using anabolic steroids. *Br J Sports Med.* 1986;20:151–152.
16. Urhausen A, Holpes R, Kindermann W. One and two-dimensional echocardiography in body builders using anabolic steroids. *Eur J Appl Physiol.* 1989;58:633–640.
17. Sullivan M, Martinez C, Gallagher J. Atrial fibrillation and anabolic steroids. *J Emerg Med.* 1999;17(5):851–857.
18. Urhausen A, Albers T, Kindermann W. Are the cardiac effects of anabolic steroid abuse in strength athletes reversible? *Heart.* 2004;90(5):496–501.
19. Clark BM, Schofield RS. Dilated cardiomyopathy and acute liver injury associated with combined use of ephedra, gamma-hydroxybutyrate, and anabolic steroids. *Pharmacotherapy.* 2005;25(5):756–761.
20. Cocaine and opiates found in Caminiti's body. November 1, 2004, ESPN.com.
21. Corrigan B. DHEA and sport. *Clin J Sport Med.* 2002;12:236–241.
22. Holden C. Interest grows in anti-aging drug. *Science.* 1995;269:33.
23. Di Pasquale MG. Dehydroepitestosterone (DHEA). *Drugs Sport.* 1994;2:2–3.
24. Issajenko A. *Running Risks.* Macmillan, Canada. 1990:146.
25. Deyssig R. Frisch H. Blum WF, et al. Effect of growth hormone treatment on hormonal parameters, body composition and strength in athletes. *Acta Endocrinol.* 1993;128:313–318.
26. Bidlingmaier M, Wu Z, Strasburger CJ. Test method: GH. *Bailliere's Clin Endocrinol Metab.* 2000;14:99–109.
27. Dean H. Does exogenous growth hormone improve athletic performance? *Clin J Sport Med.* 2002;12:250–253.
28. Rogol A. Sex steroid and growth hormone supplementation to enhance performance in adolescent athletes. *Curr Opin Pediatr.* 2000;12:382–387.
29. Colao A, Marzullo P, Di Somma C, et al. Growth hormone and the heart. *Clin Endocrinol.* 2001;54:137–154.
30. Audran M, Gareau R, Matecki S, et al. Effects of erythropoietin administration in training athletes and possible indirect detection in doping control. *Med Sci Sport Exerc.* 1999;31:639–645.
31. Vergouwen PC, Collee T, Marx JJ. Haematocrit in elite athletes. *Int J Sports Med.* 1999;20:538–541.

32. Noakes TD. Tainted glory. Doping and athletic performance. *N Engl J Med.* 2004;151:847–849.
33. World Anti-Doping Agency. *The World Anti-Doping Code – The 2009 prohibited list, International Standard.* Lausanne: WADA; 2008. Web site http://www.wada-ama.org.
34. George A. Central nervous system stimulants. *Bailliere's Clin Endocrinol Metab.* 2000;14:79–88.
35. Cregler L. Substance abuse in sports: The impact of cocaine, alcohol, steroids, and other drugs on the heart. In: Williams RA, ed. *The Athlete and Heart Disease: Diagnosis, Evaluation and Management.* Philadelphia: Lippincott, Williams and Wilkins; 1999:131–153.
36. Billman GE. Cocaine: a review of its toxic actions on cardiac function. *Crit Rev Toxicol.* 1995;25:113–132.
37. Shekelle PG, Hardy ML, Morton SC, et al. Efficacy and safety of ephedra and ephedrine for weight loss and athletic performance: a meta-analysis. *JAMA.* 2003;289:1537–1545.
38. Williams AD, Cribb PJ, Cooke MB, et al. The effect of ephedra and caffeine on maximal strength and power in resistance-trained athletes. *J Strength Cond Res.* 2008;22:464–470.
39. Malek MH, Housh TJ, Coburn JW, et al. Effects of eight weeks of caffeine supplementation and endurance training on aerobic fitness and body composition. *J Strength Cond Res.*2006; 20(4):751–755.
40. Pipe A, Ayotte C. Nutritional supplements and doping. *Clin J Sport Med.* 2002;12:245–249.
41. Clauson KA, Shields KM, McQueen CE, et al. Safety issues associated with commercially available energy drinks. *J Am Pharm Assoc.* 2008;48(3):e55–e63.
42. Graham TE, Spriet LL. Caffeine and exercise performance. *Sport Sci Exerc.* 1996;9:1.
43. Australia New Zealand Food Authority. Report of the expert group on the safety aspects of dietary caffeine ANZFA, Canberra. 2000.
44. http://www.ncaa.org.
45. Ellison RC, Singer MR, Moore LL. Current caffeine intake of young children; amount and sources. *J Am Diet Assoc.* 1995;95:802–803.
46. Morgan KJ, Stults VJ, Zabik ME. Amount and dietary sources of caffeine and saccharin intake by individuals 5–18 years. *Regul Toxiol Pharmacol.* 1982;2:296–307.
47. Nawrot P, Jorden S, Eastwood J, Rostein J, Hugenholtz A, Feeley M. Effects of caffeine on human health Food Addit Contam 2003;20:1–30.
48. Frary CD, Johnson RK, Wang MQ. Food sources and intakes of caffeine in the diets of persons in the United States. *J Am Diet Assoc.* 2003;103:1326–1331.
49. Santa Maria A, Lopez A, Diaz M, et al. Evaluation of toxicity of guarana with invitro bioassays. *Ecotoxicol Environ Saf.* 1998;39:164–167.

Suggested Web sites

American College of Cardiology – http://www.acc.org
American College of Sports Medicine – http://www.acsm.org
National Collegiate Athletic Association – http://www.ncaa.org
United States Anti-Doping Agency – http://www.usada.org
World Anti-Doping Agency – http://www.wada-ama.org

Chapter 21
Return-to-Play Decisions in Athletes with Cardiac Conditions: Guidelines and Considerations

Christine E. Lawless

Introduction

Clinicians who treat the more than 20 million competitive and recreational athletes in the USA are confronted by a variety of return-to-play (RTP) decisions [1, 2]. The main objective of these decisions is to prevent sudden cardiac death (SCD) during sports participation, while allowing all individuals to experience the benefits of exercise and physical activity. Specific goals are to (1) detect unsuspected underlying heart disease through preparticipation screening; (2) determine the risk of participating in competitive sports for athletes with known underlying heart disease; and (3) provide recommendations for physical activity and recreational sports participation for those athletes with underlying heart disease considered to be too high risk for participation in competitive sports. This chapter reviews existing guidelines from large professional organizations and describes key considerations when making RTP decisions. Case studies are provided to illustrate challenging RTP decisions.

Guidelines for Sports Participation for Athletes with Known Cardiac Conditions

Major guidelines for sports participation for athletes with known cardiac conditions are listed in Table 21.1 [3–9] and reviewed in greater detail elsewhere[2]. Among the most widely used guidelines are the 36th Bethesda Conference Eligibility Recommendations for Competitive Athletes with Cardiovascular Abnormalities [4]. In the USA, the 36th Bethesda Guidelines are considered the "gold standard" for determining RTP; key recommendations for the most common causes of SCD in athletes are summarized in Table 21.2.

C.E. Lawless (✉)
Sports Cardiology Consultants, LLC, Clinical Associate Faculty, University of Chicago Consulting Cardiologist, Major League Soccer Team Physician, US Figure Skating World Teams, 360 West Illinois Street #7D, Chicago, IL 60654, USA
e-mail: christine.lawless@yahoo.com

C.E. Lawless (ed.), *Sports Cardiology Essentials: Evaluation, Management and Case Studies*, DOI 10.1007/978-0-387-92775-6_21,

Table 21.1 Guidelines for sports participation for athletes with known cardiac conditions [3–9]

Guideline	Comment
AHA 2007 update	• Twelve-element focused examination as part of preparticipation examination • Can help to identify athletes with preexisting conditions or suspected cardiac disease • Does NOT recommend routine ECG screening
36th Bethesda Conference Recommendations	• Gold standard for RTP in the USA • Classifies sports by static and dynamic components; 1A sports are low static/low dynamic • See Table 21.2 for summary
European Society of Cardiology	• Similar to the Bethesda Guidelines • Some notable differences
AHA Consensus for Young Patients with Genetic CVD	• Includes grading system for exercise • Consistent with the Bethesda Guidelines • Useful for prescribing exercise for athletes with high-risk conditions
NASPE policy conference on arrhythmias and the athlete	• Favored by EP community • Older, but similar to the Bethesda Guidelines • One exception is postablation RTP; this technique is now more common and athletes can RTP sooner than described by NASPE guidelines
WHF, IFSM, AHA Consensus on Masters Athletes	• Similar to Bethesda Guidelines • Athletes >40 years of age • Range of conditioning from elite athletes to walk-up athletes

AHA American Heart Association, *CVD* cardiovascular disease, *NASPE* North American Society for Pacing and Electrophysiology (now the Heart Rhythm Society), *WHF* World Heart Federation, *IFSM* International Federation of Sports Medicine, *EP* electrophysiology, *RTP* return-to-play

It should be noted that the older 26th Bethesda Guidelines were used in a court case in the 1990s to support disqualification of a college athlete. This case set a precedent for the use of the guidelines in a court of law [4]. As a result, physicians should be prepared to defend any decisions they make that deviate from the Bethesda Guideline recommendations.

The European Society of Cardiology offered guidelines similar to the 36th Bethesda Guidelines [5, 6]. However, there are notable differences between the two documents, including recommendations regarding genotype positive-phenotype negative hypertrophic cardiomyopathy (HCM) and dilated cardiomyopathy (DCM) [10]. These differences are reviewed elsewhere [2, 10]. However, clinicians treating athletes with such conditions may consider the recommendations of both panels.

Recommendations for Young Patients with Genetic Cardiovascular Diseases

The American Heart Association (AHA) has published recommendations regarding participation of young patients (≤40 years of age) with genetic cardiovascular diseases in recreational sports. Cited conditions included inherited cardiomyopathies, ion-channel

Table 21.2 Summary of 36th Bethesda Guidelines Recommendations for sports participation for athletes with underlying heart disease known to predispose to sudden cardiac death [4]

	HCM	Anomalous coronary	ARVC	DCM	Long QT syndrome	Marfan's syndrome
Participation in all sports allowed	No	No	No	No	No	IA–IIA sports, with certain restrictions, depending on the size of aorta (≤40 mm), the absence of family history of dissection, and the absence of significant valve disease)
Participation allowed if genotype +, phenotype -	Yes	N/A	Not specified in Bethesda Guidelines	N/A	Yes, but no swimming allowed for Long QT1	Not specified
Participation allowed after corrective surgery	No	Yes	N/A	Yes, postheart transplant, provided no coronary luminal narrowing or ischemia	N/A	Low intensity (IA) sports only
Participation allowed with ICD	No	No	No	No	No	N/A
Participation allowed with beta blockers	No	Not specifically addressed	Not specifically addressed	Not addressed. If ejection fraction has normalized, no specific comment made	Not specifically addressed	Not specifically addressed

ARVC arrhythmogenic right ventricular cardiomyopathy, *DCM* dilated cardiomyopathy, *HCM* hypertrophic cardiomyopathy, *ICD* implantable cardioverter defibrillator, *LVEF* left ventricular ejection fraction
Reproduced with permission from *The Physician and Sportsmedicine*

diseases [e.g., long QT syndrome (LQTS), Brugada syndrome], and connective tissue disorders (e.g., Marfan's syndrome) [7]. The authors also proposed a convenient grading system that ranks common forms of exercise a scale of 0–5 (Table 21.3). Overall, these guidelines are consistent with the 36th Bethesda Guidelines.

Table 21.3 Summary of recommendations for acceptability of recreational (Noncompetitive) sports activities and exercise in patients with genetic cardiovascular diseases [7]

Intensity level	HCM[a]	LOTS[a]	Marfan syndrome[b]	ARVC	Brugada syndrome
High					
Basketball					
Full court	0	0	2	1	2
Half court	0	0	2	1	2
Body building[c]	1	1	0	1	1
Ice hockey[c]	0	0	1	0	0
Racquetball/squash	0	2	2	0	2
Rock climbing[c]	1	1	1	1	1
Running (sprinting)	0	0	2	0	2
Skiing (downhill)[c]	2	2	2	1	1
Skiing (cross-country)	2	3	2	1	4
Soccer	0	0	2	0	2
Tennis (singles)	0	0	3	0	2
Touch (flag) football	1	1	3	1	3
Windsurfing[d]	1	0	1	1	1
Moderate					
Basketball/softball	2	2	2	2	4
Biking	4	4	3	2	4
Modest hiking	4	5	5	2	4
Motorcycling[c]	3	1	2	2	2
Jogging	3	3	3	2	5
Sailing[d]	3	3	2	2	4
Surfing[d]	2	0	1	1	1
Swimming (lap)[d]	5	0	3	3	4
Tennis (doubles)	4	4	4	3	4
Treadmill/stationary bicycle	5	5	4	3	5
Weightlifting (free weights)[c,e]	1	1	0	1	1
Hiking	3	3	3	2	4
Low					
Bowling	5	5	5	4	5
Golf	5	5	5	4	5
Horseback riding[c]	3	3	3	3	3
Scuba diving[d]	0	0	0	0	0
Skating[f]	5	5	5	4	5
Snorkeling[d]	5	0	5	4	4
Weights (nonfree weights)	4	4	0	4	4
Brisk walking	5	5	5	5	5

Note: 0–1 generally not advised, 2–3 to be assessed individually, and 4–5 probably permitted

(continued)

Table 21.3 (continued)

Recreational sports are categorized with regard to high, moderate, and low levels of exercise and graded on a relative scale (from 0 to 5) for eligibility with 0–1 indicating generally not advised or strongly discouraged; 4–5 indicating probably permitted; and 2–3 indicating intermediate and to be assessed clinically on an individual basis; The designations of high, moderate, and low levels of exercise are equivalent to estimated >6, 4–6, and <4 metabolic equivalents.

[a] Assumes absence of laboratory DNA genotyping data; therefore, limited to clinical diagnosis

[b] Assumes no or only mild aortic dilatation

[c] These sports involve the potential for traumatic injury, which should be taken into consideration for individuals with a risk for impaired consciousness

[d] The possibility of impaired consciousness occurring during water-related activities should be taken into account with respect to the clinical profile of the individual patient. Barotrauma is a primary risk associated with the use of the scuba apparatus in Marfan syndrorne

[e] Recommendations generally differ from those for weight-training machines (nonfree weights), based largely on the potential risks of traumatic injury associated with episodes of impaired consciousness during bench-press maneuvers. Otherwise, the physiological effects of all weight-training activities are regarded as similar with respect to the present recommendations

[f] Individual sporting activity not associated with the team sport of ice hockey

Recommendations for Masters Athletes

A collaborative effort of several international and US organizations produced a set of recommendations for masters athletes [9]. Masters athletes are defined as those older 40 years of age at various levels of conditioning. The incidence of SCD is higher in masters athletes compared with younger athletes; the risk of SCD in masters joggers and marathon participants is estimated to be 1/15,000 and 1/50,000, respectively [9, 11, 12]. The recommendations note that 12-lead ECG should be used for preparticipation screening of all masters athletes. However, preparticipation exercise testing should be reserved for men >40–45 years of age and women >50–55 years of age with moderate to high cardiovascular risk. The probability of an exercise-induced cardiac event is greater in athletes with atherosclerotic coronary disease and left ventricular dysfunction. Therefore, masters athletes should be discouraged from participation in high-intensity sports if they have left ventricular ejection fraction <50% or evidence of exercise-induced ischemia, ventricular arrhythmia, or systolic hypotension [9].

Return-to-Play: General Considerations

Implanted Defibrillators

Implanted cardiac defibrillators (ICDs) are generally effective in preventing SCD in nonathletes with diagnoses such as HCM [13]. However, the fluid shifts, electrolyte abnormalities, and catecholamine excess that occur during vigorous activity may alter defibrillation thresholds, and it cannot be assumed that ICD will reliably defibrillate under such conditions [14–16]. According to the Bethesda Guidelines, athletes with high-risk conditions such as HCM should not participate in vigorous sports, even when an ICD is present [4]. Indeed, ICDs have not been proven to prevent SCD during athletics. Nevertheless, clinical practice often differs from this recommendation. Surveys of implanting physicians and team physicians suggest that as many as 70% of athletes with ICDs and underlying cardiac conditions continue to participate in sports[14–16]. The Sports ICD Registry was created in 2006 to address issues surrounding the safety of ICDs in athletics and actively exercising individuals (see Chapters 10 and 18).

Ablations

Ablations are relatively common procedures for the diagnosis of conditions such as atrial flutter, atrial fibrillation, right ventricular outflow tract tachycardias, reentrant AV nodal tachycardias, and Wolff–Parkinson–White (WPW) syndrome. Athletes who are *symptomatic* with such conditions should be considered for electrophysiologic testing and treatment with radiofrequency ablation (RFA). The determination of RTP hinges on the length of recovery following ablation procedures and the use of anticoagulation.

Beta Blockers

Clinicians may wish to allow play for athletes with HCM or LQTS who are taking beta blockers. Although beta blockers appear to reduce the incidence of SCD episodes in nonathletic populations [17, 18], their effectiveness in the context of vigorous sport has not yet been demonstrated. Furthermore, the degree of beta blockade required to prevent SCD episodes would likely impact maximal heart rate and athletic performance, making this strategy impractical for athletes [19].

Corrective Cardiac Surgery

Corrective surgery for underlying cardiac conditions may help reduce symptoms and, possibly, the risk for SCD. The RTP decision following corrective surgery depends on whether the procedure has sufficiently reduced the risk for SCD. For example, surgical myectomy or alcohol septal ablation in a patient with HCM can reduce outflow tract obstruction and relieve symptoms; however, the underlying arrhythmogenic substrate remains largely unchanged. Therefore, the history of a corrective procedure does not necessarily alter recommendations for sports participation. Conversely, surgical correction of an anomalous coronary artery results in anatomical correction of the underlying problem and likely reduces or eliminates risks of ischemia and malignant ventricular arrhythmias. According to the Bethesda Guidelines, sports participation is allowed 3 months after surgical correction so long as there is no evidence of exercise-induced LV dysfunction, arrhythmia, or ischemia [4].

The Grey-Zone Athlete

Certain athletes may have indefinite cardiac findings on preparticipation exam. These grey-zone athletes neither have a clear cardiac diagnosis nor can a cardiac diagnosis be ruled out. An example of a grey-zone athlete is one who has negative genotype for HCM, normal MRI, and inconclusive echocardiogram, but has a thickened ventricular wall and abnormal ECG. The decision to allow play for grey-zone athletes is a challenge. When a diagnosis is uncertain, it may be prudent to disallow participation, especially for high-intensity sports. However, there may be ramifications to disqualifying such athletes; they may consider legal action to pursue right to play or seek a different team or team physician. Athletes may also consider signing waivers of responsibility, although this course may not be in the best interests of the athlete.

Grey-Zone Athlete: Case Study

A 17-year-old professional soccer player underwent preparticipation physical for participation in Major League Soccer. An ECG was performed (Fig. 21.1). On questioning, the player reported becoming fatigued at an earlier point in conditioning drills compared with his colleagues. Family history was negative for HCM, syncope, chest pain, and palpitations. Examination was unremarkable, and no murmur was detected. Echocardiography suggested thickened myocardium at the left ventricular apex. Stress testing revealed a decrease in blood pressure at peak exercise. Cardiac

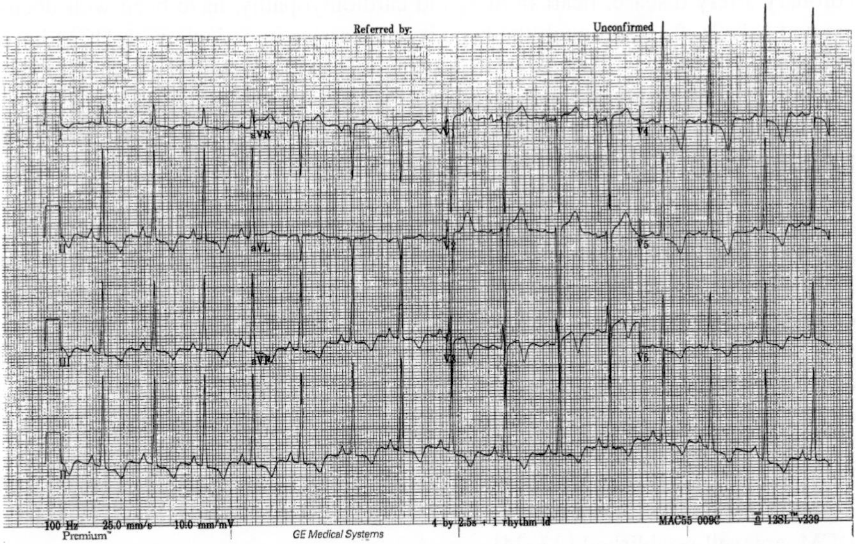

Fig. 21.1 Electrocardiogram for 17-year-old professional soccer player with features suggestive of apical HCM but with uncertain diagnosis

MRI showed apical thickening, and contrast imaging was consistent with the endomyocardial scarring seen in HCM. Genetic testing was negative for HCM. Although he was not given definitive diagnosis of HCM, consulting cardiologists felt that he was too high risk to play competitive Major League Soccer.

Specific Considerations for Conditions That Predispose to SCD Episodes

The majority of SCD episodes in young athletes are due to three categories of conditions: cardiomyopathies, anomalous coronary artery, and high-risk channelopathies.

Cardiomyopathies and Inflammatory Diseases

HCM is characterized by cardiac hypertrophy with diastolic dysfunction, which can be detected by ECG in 75–95% of cases [20]. According to the Bethesda Guidelines, all athletes with a "probable or unequivocal clinical diagnosis of HCM should be excluded from most competitive sports with the possible exception of those of low intensity [4]."

For athletes with HCM who have been disqualified from participation in competitive sports, clinicians should consider recommendations for physical activity (i.e., exercise prescription). The benefits of regular exercise for various disease states, including coronary artery disease, heart failure, and cardiomyopathy, have been well documented [11, 21–23]. Although the benefits of exercise in patients with HCM have not been studied, it is reasonable to assume that exercise would provide similar benefits for these patients. Until appropriate studies are performed, clinicians may consider recommending a level of exercise consistent with cardiac rehabilitation for patients with HCM. However, HCM patients are contraindicated from participation in competitive sports other than 1A.

DCM is characterized by ventricular chamber enlargement, systolic dysfunction, and risk for SCD. The Bethesda Guidelines recommend that athletes with DCM not participate in competitive sports, with the possible exception of 1A sports for certain patients [4]. A substantial number of athletes diagnosed with DCM may show normalization of the LV ejection fraction after treatment with angiotensin-converting enzyme inhibitors and beta blockers. Although the Bethesda Guidelines do not specifically address this dilemma, clinicians informally report making RTP decisions based on the type of sport and level of competition (Dr. A. Anderson, Dr. P. Binkley, Dr. C. Lawless, personal communication, July 2006). The benefits of cardiac-rehabilitation level of exercise for patients with heart failure, including DCM, are well established [22–24].

Arrhythmogenic right ventricular dysplasia or cardiomyopathy (ARVD or ARVC) is characterized by fibrofatty infiltration of the myocardium. The condition is estimated to account for 2.8% of the SCD in athletes in the USA [25], whereas estimates from Europe range as high as 22% [26, 27]. Athletes with this extremely high-risk cardiomyopathic condition are disqualified from sports [4]. The risks and benefits of moderate levels of exercise remain unknown, but guidelines for young athletes with genetic conditions indicate that 1A activities are probably allowed (with the exception of scuba diving) [7].

Myocarditis is an acute inflammatory disease of the myocardium. Inflammation may partially or completely resolve or progress to DCM. When probable or definite acute myocarditis is identified, the subject should be disqualified from all competitive sports. A rest period of approximately 6 months is recommended following onset. Following this rest period, sports participation may be allowed so long as left ventricular function, serum markers of inflammation, and 12-lead ECG have all returned to normal, and 24-h ambulatory monitoring and graded exercise testing detect no evidence of clinically relevant supraventricular or ventricular arrhythmias [4].

Pericarditis is an acute inflammatory disease of the pericardium that may or may not be associated with acute myocarditis. The condition is characterized by chest pain, ST-segment elevation, elevated serum markers of inflammatory, and pericardial effusion on echocardiography. A diagnosis of acute pericarditis disqualifies athletes from participation in competitive sports. However, once the condition has resolved (including all symptoms, inflammation, and effusion), RTP may be allowed. It should be noted that the presence of chronic pericardial constriction disqualifies the athlete from all competitive sports [4].

Congenital Heart Disease

Anomalous coronary artery occurs with an incidence of approximately 0.1% in the general population, but accounts for up to 19% of the SCD episodes in young athletes [25]. The most lethal variant appears to be anomalous coronary arising from the opposite sinus of Valsalva [28]. Symptoms may include exertional syncope, palpitations, chest pain, or dyspnea [28]. For symptomatic athletes with anomalous coronary artery, symptoms should be detected on PPE. The prevailing practice is to perform surgical transposition of the artery. Athletes may return to play 3 months later, so long as postoperative stress testing is negative for ischemia or arrhythmias [4].

Other congenital conditions, including congenital heart disease, Marfan's syndrome, bicuspid valve, and other forms of valvular heart disease, are discussed in detail in the Bethesda Guidelines and in corresponding chapters in this text [4].

Aortic Reconstruction: Case Study

A 27-year-old professional soccer player presented with new onset chest pain about 2 months into the competitive season. Evaluation revealed at least moderately severe aortic regurgitation, bicuspid aortic valve with dilated aorta, and aortic root diameter of 4.8 cm. Aortic root reconstruction was performed, including repair of the aortic valve without replacement. According to the Bethesda Guidelines, athletes with prior surgical aortic root reconstruction can participate only in 1A competitive sports. However, there are cases of professional athletes with a similar condition who continue to play, including Ronny Turiaf, a professional basketball player who underwent aortic root reconstruction in 2005 and continues to play in the NBA [29]. The soccer player was given all this information, and although RTP was not allowed for him in the USA, he was allowed to play in Europe after a sports cardiology consultation was obtained.

Rhythm Disturbances

Supraventricular Rhythm Disturbances

Sinus bradycardias, sinus tachycardia, premature atrial contractions (PACs), and nonsustained supraventricular arrythmias are generally manageable, nonlethal rhythm disturbances. For symptomatic athletes with no evidence of underlying high-risk heart disease, all sports are allowed. However, the Bethesda Guidelines note that athletes with pacemakers should not participate in collision sports [4].

Clinicians are referred to the NASPE and Bethesda Guidelines and the chapter on specific rhythm disturbances in this text for more complex management decisions regarding conditions such as atrial flutter and atrial fibrillation [4, 8].

AV Nodal Reentrant Tachycardia

The most common cause of sustained supraventricular tachycardia in the athlete is AV nodal reentrant tachycardia. More than 95% of cases can be successfully treated with RFA, with complication rates less than 1%. Indeed, many electrophysiologists and cardiologists recommend RFA for initial treatment [30, 31]. RTP may be considered within 2–4 weeks after successful treatment with RFA. Play may be allowed even within a few days if the rhythm disturbance cannot be induced on electrophysiologic testing [4].

Wolff–Parkinson–White Syndrome

Athletes with WPW may present with or without symptoms. The presentation of WPW may include abnormal ECG, palpitations, syncope, or rarely, ventricular fibrillation arrest [32]. The classic ECG pattern of short PR interval and delta waves may or may not be present. For symptomatic athletes, RFA is successful in more than 95% of cases, with RTP generally allowed within 2–4 weeks if repeat stimulation testing has not been performed [4]. For asymptomatic athletes, treatment and RTP guidelines are more controversial. Some electrophysiologists recommend allowing RTP, since the incidence of SCD in athletes with asymptomatic WPW is very low. However, other investigators suggest performing assessment of the refractory period of the bypass tract; for conduction rates >240 beats/min, RFA is recommended to eliminate the risk of life-threatening arrhythmias [4, 32–34].

Ventricular Rhythm Disturbances

Certain ventricular rhythm disturbances, such as premature ventricular contractions (PVCs) and frequent and complex ventricular ectopy, are common in some athletes. Greater frequency of PVC generally suggests greater likelihood of underlying heart disease [35]. Sports participation hinges on the presence or absence of underlying heart disease. When underlying disease is evident, sports participation is generally restricted by the underlying condition. In the absence of structural heart disease, participation is generally not restricted [4].

Nonsustained or Sustained Ventricular Tachycardia

Monomorphic, nonsustained ventricular tachycardia (NSVT, defined as duration <30 s) does not present a risk for SCD in the absence of underlying structural heart disease [36–39]. However, athletes with polymorphic NSVT should be considered for treatment with beta blockers and restriction of athletic activity [4]. Sustained ventricular tachycardia (defined as >30 s in duration and either monomorphic or polymorphic) occurs most often in younger athletes in the context of underlying structural heart disease. For older athletes with sustained ventricular tachycardia, ischemic heart disease should be considered. The RTP decision should be dictated by current guidelines for the underlying cardiac disease.

Arrhythmias in athletes with structurally normal hearts include ventricular tachycardia arising from the right or left ventricular outflow tract and idiopathic left ventricular tachycardia [36–40]. These conditions are often treated with RFA, and RTP is allowed in 2–4 weeks or sooner [4].

Ventricular Fibrillation

Any athlete who has experienced and survived an episode of ventricular fibrillation will likely have an ICD. As discussed previously, competitive sport at a moderate or high level of intensity is not allowed according to the Bethesda Guidelines [4].

However, participation in 1A sports is allowed for athletes with an ICD and no device therapy for ventricular flutter or fibrillation within 6 months [4].

Common Valvular Diseases

Bicuspid Aortic Valve

Among the most common valvular lesions is bicuspid aortic valve, which can be associated with progressive aortic dilatation, aortic dissection and rupture, and other congenital abnormalities such as coarctation of the aorta. Participation and RTP can be determined by the degree of aortic stenosis/insufficiency, the diameter of the aorta, and the degree of coarctation of the aorta, if present [4].

Aortic Stenosis

Sports participation for athletes with aortic stenosis depends on the severity of stenosis [4]. All sports are allowed for athletes with mild aortic stenosis, and participation in 1A, 1B, and 2A sports is allowed for athletes with moderate aortic stenosis. However, play is not allowed for athletes with severe aortic stenosis unless they have undergone a corrective procedure. RTP following surgical repair or valvuloplasty depends on the presence of a bioprosthesis or a mechanical valve or degree of aortic regurgitation. Collision sports are prohibited for athletes requiring long-term anticoagulation [4].

Aortic Insufficiency

Aortic insufficiency may occur in athletes with bicuspid aortic valve. The condition may be associated with aortic dilation, increased left ventricular size, reduced exercise tolerance, or ventricular arrhythmias. Clinicians should refer the athlete for evaluation by a cardiologist, as RTP recommendation may depend on several factors [4].

Mitral Valve Prolapse

Mitral valve prolapse (MVP) accounts for 2% of SCD in athletes [41]. There are two types of MVP: anatomic and syndromic. Anatomic MVP is characterized by myxomatous degeneration of the mitral valve and is associated with the risk for sudden death, embolism, and rhythm disturbances. In syndromic MVP, the valve appears to be normal. Symptoms due to MVP are thought to relate to neuroendocrine or autonomic dysfunction [41]. Determination of participation and RTP is based on the degree of mitral regurgitation, left ventricular dysfunction, ectopy, prior embolic event, and family history of sudden death [4].

Summary

Clinicians are often required to identify athletes at risk for cardiac events, evaluate underlying heart disease, and apply published guidelines for RTP decisions. The decision to allow play is generally based on the presence or absence of an underlying, potentially lethal cardiac condition. For athletes with cardiac conditions who undergo treatment, RTP decisions are based on the degree to which treatment has altered the underlying condition such that the risk of SCD is eliminated or significantly reduced.

References

1. Street and Smith's Sports Business Daily. Team sports participation in the US up for organized leagues. September 10, 2008; Accessed March 18, 2009. Web Page Available at: http://www.sportsbusinessdaily.com/article/123897.
2. Lawless CE. Return-to-play decisions in athletes with cardiac conditions. *Physician Sportsmed.* 2009;37:80–91.
3. Maron BJ, Thompson PD, Ackerman MJ, et al. Recommendations and considerations related to preparticipation screening for cardiovascular abnormalities in competitive athletes: 2007 update: a scientific statement from the American Heart Association Council on Nutrition, Physical Activity, and Metabolism: endorsed by the American College of Cardiology Foundation. *Circulation.* 2007;115:1643–1655.
4. Maron BJ, Zipes DP. Introduction: eligibility recommendations for competitive athletes with cardiovascular abnormalities – general considerations. *J Am Coll Cardiol.* 2005;45:1318–1321.
5. Pelliccia A, Fagard R, Bjornstad HH, et al. Recommendations for competitive sports participation in athletes with cardiovascular disease: a consensus document from the Study Group of Sports Cardiology of the Working Group of Cardiac Rehabilitation and Exercise Physiology and the Working Group of Myocardial and Pericardial Diseases of the European Society of Cardiology. *Eur Heart J.* 2005;26:1422–1445.
6. Pelliccia A, Corrado D, Bjornstad HH, et al. Recommendations for participation in competitive sport and leisure-time physical activity in individuals with cardiomyopathies, myocarditis and pericarditis. *Eur J Cardiovasc Prev Rehabil.* 2006;13:876–885.
7. Maron BJ, Chaitman BR, Ackerman MJ, et al. Recommendations for physical activity and recreational sports participation for young patients with genetic cardiovascular diseases. *Circulation.* 2004;109:2807–2816.
8. Estes NA 3rd, Link MS, Cannom D, et al. Report of the NASPE policy conference on arrhythmias and the athlete. *J Cardiovasc Electrophysiol.* 2001;12:1208–1219.
9. Maron BJ, Araujo CG, Thompson PD, et al. Recommendations for preparticipation screening and the assessment of cardiovascular disease in masters athletes: an advisory for healthcare

professionals from the working groups of the World Heart Federation, the International Federation of Sports Medicine, and the American Heart Association Committee on Exercise, Cardiac Rehabilitation, and Prevention. *Circulation*. 2001;103:327–334.
10. Pelliccia A, Zipes DP, Maron BJ. Bethesda Conference #36 and the European Society of Cardiology Consensus Recommendations revisited a comparison of U.S. and European criteria for eligibility and disqualification of competitive athletes with cardiovascular abnormalities. *J Am Coll Cardiol*. 2008;52:1990–1996.
11. Thompson PD, Franklin BA, Balady GJ, et al. Exercise and acute cardiovascular events placing the risks into perspective: a scientific statement from the American Heart Association Council on Nutrition, Physical Activity, and Metabolism and the Council on Clinical Cardiology. *Circulation*. 2007;115:2358–2368.
12. Thompson PD, Funk EJ, Carleton RA, Sturner WQ. Incidence of death during jogging in Rhode Island from 1975 through 1980. *JAMA*. 1982;247:2535–2538.
13. Maron BJ, Shen WK, Link MS, et al. Efficacy of implantable cardioverter–defibrillators for the prevention of sudden death in patients with hypertrophic cardiomyopathy. *N Engl J Med*. 2000;342:365–373.
14. Lampert R, Cannom D, Olshansky B. Safety of sports participation in patients with implantable cardioverter defibrillators: a survey of heart rhythm society members. *J Cardiovasc Electrophysiol*. 2006;17:11–15.
15. Lawless CE. Implantable cardioverter defibrillators in athletes: rationale for use and issues surrounding return to play. *Curr Sports Med Rep*. 2008;7:86–92.
16. Lawless CE, Lampert R, Olshansky B, Cannom D. Safety and efficacy of implantable defibrillators and automatic external defibrillators in athletes: results of a nationwide survey among AMSSM members. *Clin J Sports Med*. 2005;15:386–391.
17. Moss AJ, Zareba W, Hall WJ, et al. Effectiveness and limitations of beta-blocker therapy in congenital long-QT syndrome. *Circulation*. 2000;101:616–623.
18. Priori SG, Napolitano C, Schwartz PJ, et al. Association of long QT syndrome loci and cardiac events among patients treated with beta-blockers. *JAMA*. 2004;292:1341–1344.
19. Vanhees L, Defoor JG, Schepers D, et al. Effect of bisoprolol and atenolol on endurance exercise capacity in healthy men. *J Hypertens*. 2000;18:35–43.
20. Savage DD, Seides SF, Clark CE, et al. Electrocardiographic findings in patients with obstructive and nonobstructive hypertrophic cardiomyopathy. *Circulation*. 1978;58:402–408.
21. Thompson PD, Buchner D, Pina IL, et al. Exercise and physical activity in the prevention and treatment of atherosclerotic cardiovascular disease: a statement from the Council on Clinical Cardiology (Subcommittee on Exercise, Rehabilitation, and Prevention) and the Council on Nutrition, Physical Activity, and Metabolism (Subcommittee on Physical Activity). *Circulation*. 2003;107:3109–3116.
22. Passino C, Severino S, Poletti R, et al. Aerobic training decreases B-type natriuretic peptide expression and adrenergic activation in patients with heart failure. *J Am Coll Cardiol*. 2006;47:1835–1839.
23. Pina IL, Apstein CS, Balady GJ, et al. Exercise and heart failure: a statement from the American Heart Association Committee on exercise, rehabilitation, and prevention. *Circulation*. 2003;107:1210–1225.
24. O'Connor CM, Whellan DJ, Lee KL, et al. Efficacy and safety of exercise training in patients with chronic heart failure: HF-ACTION randomized controlled trial. *JAMA*. 2009;301:1439–1450.
25. Maron BJ. Sudden death in young athletes. *N Engl J Med*. 2003;349:1064–1075.
26. Corrado D, Thiene G, Nava A, Rossi L, Pennelli N. Sudden death in young competitive athletes: clinicopathologic correlations in 22 cases. *Am J Med*. 1990;89:588–596.
27. Thiene G, Nava A, Corrado D, Rossi L, Pennelli N. Right ventricular cardiomyopathy and sudden death in young people. *N Engl J Med*. 1988;318:129–133.
28. Angelini P, Velasco JA, Flamm S. Coronary anomalies: incidence, pathophysiology, and clinical relevance. *Circulation*. 2002;105:2449–2454.
29. Mannix, C. The cardiac kid. *Sports Illustrated*. March 20, 2006; Accessed May 3, 2010. Web Page Available at: http://www.sportsillustrated.cnn.com/vault/article/magazine/MAG1110124/index.htm.

30. Calkins H, Yong P, Miller JM, et al. Catheter ablation of accessory pathways, atrioventricular nodal reentrant tachycardia, and the atrioventricular junction: final results of a prospective, multicenter clinical trial. The Atakr Multicenter Investigators Group. *Circulation*. 1999;99:262–270.
31. Naccarelli GV, Shih HT, Jalal S. Catheter ablation for the treatment of paroxysmal supraventricular tachycardia. *J Cardiovasc Electrophysiol*. 1995;6:951–961.
32. Klein GJ, Bashore TM, Sellers TD, Pritchett EL, Smith WM, Gallagher JJ. Ventricular fibrillation in the Wolff–Parkinson–White syndrome. *N Engl J Med*. 1979;301:1080–1085.
33. Pappone C, Santinelli V, Rosanio S, et al. Usefulness of invasive electrophysiologic testing to stratify the risk of arrhythmic events in asymptomatic patients with Wolff–Parkinson–White pattern: results from a large prospective long-term follow-up study. *J Am Coll Cardiol*. 2003;41:239–244.
34. Pappone C, Santinelli V, Manguso F, et al. A randomized study of prophylactic catheter ablation in asymptomatic patients with the Wolff–Parkinson–White syndrome. *N Engl J Med*. 2003;349:1803–1811.
35. Biffi A, Pelliccia A, Verdile L, et al. Long-term clinical significance of frequent and complex ventricular tachyarrhythmias in trained athletes. *J Am Coll Cardiol*. 2002;40:446–452.
36. Cole CR, Marrouche NF, Natale A. Evaluation and management of ventricular outflow tract tachycardias. *Card Electrophysiol Rev*. 2002;6:442–447.
37. Lerman BB, Stein KM, Markowitz SM, Mittal S, Slotwiner DJ. Ventricular arrhythmias in normal hearts. *Cardiol Clin*. 2000;18:265–291.
38. Maruyama M, Tadera T, Miyamoto S, Ino T. Demonstration of the reentrant circuit of verapamil-sensitive idiopathic left ventricular tachycardia: direct evidence for macroreentry as the underlying mechanism. *J Cardiovasc Electrophysiol*. 2001;12:968–972.
39. Nogami A. Idiopathic left ventricular tachycardia: assessment and treatment. *Card Electrophysiol Rev*. 2002;6:448–457.
40. Ouyang F, Cappato R, Ernst S, et al. Electroanatomic substrate of idiopathic left ventricular tachycardia: unidirectional block and macroreentry within the purkinje network. *Circulation*. 2002;105:462–469.
41. Jacobs W, Chamoun A, Stouffer GA. Mitral valve prolapse: a review of the literature. *Am J Med Sci*. 2001;321:401–410.

Index

C.E. Lawless (ed.), *Sports Cardiology Essentials: Evaluation, Management and Case Studies*, DOI 10.1007/978-0-387-92775-6,

I

L

T

V

W